# Almond Flour Cookbook

## Gluten-Free Low Carb Almond Flour Recipes

MARIA SOBININA

BRILLIANTkitchenideas.com

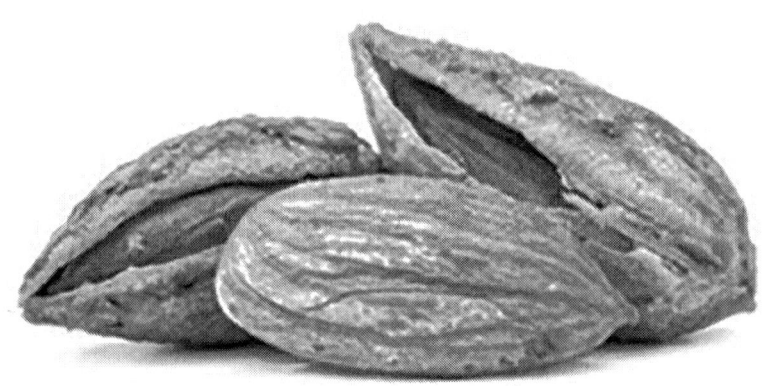

Second Edition

Copyright © 2019 MARIA SOBININA
BRILLIANT kitchen ideas

All rights reserved.

ISBN: 9781097586677

# DEDICATION

This book is dedicated to my beautiful family and friends, as well as to you, my reader. I am happy to share the amazing joy of preparing healthy meals with you.

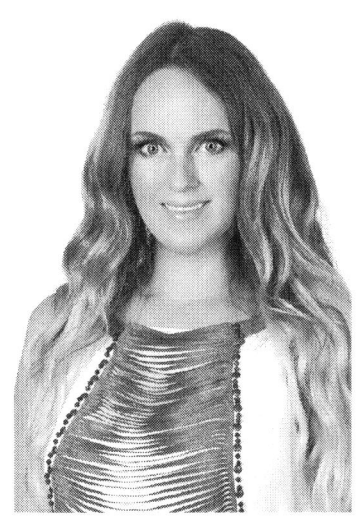

*MARIA XOXO*

# TABLE OF CONTENTS

About Almond Flour    4

Almond Flour Banana Bread    7

Almond Flour Coconut Bread    9

Almond Flour Pumpkin Bread    12

Almond Flour Pancakes    16

Almond Flour Coconut Pancakes    18

Almond Flour Waffles    21

Almond Flour Dessert Crepe    24

Almond Flour Cookies    27

Almond Flour Coconut Cookies    30

Almond Flour Cake    34

Carrot Sweet Potato Cheesecake    37

Carrot Almond Bundt Cake    44

Marzipan Icing    50

Almond Butter    52

Almond Chocolate Squares    53

Almond Coconut Balls    57

Almond Flour Naan With Fruits & Nuts    61

Almond Flour Stuffed Mushrooms    64

Sweet Potato Crust Almond Pizza    67

Almond Flour Crust Pizza    72

Almond Flour Crab Cakes    78

## Almond Flour Crusted Salmon 81

# About Almond Flour

Almond flour has high **nutritional content**, and it is **low on carbohydrates**. It is a popular **gluten-free** substitute for wheat flour. Almond flour is used one to one to substitute wheat flour in a recipe. Almond flour requires using more binding agents.

Almond flour has more calories than coconut flour. It also has fewer carbs and less fiber than coconut flour. Almond flour is a good source of **magnesium, iron, potassium, calcium,** and **vitamin E.**

Consumption of almonds, whether you consume them raw, or as almond flour or almond meal, boosts the level of **antioxidants, enhances blood flow** and **normalizes blood pressure.**

Almond flour, also aids **in reducing bad (LDL) cholesterol** and **insulin resistance.** Furthermore, as research studies show, almond flour **promotes weight loss** in obese individuals.

Almond flour has a **low glycemic index.** It also **helps to regulate blood sugar** for people with diabetes.

The glycemic index (GI) is a ranking of carbohydrates on a scale from 0 to 100 (from low to high) based on how much they elevate blood sugar levels after consumption of food.

High GI foods are quickly absorbed and rapidly elevate blood sugar. Low GI foods have slower absorption and a more gradual effect on blood sugar.

Consumption of almonds may also **decrease the risk of certain cancers**. It also **reduces the risk of coronary heart disease.**

You can purchase almond flour at a local food store or online. Make sure you select almond flour that contains **one only ingredient: almonds.**

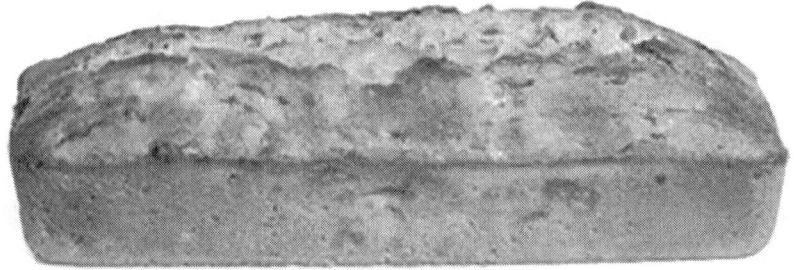

*Almond Flour Banana Brea*

# Almond Flour Banana Bread

**INGREDIENTS:**

3 cups **Almond Flour**

2 **Bananas**, ripe, mashed

½ cup **Almond Milk**

¼ cup **Honey**, raw

¼ cup **Olive Oil**, virgin, first cold pressed

4 tablespoons **Water**, hot

2 tablespoons **Flax Seeds**, ground

1 teaspoon **Baking Soda**

1 teaspoon **Vanilla**, extract, pure

¼ teaspoon **Salt,** fine, pink, Himalayan

**Cooking Spray** for greasing the baking tray

**EQUIPMENT:**

*Rectangular bread baking tray, Stand or hand mixer fitted with the paddle attachment, Measuring cups, Cup,*

*Fork, Wire cooling racks, Parchment paper (optional), Cake decorating piping tips and bags (optional).*

## PREPARATION:

**Step 1:** Prepare egg replacement: add flax seeds into a cup and cover it with hot water. Place flax seeds onto a countertop and wait until flax seeds become gelatin-like.

**Step 2:** Grease the bottom and sides of the baking tray with a cooking spray. Line the bottom of the tray with parchment paper (optional).

**Step 3:** In a bowl of a stand mixer, mash bananas with a fork. Add flax eggs, almond flour, almond milk, olive oil, honey, baking soda, salt, and vanilla extract. Process everything on low-medium speed until all is combined.

**Step 4:** Pour the batter into the baking tray. Bake for about 40 minutes or until a wooden skewer comes out clean.

**Step 5:** Place on a cooling rack and let it cool for an hour. Decorate with decorating tools before serving. *(Optional)*

*Almond Flour Banana Bread will keep for a week in a fridge or one month in a freezer.*

# Almond Flour Coconut Bread

## INGREDIENTS:

2 cups **Almond Flour**

1 cups **Coconut Flour**

1 cup **Apple Puree**

½ cup **Almond Milk**

¼ cup **Honey**, raw

¼ cup **Olive Oil**, virgin, first cold pressed

4 tablespoons **Water**, hot

2 tablespoons **Flax Seeds**, ground

1 teaspoon **Baking Soda**

1 teaspoon **Vanilla**, extract, pure

¼ teaspoon **Salt,** fine, pink, Himalayan

**Cooking Spray** for greasing the baking tray

## EQUIPMENT:

*Rectangular bread baking tray, Stand or hand mixer fitted with the paddle attachment, Measuring cups, Cup, Fork, Wire cooling racks, Parchment paper (optional), Cake decorating piping tips and bags (optional).*

## PREPARATION:

**Step 1:** Prepare egg replacement: add flax seeds into a cup and cover it with hot water. Place flax seeds onto a countertop and wait until flax seeds become gelatin-like.

**Step 2:** Grease the bottom and sides of the baking tray with a cooking spray. Line the bottom of the tray with parchment paper (optional).

**Step 3:** In a bowl of a stand mixer add apple puree, flax eggs, almond flour, coconut flour, almond milk, olive oil, honey, baking soda, salt, and vanilla extract. Process everything on low-medium speed until all is combined.

**Step 4:** Pour the batter into the baking tray. Bake for about 40 minutes or until a wooden skewer comes out clean.

**Step 5:** Place on a cooling rack and let it cool for an hour. Decorate with decorating tools before serving. *(Optional)*

*Almond Flour Coconut Bread will keep for a week in a fridge or one month in a freezer.*

# Almond Flour Pumpkin Bread

**INGREDIENTS:**

2 cups **Almond Flour**

½ cup **Coconut Flour**

1 cup **Pumpkin**, puree

½ cup **Almond Milk**

¼ cup **Honey**, raw

¼ cup **Olive Oil**, virgin, first cold pressed

4 tablespoons **Water**, hot

2 tablespoons **Flax Seeds**, ground

1 teaspoon **Baking Soda**

1 teaspoon **Vanilla**, extract, pure

½ teaspoon **Pumpkin Pie Spice**

½ teaspoon **Cinnamon,** powder

¼ teaspoon **Salt,** fine, pink, Himalayan

**Cooking Spray** for greasing the baking tray

## EQUIPMENT:

*Rectangular bread baking tray, Stand or hand mixer fitted with the paddle attachment, Measuring cups, Cup, Fork, Wire cooling racks, Parchment paper (optional), Cake decorating piping tips and bags (optional).*

## PREPARATION:

Preheat the oven to 365°F.

**Step 1:** Cut the raw pumpkin, remove the seeds.

Place pumpkin pieces onto a baking tray. Bake the pumpkin for approximately forty minutes until it is soft. Set aside to cool. Place cooled pumpkin into the food processor. Process until smooth. Set aside.

**Step 2:** Prepare egg replacement: add flax seeds into a cup and cover it with hot water. Place flax seeds onto a countertop and wait until flax seeds become gelatin-like.

*Alternatively, you can use 3-4 eggs.*

**Step 3:** Preheat the oven to 355°F. Grease bottom and sides of the baking tray with a cooking spray. Line the bottom of the tray with parchment paper (optional).

**Step 4:** In a bowl add flax eggs, pumpkin puree, almond flour, coconut flour, almond milk, honey, olive oil, baking soda, salt, and spices. Process everything on low-medium speed until all is combined.

**Step 5:** Pour the batter into the baking tray. Bake for about 40 minutes or until a wooden skewer comes out clean.

**Step 6:** Place on a cooling rack and let it cool for an hour. Decorate with decorating tools before serving. *(Optional)*

*Banana Flour Pumpkin Bread will keep for a week in a fridge or one month in a freezer.*

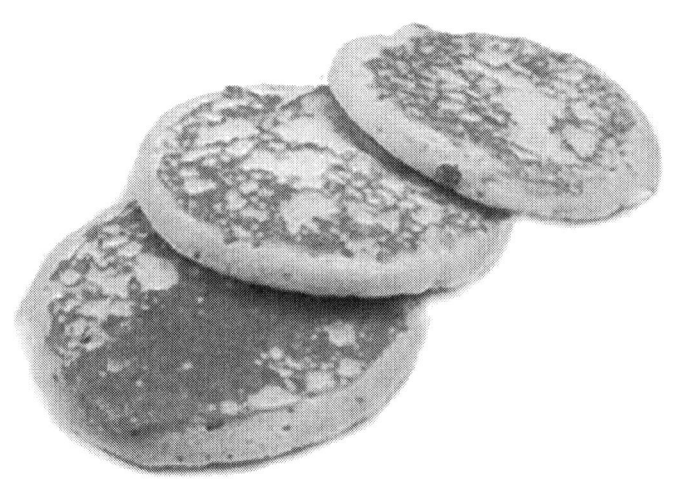

*Almond Flour Pancakes*

# Almond Flour Pancakes

**INGREDIENTS:**

2 cups **Almond Flour**

¾ cup **Almond Milk**

¼ cup **Agave Nectar**

¼ cup **Olive Oil**, virgin, first cold pressed

4 tablespoons **Water**, hot

2 tablespoons **Flax Seeds**, ground

1 teaspoon **Baking Soda**

1 teaspoon **Vanilla**, extract, pure

¼ teaspoon **Salt,** fine, pink, Himalayan

**Cooking Spray** for greasing the baking tray

**EQUIPMENT:**

*Medium size skillet, Stand or hand mixer fitted with the paddle attachment, Measuring cups, Cup, Spatula, Cake decorating piping tips and bags (optional).*

## PREPARATION:

**Step 1:** Prepare egg replacement: add flax seeds into a cup and cover it with hot water. Place flax seeds onto a countertop and wait until flax seeds become gelatin-like.

**Step 2:** In a bowl of a stand mixer add flax eggs, almond flour, almond milk, olive oil, agave nectar, baking soda, salt, and vanilla extract. Process everything on low-medium speed until all is combined.

**Step 3:** Grease the skillet with a cooking spray. Pour the batter into the skillet. Cook for a few minutes from each side (flip with a spatula).

*Almond Flour Coconut Pancakes will keep for a few days in a fridge or one month in a freezer.*

# Almond Flour Coconut Pancakes

**INGREDIENTS:**

1 cup **Almond Flour**

1 cup **Coconut Flour**

¾ cup **Almond Milk**

¼ cup **Agave Nectar**

¼ cup **Olive Oil**, virgin, first cold pressed

4 tablespoons **Water**, hot

2 tablespoons **Flax Seeds**, ground

1 teaspoon **Baking Soda**

1 teaspoon **Vanilla**, extract, pure

¼ teaspoon **Salt,** fine, pink, Himalayan

**Cooking Spray** for greasing the baking tray

**EQUIPMENT:**

*Medium size skillet, Stand or hand mixer fitted with the paddle attachment, Measuring cups, Cup, Spatula, Cake decorating piping tips and bags (optional).*

## PREPARATION:

**Step 1:** Prepare egg replacement: add flax seeds into a cup and cover it with hot water. Place flax seeds onto a countertop and wait until flax seeds become gelatin-like.

**Step 2:** In a bowl of stand mixer add almond flour, coconut flour, tapioca flour, almond milk, flax eggs, olive oil, agave nectar, baking soda, salt, and vanilla extract. Process everything on low-medium speed until all is combined.

**Step 3:** Grease the skillet with cooking spray. Pour the batter into the skillet. Cook for a few minutes on each side (flip with a spatula).

*Almond Flour Pancakes will keep for a few days in a fridge or one month in a freezer.*

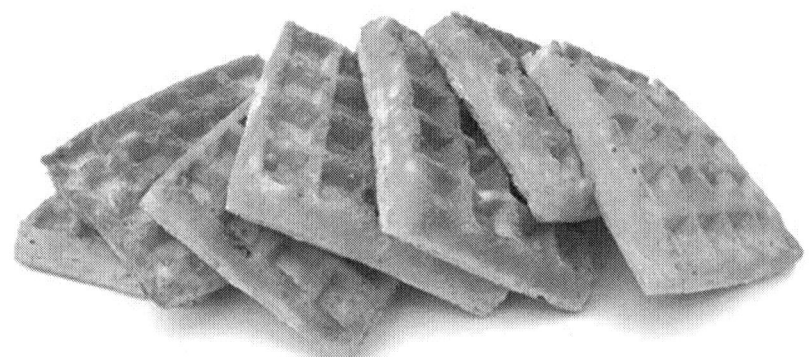

*Almond Flour Waffles*

# Almond Flour Waffles

**INGREDIENTS:**

2 cups **Almond Flour**

4 **Eggs**

¼ cup **Almond Milk**

½ cup **Honey**, raw

¼ cup **Olive Oil**, virgin, first cold pressed

1 teaspoon **Baking Soda**

1 teaspoon **Vanilla**, extract, pure

¼ teaspoon **Salt,** pink, Himalayan

**Cooking Spray** for greasing the baking tray

**EQUIPMENT:**

*Waffle maker, Medium mixing bowl, Whisk, Measuring cups, Cup, Spatula, Cake decorating piping tips and bags (optional).*

**PREPARATION:**

**Step 1:** In a medium mixing bowl add eggs, almond flour, almond milk, olive oil, honey, baking soda, salt, and vanilla extract. Whisk everything together until all is well combined.

**Step 2:** Grease the waffle maker with a cooking spray. Pour the batter into the hot waffle maker. Cook for a few minutes from each side until it is lightly golden.

*Almond Flour Waffles will keep for a few days in a fridge or one month in a freezer.*

Almond Flour: Gluten Free Almond Flour Dishes

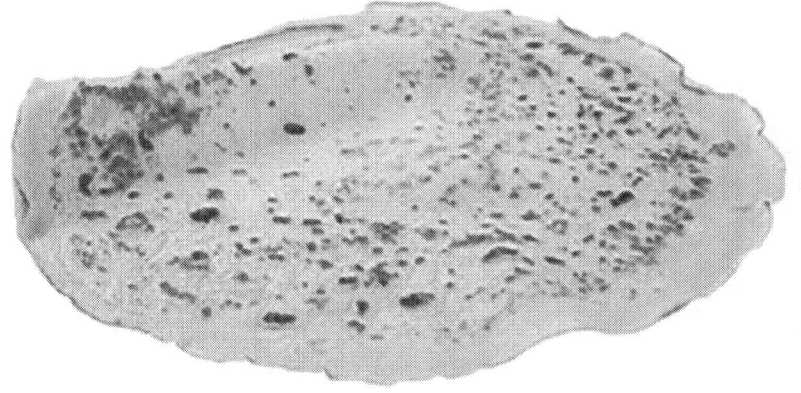

*Almond Flour Crepe*

# Almond Flour Dessert Crepe

**INGREDIENTS:**

1 cup **Tapioca Flour**

1 cup **Almond Flour**

1 cup **Almond Milk**

4 tablespoons **Agave Nectar**

2 tablespoons **Olive Oil**, virgin, first cold pressed

1 teaspoon **Baking Soda**

1 teaspoon **Vanilla**, extract, pure

¼ teaspoon **Salt,** pink, Himalayan

**Cooking Spray** for greasing the skillet

**EQUIPMENT:**

*Medium size skillet, Stand or hand mixer fitted with the paddle attachment, Measuring cups, Cup, Spatula, Cake decorating piping tips and bags (optional).*

## PREPARATION:

**Step 1:** In a bowl of a stand mixer add almond flour, tapioca flour, almond milk, olive oil, agave nectar, baking soda, salt, and vanilla extract. Process everything on low-medium speed until all is combined.

**Step 2:** Grease the skillet with a cooking spray. Pour the batter into the skillet. Spread as thin as you can (or to taste). Cook for a one to two minutes on each side (flip with a spatula).

*Almond Flour Dessert Crepe will keep for a few days in a fridge or one month in a freezer.*

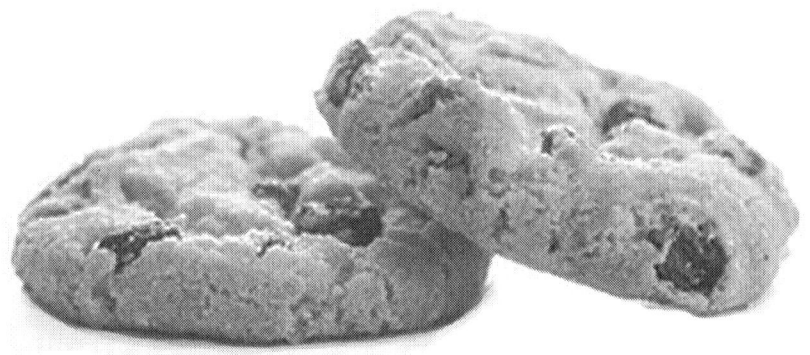

*Almond Flour Cookies*

# Almond Flour Cookies

**INGREDIENTS:**

2 cups **Almond Flour**

½ cup **Raisins**, brown

¼ cup **Maple Syrup,** raw

2 tablespoons **Coconut oil**, virgin, cold pressed

4 tablespoons **Water**, hot

2 tablespoons **Flax Seeds**, ground

1 teaspoon **Baking Soda**

1 teaspoon **Vanilla**, extract, pure

¼ teaspoon **Salt,** fine, pink, Himalayan

**Cooking Spray** for greasing the baking tray

**EQUIPMENT:**

*Cup, Large and medium mixing bowls, Baking tray, Measuring cups, Spatula, Wire cooling rack, Parchment paper, Cake decorating piping tips and bags (optional).*

## PREPARATION:

**Step 1:** Prepare egg replacement: add flax seeds into a cup and cover it with hot water. Place flax seeds onto a countertop and wait until flax seeds become gelatin-like.

**Step 2:** In a large bowl add coconut oil and maple syrup. Whisk the ingredients to combine and add flax seeds and vanilla extract. Whisk again.

**Step 3:** In a medium bowl add almond flour, baking soda, and salt. Whisk all together.

Add dry mixture to the wet mixture. Stir all together. Add olive oil. Add raisins and fold them into the mixture to incorporate. Set aside.

**Step 4:** Preheat the oven to 365°F. Grease the baking tray with a baking spray. Line the baking tray with parchment paper.

Scoop the almond cookie dough with a tablespoon and place it onto the baking tray. Space two inches apart.

**Step 5:** Bake the cookies for approximately 10 minutes or until the edges are golden brown.

Remove from the oven and transfer cookies onto a wire cooling rack to cool.

*Almond Flour Cookies will keep for a few days in a fridge or one month in a freezer.*

# Almond Flour Coconut Cookies

**INGREDIENTS:**

1 ½ cups **Almond Flour**

½ cup **Coconut Flour**

1 cup **Coconut**, shredded, unsweetened

¼ cup **Maple Syrup,** raw

2 tablespoons **Coconut oil**, virgin, cold pressed

4 tablespoons **Water**, hot

2 tablespoons **Flax Seeds**, ground

1 teaspoon **Baking Soda**

1 teaspoon **Vanilla**, extract, pure

¼ teaspoon **Salt,** fine, pink, Himalayan

**Cooking Spray** for greasing the baking tray

**EQUIPMENT:**

*Cup, Large and medium mixing bowls, Baking tray, Measuring cups, Spatula, Wire cooling rack, Parchment paper, Cake decorating piping tips and bags (optional).*

## PREPARATION:

**Step 1:** Prepare egg replacement: add flax seeds into a cup and cover it with hot water. Place flax seeds onto a countertop and wait until flax seeds become gelatin-like.

*Alternatively, you can substitute flaxseed eggs for 3 chicken eggs.*

**Step 2:** In a large bowl combine coconut oil and maple syrup. Whisk together and add flax seeds and vanilla extract. Whisk again.

**Step 3:** In a medium bowl add almond flour, coconut flour, baking soda, and salt. Whisk all together.

Add dry mixture to the wet mixture. Stir all together. Add shredded coconut and fold it into the mixture to incorporate. Set aside.

**Step 4:** Preheat the oven to 365°F. Grease the baking tray with a baking spray. Line the tray with parchment paper.

Scoop the almond cookie dough with a tablespoon and place it onto the baking tray. Space two inches apart.

**Step 5:** Bake for approximately 10 minutes or until

the edges are golden brown. Remove cookies from the oven and transfer cookies onto a wire cooling rack to cool.

*Almond Flour Coconut Cookies will keep for a few days in a fridge or one month in a freezer.*

Almond Flour: Gluten Free Almond Flour Dishes

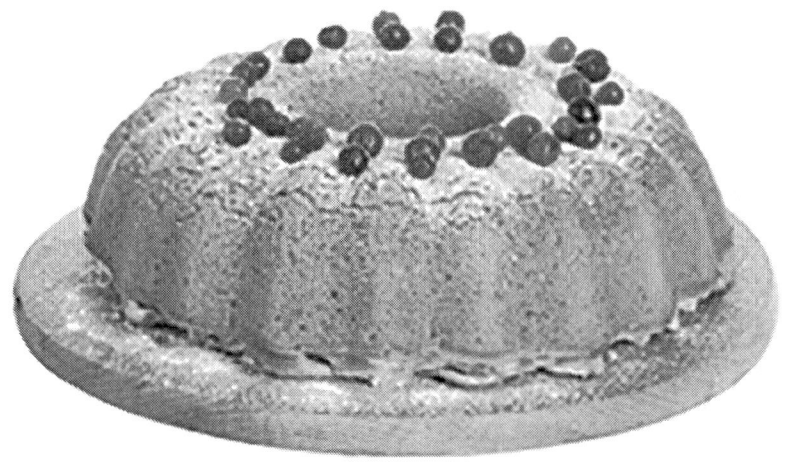

*Almond Flour Cake*

# Almond Flour Cake

**INGREDIENTS:**

1 ½ cups **Almond Flour**

¼ cup and ¼ cup **Sugar**, coconut

4 **Eggs**, separated on yoks and whites

¾ cup **Almond Milk**

¼ cup **Olive Oil**, virgin, first cold pressed

1 teaspoon **Baking Soda**

1 teaspoon **Vanilla**, extract, pure

¼ teaspoon **Salt,** fine, pink, Himalayan

**Cooking Spray** for greasing the baking tray

**EQUIPMENT:**

*Small and medium size mixing bowls, 10-inch cake baking tray, Stand or hand mixer fitted with the paddle attachment, Measuring cups, Cake decorating piping tips and bags (optional).*

**PREPARATION:**

**Step 1:** In a medium mixing bowl add egg yolks, ¼

cup of coconut sugar, vanilla extract and beat the ingredients with a hand mixer or a whisk. Set the egg yolks mixture aside.

**Step 2:** In a bowl of a stand mixer add egg whites and beat them until they start forming soft peaks. Add ¼ cup of coconut sugar. Process everything on low-medium speed until all is combined.

**Step 3:** In a small mixing bowl combine dry ingredients: flour, baking soda, and salt. Add to the egg yolks mixture and mix together. Fold in the egg whites mixture and mix it together until it forms a smooth batter. Add almond milk and olive oil and mix again to incorporate.

Preheat the oven to 355°F.

**Step 4:** Grease a baking tray with a cooking spray. Pour the batter into the baking tray. Bake for about 40 minutes until a wooden skewer comes out clean.

**Step 5:** Place on a cooling rack and let it cool for an hour. Decorate with fruits or cake decorating tools before serving. *(Optional)*

*Almond Flour Cake will keep for a few days in a fridge or one month in a freezer.*

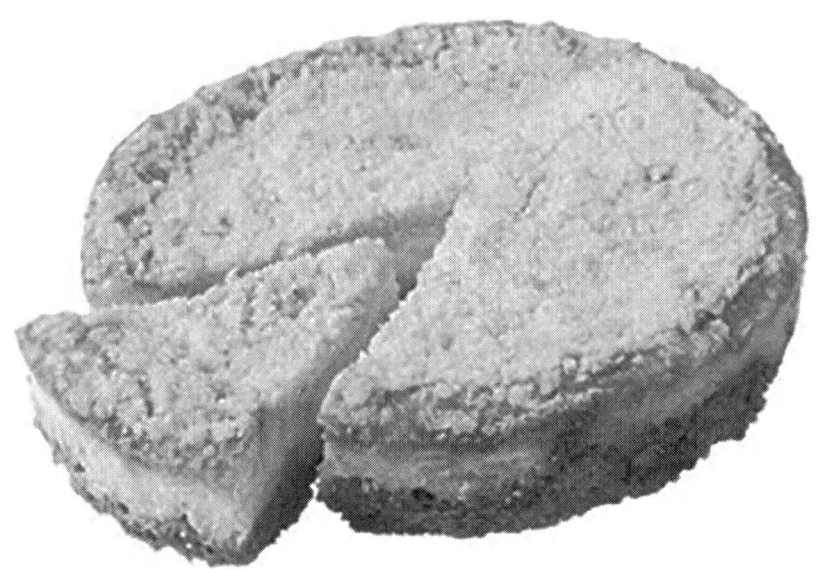

*Carrot Sweet Potato Cheesecake*

# Carrot Sweet Potato Cheesecake

**INGREDIENTS:**

**FOR THE CAKE:**

1 lbs. **Carrots**, peeled

3 **Eggs**

1 ½ cups **Almond Flour**

1 cup **Sugar,** white, powdered

1/2 cup **Sugar**, brown

1 teaspoon **Baking Powder**

3/4 teaspoon **Baking Soda**

3/4 teaspoon **Salt**

1 cup **Vegetable oil**

1 cup **Sweet Potato**, mashed

1/2 cup **Applesauce,** unsweetened

1/2 cup **Sour cream**

**Cooking spray** for greasing the springform pan

**FOR THE CHEESE:**

8 Oz **Cream cheese**

1 **Egg**

1/2 cup **Sour cream**

1/4 cup **Cranberry sauce,** canned

1 tablespoon **Almond Flour**

**For the Frosting:**

6 Oz **Farmers cheese**

6 Oz **Butter**, unsalted, softened

2 ½ cups **Sugar**, white, powdered

1/2 tablespoon **Vanilla,** extract, pure

**FOR THE DECORATIONS:**

1 cup **Cranberries,** dried

## EQUIPMENT:

*One 9-inch springform baking pan, Stand or hand mixer fitted with the paddle attachment, Medium and large mixing bowls, Food processor or hand grater, Cake decorating piping tips and bags (optional).*

## PREPARATION:

## MAKE THE CAKE:

**Step 1:** Preheat the oven to 355°F. Grease the bottom and sides of 9-inch springform pan with a cooking spray. Line the bottom with parchment paper (optional).

**Step 2:** Grate the carrots in a food processor (or with a hand grater).

**Step 3:** In a large bowl, combine almond flour, baking powder, baking soda, and salt.

**Step 4:** In a bowl of stand mixer fitted with the paddle attachment (you can use a bowl and a hand mixer) combine sugar and eggs.

Mix on low speed until everything is well incorporated and achieves a smooth consistency.

**Step 5**: Add vegetable oil, buttermilk, vanilla, mashed sweet potato (puree), and applesauce. Continue mixing until all is well incorporated.

**Step 6**: Separate the flour mix onto 3 or 4 parts and add them in 3 or 4 batches, using a spatula to fold the mixture in until all is incorporated. Fold in carrots with a spatula. Set aside.

## MAKE THE CHEESE:

In a bowl of a stand mixer, combine cream cheese, buttermilk, sour cream, and flour. Beat the mixture with a paddle attachment until all is evenly incorporated and the mixture becomes smooth.

Fold in cranberry sauce and mix with a spatula.

## ASSEMBLE THE CAKE:

Pour 1/3 of carrot cake batter into a greased springform pan.

Pour 1/3 of cheese over the carrot batter.

Repeat until you add all batter and cheese into the springform pan.

You can swirl it with a wooden skewer to create a "marbled" effect.

## BAKE THE CAKE:

**Step 1:** Preheat oven to 355°F. Bake the cake for about 60-65 minutes or until the center is set and not too wobbly.

**Step 2:** At 30-35 minutes into baking, cover the springform pan with aluminum foil to prevent burning of the top.

Once ready set it aside for one hour to cool. (Once it is cooled to room temperature, leave it overnight in the fridge).

## MAKE THE FROSTING:

**Step 1:** In a bowl of stand mixer fitted with the paddle attachment (you can use a bowl and a hand mixer) combine butter and powdered sugar.

Beat on medium speed for 1 to 2 minutes until all is fully incorporated and becomes fluffy and light in color.

**Step 2:** Spoon by spoon, add farmers cheese and beat on medium speed for 1 to 2 minutes until it is fully incorporated and becomes light and fluffy.

If you decorate your cake using cake decorating piping tips and bags set aside 1/3 of the frosting. Refrigerate the frosting for about one hour or until it becomes firm.

This will be cooled frosting. The rest of the frosting will be room temperature frosting.

**DECORATE THE CAKE:**

Cover the top of cheesecake with the room temperature frosting. Sprinkle with dried cranberries.

If you are decorating your cake with cake decorating tools place the cooled frosting into a piping bag and start piping borders and flowers. You can also add food coloring.

*(We recommend using natural food coloring instead of artificial colors).*

*Carrot Sweet Potato Cheesecake will keep for a few days in a fridge or one month in a freezer.*

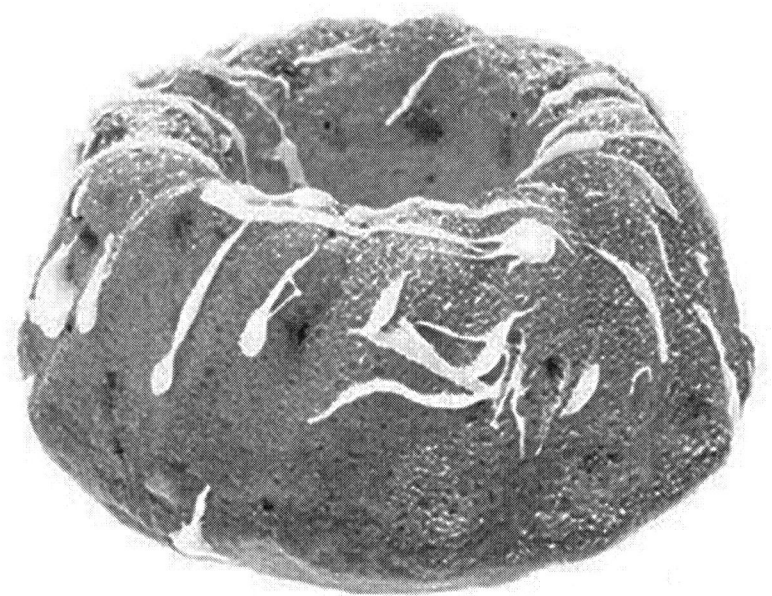

*Carrot Almond Bund Cake*

# Carrot Almond Bundt Cake

**INGREDIENTS:**

**FOR THE CAKE:**

1 lbs. **Carrots**, peeled

4 **Eggs**

1 ½ cup **Almond Flour**

½ cup **Coconut Flour**

½ cup **Coconut Milk**

1 cup **Sugar,** white, granulated

1 cup **Sugar**, brown

1 teaspoon **Baking Powder**

3/4 teaspoon **Baking soda**

3/4 teaspoon **Salt**

1 cup **Vegetable Oil,** virgin, cold pressed

1/2 cup **Pecans,** chopped

1/2 cup **Pistachios**, chopped

1/2 cup **Pineapple,** dried, diced

1/2 cup **Raisins**, golden

1/2 cup **Apricots**, dried, diced

1/2 cup **Ginger**, crystallized, diced

1 teaspoon **Cinnamon**, ground

1/2 teaspoon **Nutmeg,** ground

1/2 teaspoon **Allspice**, ground

**Cooking Spray** for greasing the pans

**FOR THE FROSTING:**

6 Oz **Farmer Cheese**

8 Oz **Butter**, unsalted, softened

3 cups **Sugar**, powdered

**EQUIPMENT:**

*Bundt baking pan, Stand or hand mixer fitted with the paddle attachment, Small, medium and large mixing bowls, 1 to 2 wire cooling racks, Food processor or hand grater, Cake decorating piping tips and bags (optional).*

## PREPARATION:

## MAKE THE CAKE:

**Step 1:** Preheat the oven to 355°F. Grease the bottom and sides of two (9-inch-round, 2-inch-deep) cake pans with a cooking spray. Line the bottoms of trays with parchment paper (optional).

**Step 2:** Grate carrots in a food processor (or with a hand grater). Chop pecans and pistachios in the food processor.

In a medium bowl, combine carrots, pecans, and pistachios. Add raisins and cubed crystallized ginger.

**Step 3:** In a small bowl combine pineapples and apricots. If dried fruits are not pre-cut, dice them into 1/2-inch pieces. Add one cup of water and leave the dried fruits for about 15 minutes to soften.

**Step 4:** In a large bowl combine almond flour, coconut flour, baking powder, baking soda, salt, cinnamon, nutmeg, and allspice.

**Step 5:** In a bowl of stand mixer fitted with the paddle attachment (you can use a bowl and a hand mixer) add white sugar, brown sugar, and eggs.

Mix on low speed until everything is well incorporated and achieves a smooth consistency.

Add vegetable oil and little by little add coconut milk. *(Add just enough of coconut milk to achieve a smooth mixture).* Continue mixing until all is well incorporated.

**Step 6**: Separate flour mix on 3 or 4 parts and add them in 3 or 4 batches, using a spatula to fold in the mixture until all is incorporated. Fold in carrots, nuts, crystallized ginger, and raisins.

Drain the water from the apricots and pineapples. Dry apricots and pineapples with a paper towel. Fold in apricots and pineapples into the flour mixture.

**Step 7:** Spread the batter into a greased Bundt cake form. Bake until firm for about 60 minutes or until a wooden skewer tester comes out clean.

**Step 8:** Transfer the crust onto a cooling rack. Let the cake cool completely.

## MAKE THE FROSTING:

**Step 1:** In a bowl of stand mixer fitted with the paddle attachment (you can use a bowl and a hand mixer) combine butter and powdered sugar.

Beat on medium speed for 1 to 2 minutes until it is fully incorporated and becomes fluffy and light in color.

**Step 2:** Spoon by spoon, add farmers cheese and beat on medium speed for 1 to 2 minutes until it is fully incorporated and becomes light and fluffy.

Add vanilla extract and beat for another 1-2 minutes. Do not overbeat.

**ASSEMBLE THE CAKE:**

If you decorate your cake using cake decorating piping tips and bags set aside and refrigerate 1/3 of the frosting for about one hour or until it becomes firm.

This will be your cooled frosting. The rest of the frosting will be the room temperature frosting.

Spread the room temperature frosting over your cake.

Use cooled frosting to decorate the cake using piping tips and bags. (Optional).

**DECORATE THE CAKE:** *(optional)*

Once you are ready to decorate your cake using piping tips and bags remove the cooled frosting from the fridge.

Place the cooled frosting into a piping bag and start piping borders and flowers. You can also add food coloring.

*(We recommend using natural food coloring instead of artificial colors).*

*Carrot Almond Bundt Cake will keep for a few days in a fridge or one month in a freezer.*

# Marzipan Icing

**INGREDIENTS:**

2 cups **Sugar**, powdered

½ Lbs. **Almonds**, blanched, finely ground

2 **Egg whites,** pasteurized

1/2 teaspoon **Salt**

1/2 teaspoon **Almond**, pure, extract

**EQUIPMENT:**

*Stand or hand mixer fitted with the paddle attachment, Plastic wrap, Cake decorating piping tips and bags (optional).*

**PREPARATION:**

**Step 1:** In a bowl of stand mixer fitted with the paddle attachment combine powdered sugar and egg whites. Beat on medium speed until the mixture becomes smooth and foamy.

**Step 2:** Add finely ground almonds, salt, and almond extract. Beat on medium speed until perfectly blended.

Cover with a plastic wrap and leave in the fridge for

24 hours to harden.

*Marzipan Icing will keep in the fridge for up to one week.*

*This recipe contains raw egg. We recommend that pregnant women, young children, the elderly, and the infirm do not consume raw eggs.*

# Almond Butter

**INGREDIENTS:**

3 cups **Almonds,** raw

½ teaspoon **Vanilla**, extract, pure

**EQUIPMENT:**

*Measuring cups, High-powered food processor.*

**PREPARATION:**

In a food processor combine almonds and vanilla extract. Process until it becomes smooth. Stop the food processor several times to scrape the sides of the food processor.

It will take 15 to 20 minutes to achieve a store-like consistency.

*Almond Butter will keep in the fridge for five days.*

# Almond Chocolate Squares

INGREDIENTS:

FOR ALMOND LAYER:

1 cup **Almond Butter***

½ cups **Almond Flour**

¼ cup **Maple Syrup**, pure

FOR CHOCOLATE LAYER:

1 cup **Chocolate Chips**, dark, bakers

½ cup **Almond Butter***

*FOR ALMOND BUTTER:

3 cups **Almonds**, raw

½ teaspoon **Vanilla**, extract, pure

EQUIPMENT:

*Small size sauce pan (for water bath), Medium bowl, Medium size silicone form, Measuring cups, High-powered food processor, Heat-proof bowl, Whisk, Spatula, Parchment paper (optional).*

## PREPARATION:

## MAKE THE ALMOND BUTTER:

In a food processor combine almonds and vanilla extract. Process until it becomes smooth. Stop the food processor several times to scrape the sides of the food processor.

It will take 15 to 20 minutes to achieve a store-like consistency. Transfer the mixture into a medium bowl.

## MAKE THE CHOCOLATE SQUARES:

**Step 1:** Prepare a medium size silicone form. *(You can use any other form or tray of your choice. If you are not using a silicone form line up your tray with parchment paper).*

In the bowl with almond butter add maple syrup and almond flour. Whisk until all is combined and forms a thick batter.

Scrape the leftovers from the whisk using a spatula. Mix the batter again.

Pour the batter into a silicone form. Smooth with the spatula to create an even layer. Set aside.

**Step 2:** Place chocolate chips and ½ cup of almond

butter into a heat-proof bowl. Heat the mixture over a water-bath until the chocolate melts. Stir the mixture until all is melted and evenly incorporated.

Pour the chocolate mixture over the almond mixture. Level evenly with a spatula.

**Step 3:** Cover the form with a plastic wrap and place it into the freezer. Freeze for 2-3 hours or until it hardens. Remove the chocolate from the freezer and slice it into even squares.

Store in an airtight container in the freezer.

*Almond Chocolate Squares will keep for several months in the freezer.*

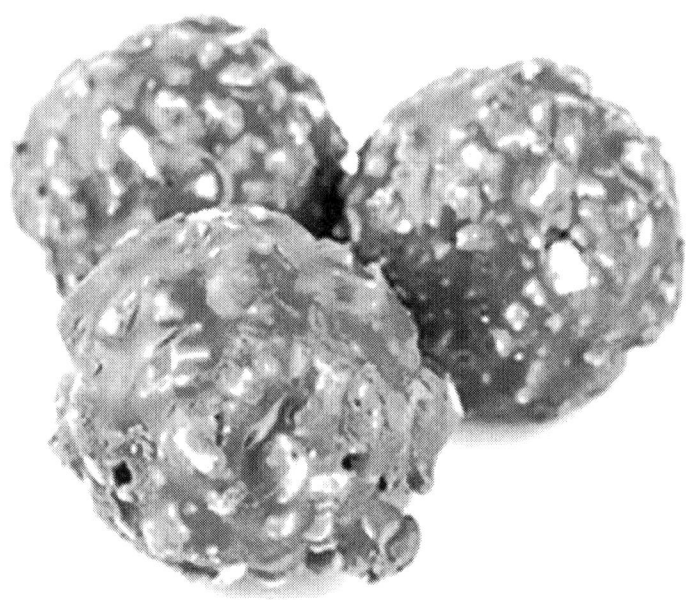

*Almond Coconut Balls*

# Almond Coconut Balls

**INGREDIENTS:**

**FOR ALMOND LAYER:**

1 cup **Almond Butter***

½ cups **Almond Flour**

¼ cup **Maple Syrup**, pure

½ cup **Chocolate Chips**, white, bakers

¾ cup and ½ cup **Coconut**, shredded, unsweetened

***FOR ALMOND BUTTER:**

3 cups **Almonds,** raw

½ teaspoon **Vanilla**, extract, pure

**EQUIPMENT:**

*Small size sauce pan (for water bath), Medium bowl, Silicone tray, Measuring cups, High-powered food processor, Heat-proof bowl, Whisk, Spatula, Parchment paper (optional).*

**PREPARATION:**

**MAKE THE ALMOND BUTTER:**

**Step 1:** In a food processor combine almonds and

vanilla extract. Process until it becomes smooth. Stop the food processor several times to scrape the sides of the food processor.

It will take 15 to 20 minutes to achieve a store-like consistency. Transfer the mixture into a medium bowl.

**Step 2:** Add maple syrup and almond flour into the bowl with almond butter. Whisk until all is combined and forms a thick batter. Scrape the leftover batter from the whisk using a spatula. Mix the batter again. Set aside.

**Step 3:** Place white chocolate chips and ½ cup of almond butter into a heat-proof bowl. Heat the mixture over a water-bath until the chocolate melts. Stir the mixture until the chocolate fully melts and all is evenly incorporated.

Pour the chocolate mixture into the bowl with almond butter. Mix it with a spatula. Fold in ¾ cup of shredded coconut. Mix it with a spatula to incorporate and mix evenly to create a thick batter.

**Step 4:** Prepare a silicone tray. *(You can use any other tray of your choice. If you are not using a silicone tray, line up your tray with parchment paper).*

Add ½ cup of shredded coconut into a plate. Make

even-size balls from the almond-coconut batter. Roll each ball in the shredded coconut. Place the balls into the silicone tray.

**Step 5:** Cover the form with a plastic wrap and place it into the freezer. Freeze for 2-3 hours or until it is hardened.

Store in the freezer in an airtight container.

*Almond Coconut Balls will keep for a few days in a fridge or one month in a freezer.*

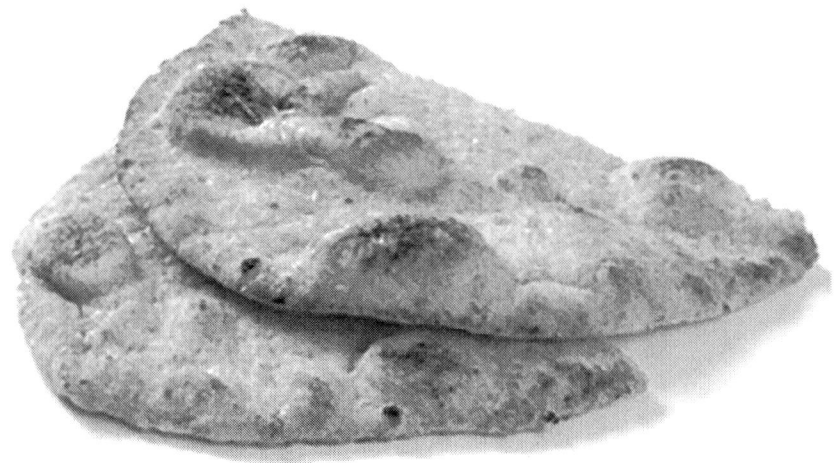

*Almond Flour Naan With Fruits & Nuts*

# Almond Flour Naan With Fruits & Nuts

**INGREDIENTS:**

1 cup **Tapioca Flour**

1 cup **Almond Flour**

¾ cup **Almond Milk**

½ cup **Apricots**, dried, chopped

½ cup **Walnuts**, raw, chopped

4 tablespoons **Agave Nectar**

2 tablespoons **Olive Oil**, virgin, first cold pressed

1 teaspoon **Baking Soda**

1 teaspoon **Vanilla**, extract, pure

¼ teaspoon **Salt,** fine, pink, Himalayan

**Cooking Spray** for greasing the baking tray

**EQUIPMENT:**

*Medium size baking tray, Stand or hand mixer fitted with the paddle attachment, Measuring cups, Spatula, Cake decorating piping tips and bags (optional).*

## PREPARATION:

**Step 1:** Chop walnuts and apricots.

**Step 2:** In a bowl of a stand mixer add almond flour, tapioca flour, almond milk, agave nectar, olive oil, baking soda, salt, and vanilla extract. Process everything on low-medium speed until all is combined and forms a soft dough. Roll the dough into a ball. Cover and set aside for one hour.

*Sprinkle the working surface with almond flour.*

**Step 3:** Cut the dough ball in half and cut each of the halves into four parts. Form smaller balls and roll each ball into a circle.

Place chopped apricots and walnuts on one side of each of the circles. Cover it with the other side of the circle. You will have half-circle shaped naans.

Preheat the oven to 355°F.

**Step 4:** Grease the baking tray with a cooking spray. Place the naans onto the baking tray. Bake for 15 minutes on each side (flip with a spatula).

*Almond Flour Naans will keep for a few days in a fridge or one month in a freezer.*

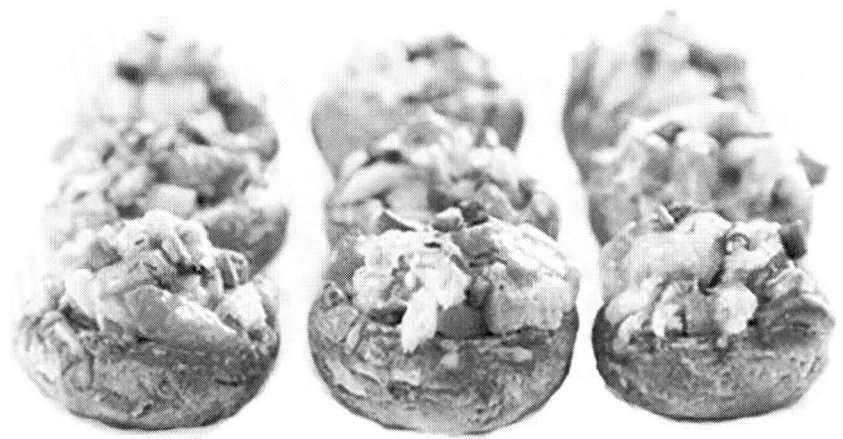

*Almond Flour Stuffed Mushrooms*

# Almond Flour Stuffed Mushrooms

**INGREDIENTS:**

16 **Mushrooms**, button, whole

½ cup **Almond Flour**

½ cup **Walnuts**, raw

6 tablespoons **Almond Milk**

4 tablespoons **Olive Oil**, virgin, first cold pressed

¼ teaspoon **Salt,** fine, pink, Himalayan

½ teaspoon **Garlic**, powder

**Black Pepper**, ground, to taste

**Cooking Spray** for greasing the baking tray

**EQUIPMENT:**

*Medium baking tray, Medium mixing bowl, Measuring cups, Food processor equipped with S-blade, Parchment paper (optional), Cake decorating piping tips and bags (optional).*

**PREPARATION:**

**PREPARE THE FILLING:**

**Step 1:** Separate mushrooms onto cups and stems.

Place walnuts into a food processor. Pulse walnuts until coarsely chopped, add mushroom stems and pulse again to combine.

**Step 2:** Transfer the mixture into the mixing bowl. Add almond flour, almond milk, olive oil, garlic powder, salt, and pepper.

**Step 3:** Preheat the oven to 355°F. Grease the bottom and sides of the baking tray with a cooking spray. Line the bottom of the tray with parchment paper (optional).

**STUFF THE MUSHROOMS:**

Spoon the mixture into the mushroom caps. Place the mushroom cups onto the baking tray. Baste the mushrooms with olive oil and bake for approximately 30 minutes. Serve warm.

*Almond Flour Stuffed Mushrooms will keep one day in a fridge or one month in a freezer.*

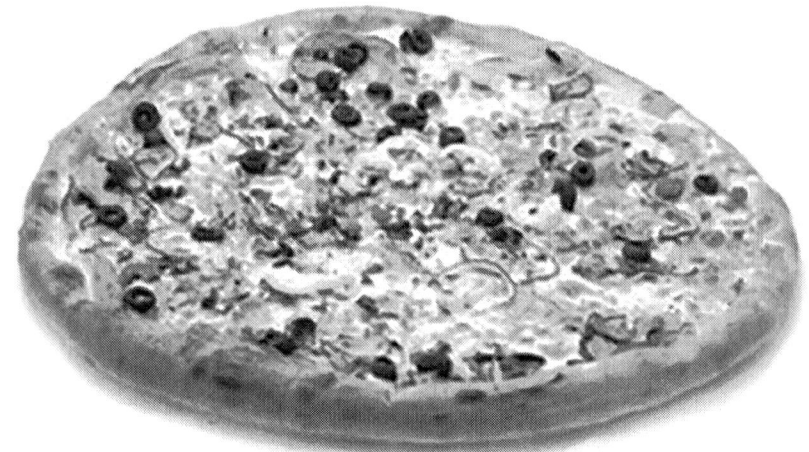

*Sweet Potato Crust Almond Pizza*

# Sweet Potato Crust Almond Pizza

INGREDIENTS:

FOR THE PIZZA CRUST:

1 ½ Lbs. **Sweet Potatoes**, peeled

2 tablespoons **Almond Flour**

2 tablespoons **Oat Flour**, raw

2 tablespoons **Nutritional yeast**

1 tablespoon **Olive Oil**, virgin, cold pressed

½ teaspoon **Oregano**, dried

½ teaspoon **Italian Spice**

3 **Garlic**, cloves, minced

¾ teaspoon **Salt**, Himalayan, pink, fine

6 tablespoons **Water**, hot

2 tablespoons **Flax Seeds**, raw, ground

**Cooking Spray** for greasing the tray

FOR THE ALMOND SPREAD:

3 cups **Almonds**, raw

½ teaspoon **Vanilla**, extract, pure

1/3 cup **Olive Oil**, unrefined

¾ teaspoon **Salt,** Himalayan, pink

## FOR THE PIZZA TOPPINGS:

1 cup **Plums,** dried, pitted, cut in halves

1 cup **Pineapple,** raw, cubed

1 **Onion**, raw

½ cup **Olives,** black, pitted

½ cup **Spinach,** fresh

½ cup **Arugula,** fresh

¾ teaspoon **Salt,** fine, Himalayan, pink

¼ cup **Coconut Oil**, cold pressed

**Cooking Spray** for greasing the tray

**Balsamic Vinegar**, to taste

**Black Pepper**, freshly ground, to taste

## EQUIPMENT:

*Food processor equipped with S-blade, Medium mixing bowl, Rolling pin (optional), Round pizza baking tray, Medium baking tray, Measuring cups, Kitchen knife, Spatula, Parchment paper.*

## PREPARATION:

## MAKE THE PIZZA:

Preheat the oven to 400°F.

**Step 1:** Place sweet potatoes on a baking tray. Bake for one hour or until tender when pierced with a fork. Set aside to cool.

**Step 2:** Prepare egg replacement: add flax seeds into a cup and cover it with hot water. Place flax seeds onto a countertop and wait until flax seeds become gelatin-like.

**Step 3:** Peel sweet potatoes. Place peeled sweet potatoes into the food processor and process until smooth.

**Step 4:** Transfer sweet potatoes into a mixing bowl, add almond flour, oat flours, flaxseed egg, olive oil, nutritional yeast, spices, garlic, and salt. Mix well and roll into a ball. Set aside for 10 minutes to rest at room temperature.

**Step 5:** Line up the pizza tray with parchment paper. Grease the paper with a cooking spray. Spread the sweet potato dough into the pizza tray in shape of a pizza.

Bake for 30 minutes or until the crust is well set and

the edges are golden brown. Cover the crust with another piece of parchment paper and flip it. Peel away the first sheet of paper. Bake the crust for another 5-7 minutes. Set aside to cool.

**MAKE THE VEGAN PARMESAN CHEESE:**

Add cashews, yeast, garlic powder, and fine pink salt to a food processor equipped with S-blade. Pulse until coarsely chopped.

**MAKE THE ALMOND SPREAD:**

In a food processor combine almonds, vanilla extract, olive oil, and salt. Pulse until all ingredients are coarsely chopped. Set aside.

**ASSEMBLE THE PIZZA:**

Preheat the oven to 365°F.

Cut pineapple into small cubes, cut plums in halves, and finely chop onions. Spread the almond butter over the pizza crust. Sprinkle with vegan parmesan cheese. Place the toppings on top of the crust.

Baste pineapple cubes and onions with coconut oil. Place pizza into the oven and bake it for 20-25 minutes. Sprinkle pizza with more parmesan cheese and balsamic vinegar. Serve warm.

*Sweet Potato Crust Almond Pizza will keep for three days in a fridge or one month in a freezer.*

# Almond Flour Crust Pizza

**INGREDIENTS:**

**FOR THE PIZZA CRUST:**

2 cups **Almond Flour**

2 tablespoons **Coconut Flour**

½ cup **Almond Milk**

¼ cup **Olive Oil**, virgin, first cold pressed

1 teaspoon **Baking Soda**

1 teaspoon **Vanilla**, extract, pure

¼ teaspoon **Salt,** fine, pink, Himalayan

**Cooking spray** for greasing the baking tray

**FOR THE FLAX SEED EGG REPLACEMENT:**

4 tablespoons **Water**, hot

2 tablespoons **Flax Seeds**, ground

**FOR THE VEGAN PARMEZAN CHEESE:**

1 cup **Cashews**, raw

6 tablespoons **Yeast,** dry, active

¾ teaspoon **Salt,** fine, Himalayan, pink

½ teaspoon **Garlic**, powder

## FOR THE SAUCE:

1 can **Tomato**, sauce, organic

¼ cup **Basil**, leaves, fresh

½ teaspoon **Oregano**, dried

½ teaspoon **Garlic**, powder

¾ teaspoon **Salt,** fine, Himalayan, pink

## FOR THE PIZZA TOPPINGS:

1 **Pepper**, red, raw

1 **Onion**, raw

½ **cup Olives,** black, pitted

½ cup **Spinach,** fresh

½ cup **Arugula,** fresh

¾ teaspoon **Salt,** Himalayan, pink, fine

¼ cup **Coconut Oil**, cold pressed

**Cooking Spray** for greasing the tray

**Balsamic Vinegar**, to taste

**Black Pepper**, freshly ground, to taste

## EQUIPMENT:

*Food processor equipped with S-blade, Medium mixing bowl, Rolling pin, Round pizza baking tray, Medium baking tray, Measuring cups, Kitchen knife, Spatula, Parchment paper.*

## PREPARATION:

## MAKE THE PIZZA:

**Step 1:** Prepare egg replacement: add flax seeds into a cup and cover it with hot water. Place flax seeds onto a countertop and wait until flax seeds become gelatin-like.

*Alternatively, you can substitute flaxseed eggs for 3 chicken eggs.*

**Step 2:** In a medium mixing bowl combine all dry ingredients. Add wet ingredients. Mix them together to form a soft dough.

**Step 3:** Sprinkle the working surface with almond flour. Transfer the dough to the working surface. Roll the dough ¼ inch thick with a rolling pin.

**Step 4:** Preheat the oven to 350°F.

Prepare the baking tray. Grease the tray with a cooking spray. Line the tray with parchment paper.

Place the crust onto the baking tray. Bake it for approximately 20 minutes. Once it is ready, cover it with another piece of parchment paper and flip it. Peel away the first sheet of paper. Bake for another 5-7 minutes. Set aside to cool.

**MAKE THE VEGAN PARMEZAN CHEESE:**

Add cashews, yeast, garlic powder, and fine pink salt into a food processor equipped with S-blade. Pulse until coarsely chopped.

**MAKE THE SAUCE:**

Combine all ingredients in a food processor. Process until all ingredients are combined. Set aside.

**ASSEMBLE THE PIZZA:**

Preheat the oven to 365°F.

Spread the sauce over the pizza crust. Sprinkle with vegan parmesan cheese. Place the toppings on top of the crust, baste the toppings with coconut oil.

Place pizza into the oven and bake it for 10-15 minutes. Once ready, sprinkle the pizza with more parmesan cheese and balsamic vinegar. Serve warm.

*Almond Flour Crust Pizza will keep for three days in a fridge or one month in a freezer.*

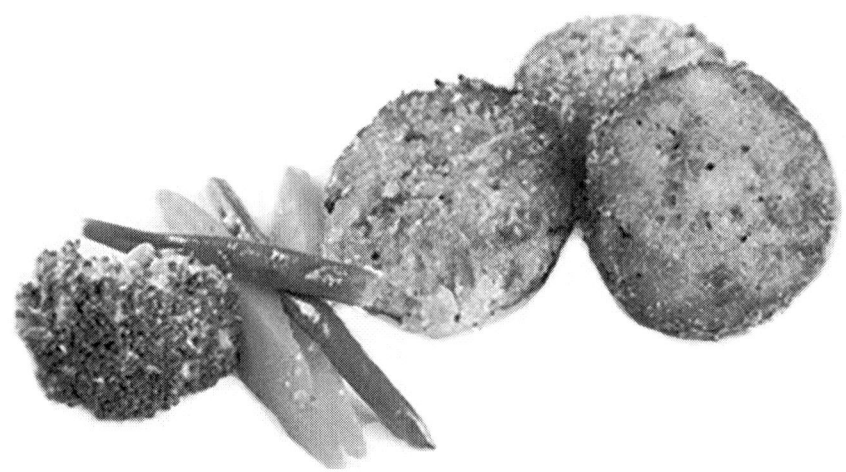

*Almond Flour Crab Cakes*

# Almond Flour Crab Cakes

INGREDIENTS:

1 Lbs. **Crabmeat**, fresh, lump

¼ cup **Almond Flour**

1 **Egg,** large

1 tablespoon **Parsley**, fresh, chopped

1 teaspoon **Lemon**, juice of

1 teaspoon **Mustard**

1 teaspoon **Horseradish**

1 teaspoon **Seafood Seasoning**

1 teaspoon **Salt,** fine, pink, Himalayan

EQUIPMENT:

*Small mixing bowl, Plate, Medium mixing bowl, Medium baking tray, Measuring cups, Kitchen knife, Spatula, Parchment paper.*

PREPARATION:

**Step 1:** In a small mixing add egg, lemon juice, mustard, and horseradish. Whisk together.

**Step 2:** In a medium mixing bowl add crab meat. Fold in almond flour, finely chopped parsley, seafood seasoning, and salt. Combine all ingredients with a spatula and add the egg mixture. Mix well. Separate the mixture into six patties. Set aside.

**Step 3:** Add 1/3 cup of almond flour into a plate. Dip each of the patties into almond flour from both sides.

**Step 4:** Preheat the oven to 365°F.

Prepare the baking tray. Line up the tray with parchment paper. Grease the paper with a cooking spray. Place crab cake patties onto the tray. Bake for 20-30 minutes until golden brown. Serve warm.

*Almond Flour Crab Cakes will keep for three days in a fridge or one month in a freezer.*

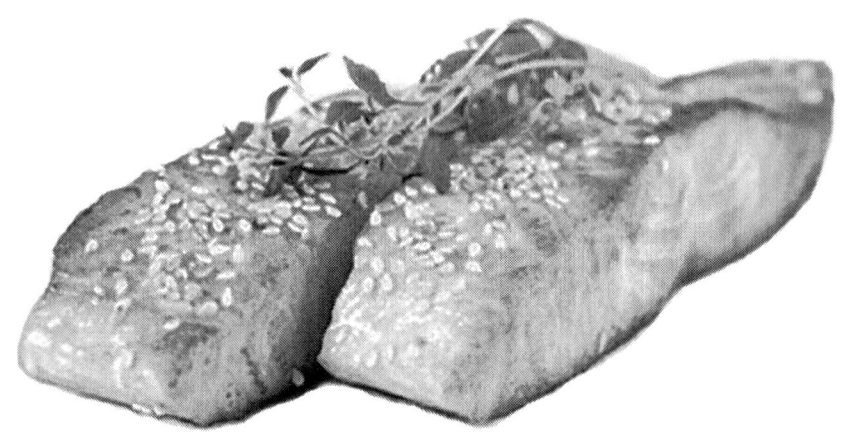

*Almond Flour Crusted Salmon*

# Almond Flour Crusted Salmon

**INGREDIENTS:**

2 Lbs. **Salmon,** fillets

1 cup **Almond Flour**

1 **Lemon,** juice of

1 teaspoon **Mustard**

1 teaspoon **Seafood Seasoning**

1 teaspoon **Salt,** fine, pink, Himalayan

**EQUIPMENT:**

*Lemon squeezer, Small mixing bowl, Plate, Medium baking tray, Measuring cups, Kitchen knife, Spatula, Parchment paper.*

**PREPARATION:**

**Step 1:** In a small mixing bowl squeeze the juice out of one lemon. Add mustard, seafood seasoning, and salt. Whisk all together.

**Step 2:** Preheat the oven to 365°F.

Prepare the baking tray. Grease the tray with a cooking spray. Line the tray with parchment paper.

Clean and portion salmon fillets. Dip the fillets into the bowl with the lemon mixture to cover them with the mixture.

**Step 3:** Add 1/3 cup of almond flour on a plate. Dip each of the salmon fillets into almond flour from both sides.

**Step 4:** Place the fillets onto the baking tray. Bake for 20-30 minutes or until salmon flakes easily when tested with a fork. Serve warm with lemon wedges.

*Almond Flour Crusted Salmon will keep for three days in a fridge or one month in a freezer.*

# Thank You for Purchasing This Book!

I create and test recipes for you. I hope you enjoyed these recipes.

Your review of this book helps me succeed & grow. If you enjoyed this book, please leave me a short (1-2 sentence) review on Amazon.

Thank you so much for reviewing this book!

Do you have any questions?
Email me at: **Maria@BRILLIANTkithenideas.com**

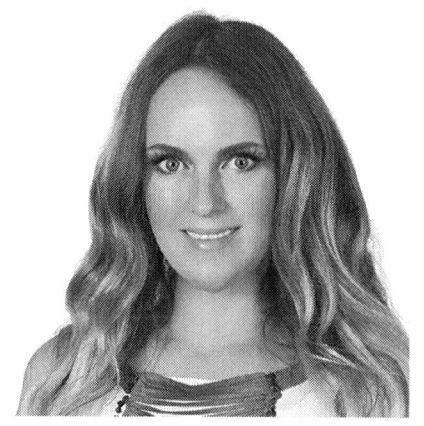

**MARIA SOBININA**
**BRILLIANT kitchen ideas**

Would you like to learn cooking techniques and tips? Visit us at:

**www. BRILLIANTkitchenideas.com**

Printed in Great Britain
by Amazon

**Books by The Winner Twins and Todd McCaffrey**

**Nonfiction:**

*The Write Path: World Building*

**Books by McCaffrey-Winner**

**Twin Soul Series:**

*TS1 - Winter Wyvern*

*TS2 - Cloud Conqueror*

*TS3 - Frozen Sky*

*TS4 - Wyvern's Fate*

*TS5 - Wyvern's Wrath*

*TS6 - Ophidian's Oath*

*TS7 - Snow Serpent*

*TS8 - Iron Air*

*TS9 - Ophidian's Honor*

*TS10 - Healing Fire*

*TS11 - Ophidian's Tears*

*TS12 - Cloud War*

*TS13 - Steel Waters*

*TS14 - Cursed Mage*

*TS15 - Wyvern's Creed*

*TS16 - King's Challenge*

*TS17 - King's Conquest*

*TS18 - King's Treasure*

*TS19 - Wyvern Rider*

*TS20 - King's Crown*

**Books by The Winner Twins**

**Nonfiction:**

*The Write Path: Navigating Storytelling*

**Science Fiction:**

*The Strand Prophecy*

*Extinction's Embrace*

*PCT: Perfect Compatibility Test*

**Poetry Books by Brianna Winner**

*Millennial Madness*

# Books by Todd McCaffrey

## Science fiction

*Ellay*

*The Jupiter Game*

*The Steam Walker*

## Collections

*The One Tree of Luna (And Other Stories)*

## Dragonriders of Pern® Series

*Dragon's Kin*

*Dragon's Fire*

*Dragon Harper*

*Dragonsblood*

*Dragonheart*

*Dragongirl*

*Dragon's Time*

*Sky Dragons*

## Non-fiction

*Dragonholder: The Life And Times of Anne McCaffrey*

*Dragonwriter: A tribute to Anne McCaffrey and Pern*

# Map

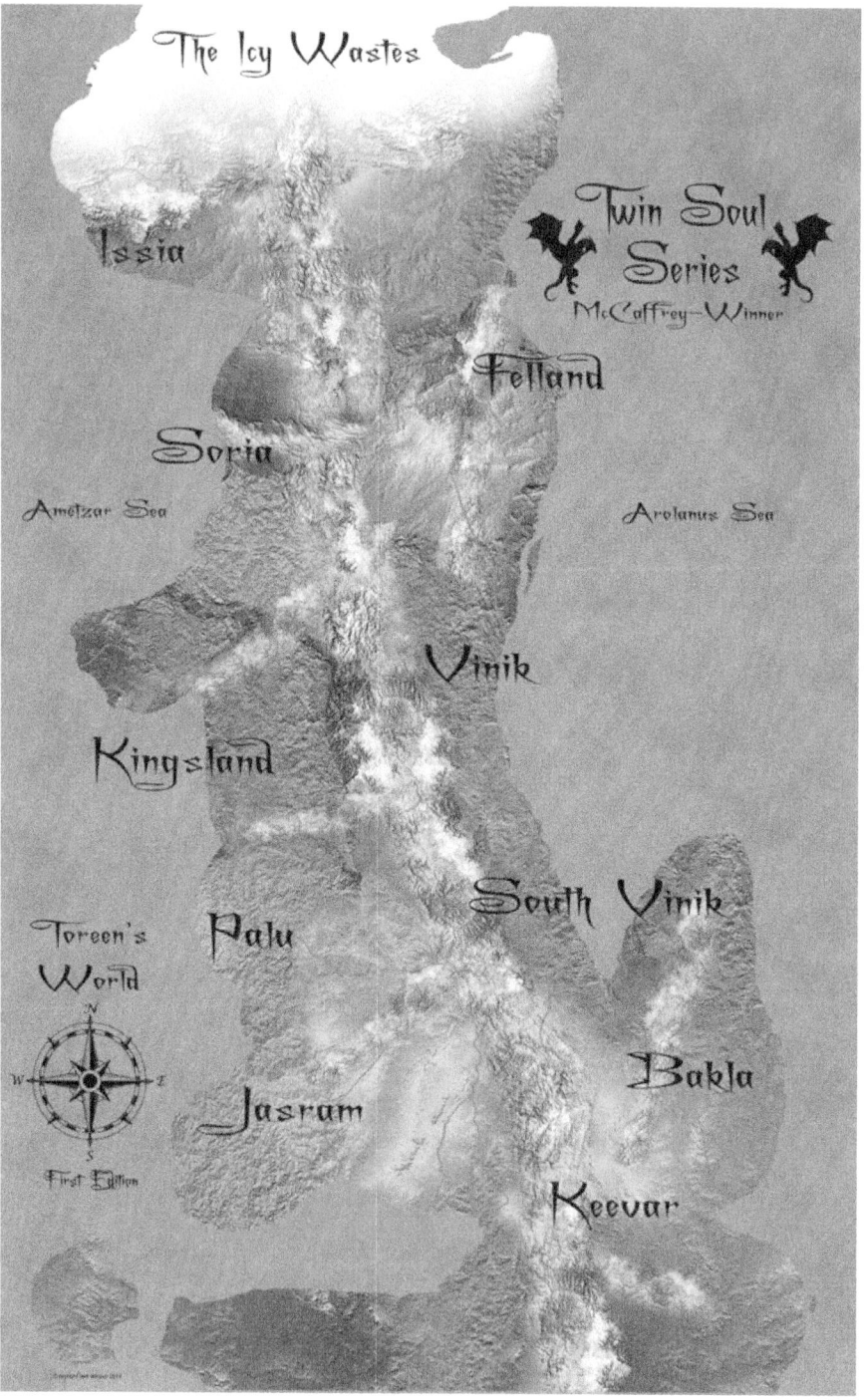

# Contents

## Twin Soul Series Omnibus 4     1

Map     6

## King's Challenge     9

Chapter One     11
Chapter Two     17
Chapter Three     25
Chapter Four     30
Chapter Five     36
Chapter Six     43

## King's Conquest     48

Chapter One     50
Chapter Two     55
Chapter Three     61
Chapter Four     66
Chapter Six     73
Chapter Seven     80
Epilog     82

## King's Treasure     84

Chapter One     86

| | |
|---|---|
| Chapter Two | 91 |
| Chapter Three | 99 |
| Chapter Four | 108 |
| Chapter Five | 115 |
| Chapter Six | 120 |
| Epilog | 127 |

# Wyvern Rider — 129

| | |
|---|---|
| Chapter One | 131 |
| Chapter Two | 136 |
| Chapter Three | 141 |
| Chapter Four | 147 |
| Chapter Five | 154 |
| Chapter Six | 161 |
| Chapter Seven | 167 |

# King's Crown — 178

| | |
|---|---|
| Prolog | 180 |
| Chapter One | 187 |
| Chapter Two | 192 |
| Chapter Three | 197 |
| Chapter Four | 202 |
| Chapter Five | 208 |
| Chapter Six | 215 |
| Chapter Seven | 224 |
| Epilog | 227 |
| Acknowledgements | 230 |
| About the Authors | 231 |

# King's Challenge

## Book 16

Twin Soul series

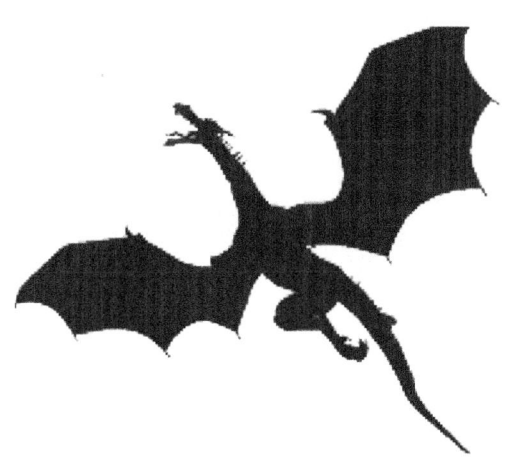

# Dedication

**For Debbie**

# Chapter One

Skara Ningan had been in many difficult situations in her short life, so this new one, while unique, was not beyond her. She was in a strange room in a strange building.

In front of her stood a strange being — dim blue lights glowed from a curved metal face with a blade nose and comical ears. The thing — a metal immortal — had a metal chest separated from its metal torso by a thin, wiry spine. The legs it stood on were thinner and more wiry than a human's but — made of metal — they were certainly stronger. As were the thin arms raised in a threatening manner. But the arms held no weapons.

Skara's arms, on the other hand, suddenly became filled with sharp pointy things. Next to her, Thomas Walpish, formerly of King Markel's cavalry, gestured for her to lower her arms.

"We mean no harm," Thomas said to the metal being. "We sought shelter here at Ibb the immortal's." He cocked his head questioningly. "Did you just arrive?"

"I have been here for some time," the mechanical said. "What is your purpose here?"

"We seek safety and shelter," Thomas said, eyeing Skara sideways and gesturing again for her to sheath her weapons. "Mage Margen suggested we could use this space without harm."

"I know nothing of this mage," the mechanical replied. "And I know nothing of you."

Thomas bowed in acknowledgement. "I am Thomas Walpish, formerly a colonel in the Kingsland cavalry." He waved a hand toward Skara. "This lady is Skara Ningan, formerly employed by mage Vistos of Kingsland as an assassin."

"'Formerly?'" the mechanical repeated.

"We left our employment under a cloud," Skara spoke up. "My former employer tried to use magic to control me and, ultimately, to kill me."

"After she was ordered to kill me," Thomas added in a dry tone.

"What has this to do with Ibb?" the mechanical asked.

"Directly: nothing," Thomas replied. "The last I heard of Ibb, he was a prisoner at the King's pleasure."

"And then?"

"I've heard that he escaped," Skara Ningan said, glancing to Thomas to see his reaction to the news. The ex-officer shrugged.

"And why are you here now?"

"The mage Vistos employs a harsh method of control," Thomas said. "We promised to make him stop."

"I doubt anything less than death would stop him," the mechanical replied, "particularly if the current situation is to his advantage." The mechanical cocked its head and sniffed. A hand rose toward Skara. "There is a miasma about you."

"Pardon?" Skara asked.

"A smell," the mechanical explained. "The smell of magic, of tainted magic."

Skara glanced to Thomas who shrugged in reply. Cautiously, Skara removed the tainted tooth from her pocket and held it up. "Is this what you smell?"

The mechanical leaned forward, sniffed again, and recoiled. "Yes," the mechanical replied. "What is it?"

"It is a tooth, an ensorceled tooth," Thomas said. "It was in her mouth."

"She should be dead," the mechanical said in a tone of surprise.

"We removed it before it could destroy her," Thomas said. "Which led us on our path here."

"I see," the mechanical said. The mechanical stood silently for a long moment. "I shall permit you to stay," the mechanical said. "It is possible that we may be able to assist each other."

"Thank you," Skara said. She extended a hand. "You know our names, may we know yours?"

"My name is unimportant," the mechanical replied. "I am Tracker, that suffices."

"Tracker?" Thomas repeated with a raised eyebrow.

"It describes my function," Tracker replied. "I track things."

"And Ibb? What does that describe?" Skara asked.

Tracker made a squeaking kind of rumble at the bottom of its chest.

"It describes a most difficult immortal," Tracker replied. "One who insists upon using a name and not a function."

"That sounds like all I've heard of Ibb," a new voice spoke up, startling all three to turn in its direction. Mage Margen stood to one side behind Skara. "I am mage Margen."

"You were not here earlier," Tracker said. "You have transported yourself through the wards just this instant."

"Indeed so," Margen replied. "And you are what appeared to be that strange barrel by the front door earlier."

"It is my dormant form," Tracker admitted. Tracker's head tilted. "Why are you here?"

"I put wards on my friends here, to protect them," Margen said.

"I did not detect such wards," Tracker said.

"Good," Margen said with a small smile.

"Here, let me help you up," Ellen Annabelle said, moving forward to the new form in front of her.

"I can get up myself!" Lisette said sharply, laying one hand on the ground to raise her torso. She failed and stopped abruptly. It was then that she looked beyond her torso to her waist. "What?"

"You were dead," Ellen Annabelle said. "We thought —"

"What happened?" Lisette cried in fear.

Ellen rushed forward. "You've got to put your legs underneath you before you can stand."

"What did you do to me?" Lisette wailed.

"You were dead," Annabelle told her. "We brought you back the only way we could."

"How?" Lisette asked. "What — why can't I see my feet?"

"Let's get you standing, first," Annabelle told her soothingly. "You'll see then."

"Help me up," Lisette said in a tone of resignation.

"We'll help you roll over," Ellen said.

"'We'?" Lisette said. "All I see is one of you but you talk funny."

"We'll explain in a bit," Ellen said. "Perhaps it's best if we —" and instantly the small girl was a wyvern who launched herself into the sky to hover over Lisette's rear. With deft work with her hind claws, Ellen rolled the new-formed person upright. She dropped down and returned to her human form immediately.

"What are you?" Lisette said. "You just turned into a — a dragon or something!"

"A wyvern, actually," Annabelle corrected pedantically. "A dragon has four feet."

Lisette tried to run away from this scary person. She took only a few steps before she halted, her legs useless.

"What's wrong with me?" she cried.

"You were dead," Ellen said. "Your mare was dying, she'd broken her legs —"

"What? How?" Lisette demanded.

"Your brother took her jumping, he says he didn't realize how hard the ground was —"

"Marie? Where is she? How is she?" Lisette demanded, turning her head toward the entrance of the stables. She took a hesitant step forward and stopped again in frustration.

"Um," Ellen said, flailing for words.

"Both her forelegs were broken," Annabelle said, taking charge of the conversation. "She would have had to be put down —"

"*No!*" Lisette shrieked in horror. Her voice broke into a horse's whinny of despair. She clapped her mouth shut in astonishment. She looked down, saw her bare torso, looked further — and stopped. Eyes bulging, she raised her head toward Ellen Annabelle.

"Marie gave us her consent," Ellen said in a small voice. "And she consented for you, too." Ellen made a sound deep in her throat. "If she was wrong —"

"What. Did. You. Do." Lisette ground out, her jaw tight with fury.

"We joined you," Annabelle said. "Two broken lives into one new whole."

"And me... what?"

"A centaur," Ellen told her. "That's why you're having trouble walking. You've got four legs now."

"Three rooms for the night!" a gruff man's voice bellowed as he entered with three youths. Helene Aubrey glanced over and made an instant decision.

"Welcome to the House of the Kind Seas," she said. "Three rooms? I'm not sure we've got that many free, kind sir, perhaps you could make do with two?"

"Moira?" the man said to the girl standing behind him. "A breath of fresh air?"

Moira smiled and waved toward the fireplace. Helene stiffened as a breeze rushed past her and the fire flared upwards. She turned back just in time to see one of the boys create a small ball of fire in his palm and smiled fiercely.

"We've just built the train station and laid tracks," the man said. "We're tired, want food, and a place for rest."

"Of course, sir!" Helene said instantly. She turned to one of her girls, saying, "You heard the man! Three rooms, clean sheets on all the beds!"

The girl gave her a startled look, looked at the four standing in the doorway and scampered away as quick as her legs could carry her.

"May we offer you food here in the dining room or would you prefer to have it served in your rooms?" Madame Aubrey asked.

"Here," the man replied. "I was told that you know a Master Hewlitt. He said that he could rely on you."

Helene's face paled and she licked her lips nervously. "Master Hewlitt? Of course. Nothing but the best for our Kingsland friends."

"Enter!" Captain Welless said when he heard a soft rap on the door to his office. A small girl opened it and glanced toward him in surprise. "What do you want?"

"Are you in charge?" the girl asked.

"What if I — wait! You're not Sorian," the captain said.

"I am Margaret Waters," the girl replied, drawing herself to her full height. "I work for the Steam Master."

"Really?" Captain Welless said mockingly. "And what do you do for him?"

A cold wind dashed past the captain's left ear and settled on his shoulders.

"I work magic," Margaret replied calmly. "I'm here to discuss the rail lines to the north and west."

"Rail lines?" Welless repeated without comprehension. "What rail lines? You can't mean for a locomotive? Those tracks weigh tons and the timbers needed —"

"I lay both of those," Margaret replied. "My men and I seek lodging until we can get resupplied —"

"That's none of my concern, young lady!" Welless growled. Another cold wind flew past his ear, the right one this time. "Stop that! Stop that magic immediately or I'll have my guards throw you in jail!"

"About the jail," Margaret replied, her lips twitching upwards, "I'm afraid we'll have to destroy it. It's on the path."

"Destroy it!" Captain Welless roared, jumping out of his seat. His explosive comment caused another door to open and a well-dressed man peered around it. "Mr. Beck! This *girl* wants to destroy your jail! Perhaps you should deal with her."

"Indeed," Hamo Beck replied. He wagged a finger toward Margaret. "Perhaps you'd care to come into my office." He glanced to the captain, whose temper was visibly cooling. "Perhaps we should get some tea?"

"I'll have my man send for it," Welless replied, glad to rid himself of this troublesome nuisance.

"Come with me then, dear," Hamo Beck said soothingly. Margaret glanced to the captain who jerked his head pointedly toward Beck's office and turned deliberately away, calling, "Nox! Nox! Tea for three, in two pots!"

"Yes sir, right away sir," a voice called from further back in the building.

Margaret followed Hamo Beck into his office. It was well appointed.

"You're Sorian?" Margaret asked, glancing toward the door behind her and the captain behind it. "He works for you?"

"The captain finds it easiest to leave civil matters to me, miss," Hamo Beck said with a small smile.

Margaret beamed and laughed at his response. "Oh, I *like* you!" she said.

"And what is it I can do for you, miss?" Hamo Beck asked as a knock interrupted them and a small, bustling soldier laid out a pot of tea and two cups from the tray he carried. "I've already seen to the captain," the man, apparently Nox, said diffidently.

"Very good, and well done," Hamo Beck said, nodding approvingly. The young private knuckled his forehead in salute and beamed, turning abruptly with tray in hand. To the girl, Hamo said, "Shall I pour?"

"Let me," Margaret said, waving her hands and smiling as she deftly sent air currents out to do the task. She smiled at him as a final wave sent his cup wafting across the mahogany table to stop just in front of his right wrist. Another gesture lifted the small milk jug and hovered it over his cup. "Milk?"

"Just sugar," Hamo Beck replied, not at all surprised at her magic. "Two, please."

Dutifully Margaret plopped two cubes of sugar into the cup and raised a spoon to stir it twice. When the spoon returned to its place beside Hamo's saucer, the man smiled gratefully and raised the cup to his lips. "Delightful!"

Margaret smiled in return and sipped her own tea appreciatively.

"That was quite the display, miss," Hamo said as he put his cup down in its saucer. "You are certainly a talented practitioner."

"I was well trained," Margaret said, her tone going tighter.

"Trained? By whom?"

"I don't know if you've heard of him," Margaret said. "In Kingsford he's called the Steam Master."

"Oh!" Hamo Beck said, surprised. "Actually, miss, I *have* heard of him."

"Really?" Margaret replied, eyebrows going up. "How?"

"I am the mayor of this town of Korin's Pass, miss," Hamo said. "Part of my job is to keep abreast of things."

"I see," Margaret said judiciously. "And what did you hear?"

"I heard that the Steam Master worked with several people to create the locomotives and the rails they ride on," Hamo replied. Thoughtfully he added, "And I'd heard rumors that there were plans to extend the lines north through Korin's Pass."

"That work has been done," Margaret said, sitting up straighter in her chair.

"Really? Now? In winter?" Hamo asked, surprised. He said softly to himself, "I wonder that I hadn't heard…"

"It was just finished this day," Margaret replied. "Which is why I'm here. My men and I need lodging and rest. Until more supplies are brought up, that is."

"Your men?" Hamo repeated thoughtfully. He looked shocked. "I'm sorry, miss, but I cannot imagine how Korin's Pass could provide lodging or food for thousands —"

"Who said anything about thousands?"

"What? I mean, your crew — it must number —"

"Thirty," Margaret said. "Thirty-three if you include the locomotive engineer and his stokers. But they'll only need food, they're staying on the train, of course. And my men can stay in tents. They'll need food and fuel for their fire." She met his eyes. "I'd like a room for myself and my sister, and another for my brother."

"With baths?"

"If possible," Margaret said. "Certainly we'll want access to a bath." She smiled at him. "My brother can provide the hot water, if that's a problem."

"We have access to coal," Hamo said, shaking his head. He glanced up. "And how long might we expect to entertain you?"

Margaret shrugged. "We need to wait until we get more rail lines and timber," she said. "Once we're ready, we'll be laying track to the west and north as quick as we can." She eyed him shrewdly. "I imagine your king will find this information of much value."

"Which king, miss?" Hamo replied, his eyes gleaming. "Recently, this town of mine has come under the rule of King Markel."

"Ah, so perhaps not, then," Margaret replied smoothly.

Hamo Beck chuckled, shaking his head. "You, miss, are quite the politician!"

"I try to be politic, nothing more," Margaret said.

"And do you, too, serve King Markel?"

"I do as my father asks," Margaret replied primly.

"As well a good child should," Hamo said agreeably. Margaret gave him a sharp look with her brows furrowed, trying to grasp the hidden meaning in his tone. Hamo saw her confusion and relented enough to say, "All children grow up, miss. And when they do, they find their own lives to lead."

"I like laying the lines, building the railways," Margaret said. Abruptly, she rose. "So, can you provide us our needs?"

Hamo rose with her. "Of course, miss," he said genially. "Korin's Pass shall be delighted to help you in your tasks." He added as he took in her doubtful look, "Your rail lines will increase trade and shall aid our profits."

"Yes," Margaret said, her agreement weak.

"Let me introduce you to our inn, miss," Hamo replied. He gave her a half bow before waving her to the door. "I am the innkeeper, so I can guarantee you the best."

# Chapter Two

"A centaur?" Lisette repeated, her eyes going wide. She twisted her neck but found her whole body twisting so she couldn't see behind her. She gave huff of annoyance and turned back to Ellen Annabelle. "Really?"

"Really," Annabelle told her. "Queen Alva and I met one when we were young." Annabelle, using Ellen's body, made a face and said, "If you try hard, you can call your brother with a whinny."

"A whinny? Like a horse?"

"No," Annabelle said. "Like a centaur." She gave Lisette a hopeful look, as she added, "Centaurs have magic, just like wyverns and other twin souls."

"You're a twin soul?" Lisette said. "Like me?"

"Different," Ellen said, capturing her voice again. "Annabelle and I are special —"

"How?"

"We can't say," Annabelle replied, looking irked with her twin soul partner. "We can change into a wyvern."

"I can change into a horse?"

"Or a human," Ellen said, exasperated at Annabelle for having hijacked the conversation. To Annabelle she added, "That's what I was trying to tell her."

"How do I change into a human?" Lisette asked.

"I would have thought that the better question would be: how do I change into a horse," Ellen said. "Right now you're just half and half. Don't you want to know what it's like to be wholly a horse?"

Lisette thought about that for a moment and nodded. "So how do I do that?"

Ellen pursed her lips and shook her head. "I haven't a clue."

"What?"

"I think Maro, Alva's mage, might," Ellen said. "That's why I thought it'd be a good idea to try to whinny and call your brother. The others will surely follow him."

"Whinny?"

"Like a horse," Ellen said.

"I *know* that!" Lisette replied angrily. "I just don't know how!"

"Try," Ellen suggested. "Let me show you how we change into a wyvern." She grinned at the new-made centaur. "Watch carefully." A moment later a large wyvern stood in front of Lisette. Lisette had to fight back an urge to flee and let out a whinny of terror. In the next instant, the human girl stood in front of her. "You learned how to whinny!"

"You scared me half to death!" Lisette raged. She started to say more but stopped as she caught movement out of the corner of her eyes. Alain, Alva, Maro, and some zwerg guards approached at a trot.

Alain stopped just in front of her, his eyes wide. He glanced at Ellen Annabelle then back to the four-legged creature. "Lisette?"

"Lisette Marie, to be precise," Annabelle said through Ellen's mouth.

Alva moved beyond the awestruck lad and moved to pat Lisette on her withers. Lisette craned her neck to see what the zwerg queen was doing but stopped when she felt gentle hands move down her forelegs.

"The break is healed," Alva said, moving back and staring up at the human half of the centaur. "How do you feel?"

"I —" Lisette started to catalog her fears and worries but stopped. "I feel great! I feel like I could run — like I could gallop forever!" She punctuated this by lifting her head up toward the skies and whinnying so loud that the ground shook. "I'm more alive than I've ever been!"

"You're not wearing anything," Alain said, stripping off his shirt and handing it to her. Lisette took the proffered, over-large shirt and draped it around herself.

"Most centaurs go bare," Maro said. "Although many prefer to paint themselves." She made a face. "I think some of it is to protect their human skin from sunburn."

"That makes sense," Queen Alva said.

"Bare?" Alain said, aghast. "But when they're older…?"

"The females appear the same as the males in their human half," Maro said. "They make no distinction there."

Alain absorbed this slowly.

"She should be able to take both forms," Ellen Annabelle said, turning to Maro, "human and horse. Can you teach her?"

Maro shook her head. "I've seen it, and I know it can be done but I'd say that Lisette —"

"Lisette Marie," Lisette corrected gently.

"— Lisette Marie, then, could learn from the other centaurs quickly enough," Maro finished with a grateful nod to the centaur for the correction. The zwerg mage glanced around and added darkly, "Although finding a centaur might be hard."

"Why?" Alain asked, his eyes narrowing.

"Because the Grand Duke is trying to kill them all," Alva said.

"He fears them," Maro added. She glanced at Lisette Marie. "And, now, he has reason to fear them."

"Reason?" Alain asked. "How?"

"Because your sister could easily lead a rebellion against him," Alva said, her head turning thoughtfully to Maro. "Between Alain Casman and Lisette Marie, they would have a strong claim, wouldn't they?"

"They would," Maro agreed. She glanced over toward Ellen Annabelle. "Was that your plan all along?"

Ellen shook her head. "Not mine," she said. "Nor Annabelle's either, I think."

"But the gods…," Lisette Marie said, glancing down to her brother and the smaller zwerg in front of her. Even though she had hardly finished her growth, she was now more than a head taller than her brother. It pleased her.

"I cannot stay here much longer," Ellen Annabelle warned. "I have to go north."

"Have to?"

"I find it wise not to argue with the gods," Annabelle said.

"Too much," Ellen added with a smirk.

"Could you take us down to the valley below?" Alain said, pointing to the wide plains that stretched to the sea.

"We should eat, rest, and plan first," Alva said. "Can you stay the night?"

"I'd like nothing better!" Annabelle said cheerfully.

"Send for more wine and food," Mage Vistos ordered the drudge attending his bath. As he scurried away, he bellowed, "And more hot water!" To himself he added, "I've been among the stench of the riffraff for too long."

He leaned back in his tub and wiped down his arm with a sponge. The water was warm, the evening cold, and he was relaxing. Finally.

He couldn't wait to get the last of the stench of the South Sea Pass from his skin. To feel clean.

The drudge returned with another. One put a small plate of food and a flagon of wine at the table beside the tub and the other added warm water, careful not to scald the mage and earn his ire.

"Better," Vistos said. "Bring towels, I'll need them soon." As the younger drudge started to scamper away, Vistos said, "Not you! You stay here." He smiled at the dirty, ragged boy, adding, "If you behave, I'll have a treat for you."

"Sir," the little boy said, his eyes downcast.

"I have a whole pocketful of the most wonderful sweets," Vistos said, reaching for his wine glass. "A little wretch like you should get some reward, eh?"

The drudge did not reply, merely glancing helplessly toward the older drudge who was all too happy to leave the room.

A drudge would hear things, Vistos knew. And a drudge with a sweet tooth would be all too willing to inform his master. A small drudge would go places a larger one would not. So the small one would do.

Mage Vistos smiled to himself and lay back in his warm bath. He could allow himself some rest. But after, when he was dressed and relaxed, he would start the search for a new apprentice. Perhaps one of Margen's brats would do. Vistos smiled to himself. Perhaps he'd sprinkle the paper-wrapped sweets around liberally and take the whole lot. Wouldn't Margen be furious when he found out. Furious and helpless. For Vistos had a god protecting him. Against his god, mage Margen was powerless. Didn't Margen have a granddaughter? Vistos smiled at the thought.

The sun was bright and warm as Ellen Annabelle landed on the Jasram Plains, gently depositing the centaur held in her claws and then moving forward and landing, allowing Alain Casmain to climb down from her shoulders.

A moment later, Ellen Annabelle stood in front of him in human form. "Whew! I wasn't quite sure I could do that," Ellen said, relieved.

"Why didn't you tell us?" Alain demanded.

'Ellen shrugged. "I didn't want to alarm you."

Alain gave her a fiery look but, before he could say anything, Lisette Marie trotted up and tapped him on the shoulder with her hand. She turned to Ellen Annabelle, placing herself in front of her brother. "We are grateful for all the help you've given us."

Alain's expression darkened but Lisette Marie tapped his foot with her hind hoof and he glanced sharply toward her then back to Ellen Annabelle. He gave her a stiff bow.

"I know nothing of these lands," Annabelle said, turning away from the brother and sister to scan the horizon.

"We grew up here," Lisette Marie assured her. Alain snorted. "Well, near here. This is the country my father ruled."

"There's a camp nearby," Annabelle said, pointing to the east. "I think it might be centaurs."

"I will scout ahead," Alain said, giving his centaur sister a cautioning look. "You stay here."

Lisette snorted and stamped her fore-hooves on the ground, hard.

"If they are not friends, and looking for centaurs," Annabelle said, "you might be in danger."

Lisette frowned, glancing between her brother and the twin souled human, looking more mulish than horse.

"If they are centaurs," Annabelle continued, "they will have seen our descent. I don't think they like wyverns."

"Because you probably eat them," Alain groused.

"Alain!" Lisette Marie chided, turning and swiftly whacking him on the shoulder.

*She likes that she's taller than him,* Ellen commented to Annabelle.

*He is afraid of women,* Annabelle responded, her tone sad.

*I think he'll get over it,* Ellen guessed. She could sense Annabelle's silent disagreement, so she explained, *He loves his sister.*

Annabelle's disagreement faded into thoughtfulness. After a moment she thought, *We must be off.*

*Yes,* Ellen agreed. She turned to look up at Lisette Marie. *I wonder what father will say.*

Annabelle was amused at the notion. *I'm sure we'll find out soon enough.*

*But you're wondering why we're needed in Kingsford,* Ellen guessed. She frowned at Lisette Marie. "We're going to have to go."

"You two were talking to each other, in your head, weren't you?" Lisette asked. When Ellen nodded, Lisette's expression grew wistful. "It's not the same with Marie."

"You should be glad. At least she's not carrying poison in her body," Annabelle replied sourly.

"I'm sorry," Marie said. "I didn't mean it like that."

"We know," Ellen said, sending a chiding thought to her older partner. "Annabelle thinks that you might find you two can communicate just like we do, only differently."

Lisette tried to smile in agreement but it was a feeble attempt.

"The sun is getting higher in the sky," Alain said, pointing to the east. He said to Ellen, "I'm sorry you must leave but I think the sooner the better."

"We'll come back," Annnabelle promised.

"I'd like that," Lisette said. Alain moved up to stand beside her, adding, "I should like to get to know you better, Ellen Annabelle."

"Maybe one day," Ellen agreed. She stepped back from the two of them, turned to the right and leaped — turning into a wyvern before her feet returned to the ground. She rose high, circled over them once and then — she just disappeared.

"That's magic," Lisette Marie said, glancing up at where the wyvern had been.

"Come on, we must be on our way," Alain said, turning to trudge eastwards.

# King's Challenge

King Markel was in the best of moods as he strode into his royal throne room, guards and courtiers falling to the side as he marched up to take his royal seat. *I wonder if the throne in Sarskal is better.*

He turned back and waved everyone to their ease. He glanced toward first minister Mannevy and nodded regally.

"Your majesty, we have some petitioners —"

"Yes, yes," Markel said, waving a languid hand. "Send them forward."

Mannevy nodded to the guards at the doors who nodded in response and opened the door to let the first petitioner in.

A well-dressed noble stepped forward, paused in front of the royal throne and went to one knee, bowing deeply.

"His Grace the Duke of Southerland," first minister Mannevy announced.

"Rise, Your Grace," King Markel said, gesturing, "and state your grievance."

"Not so much a grievance, your majesty," Duke Southerland said as he rose slowly to his feet, "but a request."

"Then state your request," Markel said, a slight bite entering his tone.

"Your majesty, we have watched from the southernmost end of your kingdom with awe and glee at your conquests," Duke Southerland began. "We are in awe of your army and its success —"

"Yes, yes," King Markel said, waving a bored hand. "State your request, my good duke."

"We were wondering, sire, when we might hope to see your great locomotives move south," the duke said succinctly. "We have a great deal of wares to sell here in the north for the profit of all the kingdom — and the royal purse in particular — and we are miserable that we cannot bring them to market here in the most efficient manner."

"You want trains going south?" King Markel asked, turning to Mannevy who nodded in agreement. Markel frowned in thought. "I see no reason —"

Beside him, his first minister coughed politely. The king stopped, glaring at his first minister. "Is there a reason?"

"Your majesty," Mannevy began, "much though it grieves me to have to say this but our treasury cannot manage expansions both northward to Soria and southwards to our lower holdings at the same time."

"It can't?"

"Not and continue our airship expansion, your majesty," Mannevy told him politely.

"Sire," the duke broke in, "if I may?"

Markel nodded permission.

The Duke of Southerland turned to the first minister and said, "I believe that the sooner your rail lines can connect all our kingdom, the sooner the treasury will benefit."

"No doubt, your grace," Mannevy returned easily, "but I was ordered to proceed on a particular course of action. If we divert our attention to building more rail lines, we'll need to recruit more magicians — and there is a lack — gather more iron, which we also lack, and cut more timbers —"

"In that, first minister, my estates in Southerland can meet your every need," His Grace broke in.

"Sadly, no," Mannevy said, shaking his head. "Your forests are marvels but they are composed mainly of the softer, lighter woods whereas the train tracks need hardier timbers to support the weight of the trains."

"Work it out," the king said. "Give him what he wants."

"Sire —" Mannevy began tentatively. "It will affect your plans, sire, and not in a good way."

"I'm sure, my good minister, that you will find a way to make both my plan and the request of my noble subject work out harmoniously."

Mannevy drew breath to protest but, catching the king's glare, let it out in a sigh. "As you wish, your majesty."

"Very good!" Markel said. He turned toward the duke. "You must join me for dinner tonight. I'm sure Mannevy will have all the details by then."

"I'll be delighted, sire!" the duke returned with a hearty laugh. He turned to Mannevy. "And I'll be most interested in your plans, my good sir."

Mannevy managed a nod but was wordless. *A plan? By evening?*

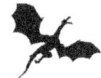

"I hope you know what you're doing," Peter Hewlitt muttered as he and first minister Mannevy entered the darkened office later that afternoon.

"I am doing the King's business, as usual," Mannevy replied. But his heart wasn't in his words.

"But I understand that the Steam Master is not one to take the unexpected lightly."

"It depends what it is," a dark voice answered from further back in the office. "And who is presenting it."

First minister Mannevy smiled. "Mr. Brookes, I am here on behalf of the king —"

"With pay, I expect," Brookes replied, moving out of the shadows and wiping his hands with a dirty rag.

"Ah…"

"No pay, no work," Brookes said, his tone going harsh. "My teams are working flat out to connect Korin's Pass with South Sea Pass. They'll want their money. And so do I."

"The payment is in process," Mannevy replied suavely.

"And you're so certain of your welcome that you brought the king's spymaster with you?"

"I asked to come along," Peter lied smoothly. "I've heard a lot about you and felt it was time to meet in person."

"I've heard more about you," Brookes said, turning to spit on the floor.

"My reputation precedes me, I see," Hewlitt said with a glance toward the gob of spit on the floor, his eyes glinting.

"So that mortals would fear you," Brookes guessed.

Hewlitt twitched his head in a quick nod.

"So, first minister, you have something to say to me?" Brookes said, turning his attention to Mannevy.

"Indeed, I do," Mannevy said. "Something for our mutual profit."

Brookes snorted. "It's always for our mutual profit and yet my coffers are still bare."

"It takes time to generate trade," Mannevy replied. "It takes time for habits to change."

"The King can change them," Brookes replied gruffly.

"And he will," Mannevy agreed smoothly. "In fact, in this new venture, he has already indicated a willingness to move quickly."

"New venture?" Brookes turned to Hewlitt. "And, spymaster, what perchance is this new venture?"

"We want to accelerate our developments to the south," Mannevy replied. "Build rail lines along the coast and inland, get more trade flowing."

Brookes snorted derisively. "I'll just bet the carters are going to *love* that!"

"Actually," Hewlitt replied, "I believe they will."

Brookes gave him an encouraging gesture with his hand.

"Mostly we transport goods by sea or river," Hewlitt said. "Carters carry them only the last little bit from the docks to the stores."

Brookes grunted in agreement and gave the spymaster a challenging look.

"We've got some roads leading to our rivers but not many and they're all bad," Hewlitt continued. "Anyone carting anything over much distance pays for that in both time and wear on their equipment."

"Which is why we use the rails," Brookes said in agreement. "But the carters won't love us, we're just more competition."

Hewlitt smiled. "If we choose to be," Peter Hewlitt said. "If we arrange it that our rails are near the warehouses, the docks, wherever carters pick up loads, then the rails will just be another stop for them. In fact, they could make a good deal of money transferring goods from the rails to the river boats and ships."

"Huh," Brookes grunted. He turned to Mannevy. "So what's in it for me?"

"You'll continue your monopoly on rail and locomotives," Mannevy said. "The King will collect a tithe."

"What else?" Torvan Brookes demanded.

"What do you want?" Mannevy asked.

"I think I'd like a title," Brookes said.

"The Steam Master is available," Peter Hewlitt murmured.

Brookes shot him a sour look. "I've already got that."

"Lord Steam?" Hewlitt suggested.

"Lord Brookes sounds better," Brookes replied. He turned his eyes to Mannevy. "When do you want this done?"

"As soon as possible," Mannevy said. "Without interfering with our other projects."

"Well… there's the problem," Brookes said. "I'll need to build more teams, find more magicians…" He gave the first minister a sly look. "I'll want the king's writ to impress whoever I want."

"The king's writ?" Mannevy said, taken aback. "I don't —"

"Everyone is fighting for mages," Brookes said. "If you want these rail lines, I'll need first pick. And no questions. I can't afford to make picks and have to fight for them later."

Mannevy shot a look at Hewlitt who shrugged, saying, "That seems fair enough."

Mannevy was more subtle. He turned to the Steam Master, "Where were you going to look?"

"I hear that one of the king's mages has been training some promising students —"

"Some of them noble!" Mannevy exclaimed.

"Which is why I want the writ," Brookes said. "I'll want no questions asked when I make my pick. I'll want my pick to be final."

"But —"

"It's that or no deal," Brookes said. Mannevy paled, his eyes darting to Hewlitt. The spymaster smiled at Brookes. Brookes nodded, pleased.

"And what else?" Hewlitt asked.

"I'll need three casks of gold, one small, two large," Brookes said.

"Three casks! But you'll be rich enough —" Mannevy spluttered in outrage.

"Not for me," Brookes cut across him, "for the steel." Mannevy looked confused, so Brookes, relenting, explained, "For the rail lines."

"The mills are working full out, the miners are hiring any able body," Hewlitt said to the first minister by way of explanation. He cut a glance toward the Steam Master. "Mr. Brookes is planning to get his supplies from outside parties."

"Where?" Mannevy asked in exasperation. "And what of the steam engines?"

Brookes leered. "Leave that to me, just give me my title, my writ, my monopoly."

"Your *way*," Hewlitt surmised.

"Yes, give me my way in this and you'll get what you want," Brookes agreed. He turned to Mannevy and extended a grimy hand. "Do we have a deal?"

Mannevy shuddered but nodded, taking the other's hand in his. "Deal."

# Chapter Three

"Line up, line up, there!" First minister Mannevy called out loudly. "Everyone, line up!"

"Sir?" one of the children, clearly someone who recognized him, said in surprise.

"We want to know what you've learned," the first minister told the child encouragingly. "Some of you may get the chance to perform great service to the King."

Beside him, the rough-hewn, harsh-faced commoner added, "A chance to show your magic!"

"What's the meaning of this?" Mage Vistos asked as he came through the doors to the classroom. He glanced first to Mannevy and then to the other man. "Oh, it's you!"

"Got a problem with that?" the commoner demanded harsher, stretching to his full height.

"There, there, gentlemen, let's have none of that!" First Minister Mannevy said soothingly. "Torvan Brookes is here on a writ from the King, mage Vistos."

"Who wants a sweet?" Vistos said, pulling a paper bag out of his robes and turning to the ranks of children lined up from the front to the back of the class. Several of the younger ones raised their hands immediately.

"There's something wrong," Bethany said, her brow furrowing.

"I'll say!" Margiss Falcon said with a hiss. She glanced to the desk at the front of the class. "Where's grandfather? And —" She broke off suddenly. Her eyes widened and she took a deep breath. With a look of dread, she asked, "Do you smell that?"

Skara and Thomas had taken turns 'accompanying' the mechanical through Ibb's place while the other dressed, ate, and spoke with mage Margen.

Margen told Skara, "I know too little of the immortals. It is said that they do not recognize the gods and certainly that they worship none of them." He frowned. "But they seem more than adept at magic, which is odd."

"I see," Skara said less in understanding than in acknowledgement of his words. "And this caravan she's tracking?"

"'She?'" Margen repeated. "I'm not sure that the immortals bother much with gender —"

"Tracker is most definitely a female," Skara asserted. Mage Margen's eyes danced with glee but he chose to dismiss the topic with a shrug.

"I know nothing of this caravan," Margen said, "expect what *she* has told us."

"I was not happy with the ease at which she entered this building," Skara said.

"Against magic, the senses are not enough," Margen said. He raised a hand as she started to say something. "And, yes, for you to do what you want, I shall have to teach you."

"Now is a good time," Skara said.

"If I teach you now, you'll have to teach your friend later," Margen warned.

"He's not my friend," Skara said, her eyes flashing.

"Companion, then," Margen allowed. When she bridled at that, he added, "You two are agreed to journey to a goal together which means you'll keep company, which makes you companions."

"However you wish," Skara said, dismissing the issue. "I'll train him." With a snort, she added, "He'd be no use guarding me if he didn't know how."

"Indeed," Margen agreed. His mood changed and he left off teasing her. "It is good that both you and he have used magic before, it makes it much easier to learn how to detect it."

"Can't everyone detect magic?"

"They can," Margen said. "But it takes training, just like it takes training to hit a target with a bow."

"Crossbow."

"Or with a crossbow," Margen agreed. He moved toward her but she stepped back, wary. "Close your eyes. Ignore your ears. Listen with your skin, taste with your brain. Tell me when you feel something. You might not feel it, exactly. It might be a smell or a tension or a flash of color."

Skara closed her eyes, took a deep breath and nodded for the mage to proceed.

Margen stood back, raised a hand and released the smallest of his spells.

"Something touched me," Skara said, not moving. "On my right shoulder."

"What?"

"Like a spider but not," Skara said after a moment's thought, her brows furrowed in concentration.

"Point to it but don't touch," Margen said. He wiggled a finger, nudging the spell. A moment later, he crooked his finger, like he was poking something.

Skara's frown deepened. "It's moving. It's got pincers. It's —" She jumped back and swatted the front of her right shoulder with her left hand. Her eyes flashed open, glaring at the mage. "It tried to bite me!"

"I did not tell you to open your eyes, nor did I tell you to move," Margen said forcefully.

"I was afraid —"

"And that will be your undoing," Margen said. "You will either learn to trust me or you will die."

Skara glowered at him furiously. She started to say something heated in response but stopped — her hand going to her lower right jaw, to the new tooth at the back — the one that had been given her by the goddess of life to replace the cursed one.

"It is hard for me to trust," Skara admitted.

"So I see," Margen agreed. "But you will have to learn to trust magic if you want to use it wisely. Did you not learn to trust your bow?"

"My crossbow," Skara corrected absently. "But I also learned not to lean too heavily on it, to know its limits."

"Yes, yes," Margen replied testily, "but before you can find its limits, you have to find *it*."

"I'm sorry," Skara said, lowering her eyes to the floor.

"You just lied to me," Margen said. Skara gave him a surprised look. "Didn't you know that whenever you lie, you lower your head?"

"It… it wasn't lying," Skara said. "Mage Vistos —"

The front door to the shop banged open loudly. The two turned toward it even as a young voice shouted, "Mage Margen, come quick! There's something wrong with Margiss!"

Margaret Waters allowed herself to luxuriate in her bath. Even Drake had been unable to find a complaint about the courtesy and hospital displayed to them by Hamo Beck, the mayor of Korin's Pass. That worthy had leaned over backwards to ensure that the three mages had all their needs met and was more than ready to aid them in relocating people and livelihoods from the necessary paths for the rail lines.

Margaret squished her toes together, delighted in the way the warm water flowed around them. *Yes, Hamo is quite the gentleman. But what's his game?*

There was something calculating about him. He seemed to handle that soldier, Captain Welless, effortlessly. He had a way of commanding without asserting himself that was to be respected. *But something about him bothers me.*

Margaret had learned to trust her feelings. She leaned back and slid deeper in the warm water, closed her eyes and thought. But the exertions of the day and the days before made her drowsy. Just at the edge of wakefulness, a thought came to her: *He seems awfully short, doesn't he?*

Margaret jerked upright and jumped out of the bath, reaching for towels, no longer sleepy at all.

"Who are you and how did you get in here?" Mage Margen demanded of the young girl who'd come rushing through the front door of Ibb's.

"The place is warded, isn't it?" Skara asked him, lowering his eyes to the girl in front of him. She seemed… "What happened? What's wrong?"

"Wrong?" Margen said, turning to her.

"I can feel it," Skara said. "Little girl, where did you come from?"

"I came from the classroom, up at the palace," the girl said. She gave Skara a quick glance, frowning. "You smell…"

"You've smelled this before?" Skara demanded, waving at Margen in expectation. "Like something *wrong*, foul yet sweet."

"He gave sweets," the girl said.

"Vistos?" Mage Margen said, his face pale. "He gave sweets to my class?"

"To Margiss," the girl said. "She tried to warn me, told me to run but he caught her by the shoulder —"

Mage Margen was no longer in the room.

The girl glanced around then looked to Skara. "He's going to need help."

"Thomas!" Skara shouted over her shoulder. She heard footsteps. "There's trouble at the palace!"

"Trouble?" Thomas Walpish strode in from the other room, the mechanical only a few paces behind him. He stopped when he spied the girl, then looked around the room. "Where's Margen?"

"He left," Skara said, throwing both her hands up and out, "just like he appeared."

"Ah, a teleportation spell," Tracker said. The mechanical closed her glowing blue eyes for a moment, opened them again. "I know where he is."

"Can you take us there?" Skara and Thomas asked in unison.

"You can't do that spell?"

"No, can you?" Skara asked in response.

"I can," said the voice of a small girl. A different small girl.

The first girl squeaked in surprise and then clapped her hands in delight. "You know Ophidian!" she squealed. She frowned. "How old are you?"

"That depends on who you're asking," the new girl said in a different tone. She turned to Skara Ningan, her face going dark. "You are an assassin. You worked for the mage."

"Vistos tried to kill her," Thomas asserted, "she's left his employ. And who are you, little girl who knows Ophidian?"

"You might say I'm his daughter," the girl replied. She nodded toward the mechanical. "You know Ibb?"

Tracker nodded.

"I've worked for him," the girl said. She turned back to Walpish. "I know you. You were at Rabel's."

"The fire?" Walpish said, surprised. "How did you know?"

"We watched you from the dragon's back," the girl said.

"You rode a dragon!" the other girl cried in surprise. Shyly she asked, "Can you do it again?"

The new girl smiled and shook her head. "Not any more," she said. She glanced toward Thomas and then, with obvious reluctance, to Skara. "I can take you to the palace."

"Quickly?" Thomas asked.

"I can show you where to go!" the other girl said. "You should take me, too!"

The new girl frowned, glancing toward Tracker. "I'm not sure I could carry four."

"Carry?" Thomas said, his expression thoughtful. Almost to himself he murmured, "'Not any more.'"

"She smells of Ophidian," the other girl said. "She knows dragons. And she can't be carried by one." She glanced at the new girl. "Are you a dragon, too?"

"Almost," the girl said. She nodded to Tracker, and spread it to include the two adults. "My name is Ellen Annabelle and I've been sent by the gods." She waved a hand to the door. "If we're going, we need to go outside."

Thomas rushed to the door and held it open, waving a hand waist-high in encouragement to Ellen Annabelle.

Skara, with one quirked eyebrow, followed the new girl and looked back to Tracker. The mechanical needed no encouragement.

"Ellen Annabelle," the little girl said as she raced to join them, "my name's Bethany. Bethany Murray."

"A pleasure," Ellen Annabelle said in a very grown-up tone.

Bethany stopped and stared at her in surprise. "It's like you're two people in one body!"

Ellen Annabelle smiled. "Exactly like!" She moved away from the door and turned to the others. As she moved to the center of the street, she called back, "Climb on!"

King Markel was taking his afternoon nap when a commotion outside his chambers interrupted him. He called for his servant but no one answered. He called again, loudly.

Nothing. Finally, with a roar of anger, he heaved himself out of his bed, crossed the distance to the double doors and slammed them open with a shout, "What is going on?"

No one answered him. The halls were deserted. Voices cried in the distance, some in worry, some in anger. With another roar, he stormed toward the commotion, determined to put an end to it in the most royal way possible. *Heads will roll!*

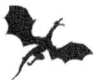

Ellen Annabelle found that she could carry them all... just. Exhausted, she deposited them on the wide marble stairs leading up to the formal halls of the king's palace. She turned back into her human form as soon as they'd all dropped from her and stumbled to fall, gasping on the ground.

"Let's... not... do... that... again!" she wheezed.

"Will you be okay?" Bethany asked, crouching down beside her and extending a hand tentatively towards her.

Ellen Annabelle took several deep breaths and nodded. Feebly, she gestured for the others to leave her. "I'll be along presently."

Tracker nodded decisively and turned to Walpish. "You were an officer here?" When Thomas nodded, she continued, "Do you know the way?"

In answer, Thomas trotted up the steps. Skara followed close behind. Tracker turned to Ellen and Bethany. To the crouching girl she said, "You go on, I'll keep watch here."

Bethany gave Ellen a troubled look but the other girl merely repeated her feeble wave. Bethany trotted rapidly up the stairs, got in front of Walpish, saying waspishly, "I know a quicker way!"

In short order the sounds of three sets of footsteps were swallowed in the immensity of the palace.

"What will they do?" Tracker asked, looking down to Ellen Annabelle. "And what would you do if you could get to them?"

Ellen shook her head, taking more deep breaths. Finally, she felt well enough to sit up, rolling over to kneel, still breathing heavily. A moment later, she rose wobbly to her feet. "I've never been here, before. Can you follow them?"

"I am Tracker," Tracker said, moving up the stairs. The mechanical glanced back at Ellen Annabelle and offered a hand. "We will go slowly, to start."

Ellen smiled. "Slow, I can manage."

# Chapter Four

Snow swirled down and coated the decks of the airship. Major Samuel Lewis blew out a breath which frosted in the night air.

"Thank you for this," he said to Captain Fawcett. "My men wouldn't survive without your help."

"That's what the King's Royal Airships are for, sir," Fawcett replied gamely, clapping the other officer on the shoulder. "Let's go back to the boiler and get ourselves warm." He glanced around in the darkness. "It's a good night for it."

"It is," Lewis agreed. Ahead of them, piercing through the darkness in rare moments, were lights far below. He pointed toward them. "What do you reckon? Another two days?"

"If that," Fawcett said with a shrug. "And then you'll have a quandary — what to do with the enemy's capital."

"We'll take it, of course," Lewis said. "You'll bring my squad over to the palace and we'll descend on it while you're firing all your guns and firing off your flares to make your ship look like twenty."

"It seems a bit chancy," Fawcett replied with a grimace. He stopped by the boiler and stretched his hands to its heat. "How many soldiers will they have in the palace?"

"It's not the palace that matters," Lewis said. "It's the king." He paused and shrugged. "And the other royals — the queen and her son, I suppose." He spread his hands towards the boiler's heat. "Capture them, make them surrender and the whole country is ours."

"And the rewards will be grand!" Fawcett said cheerfully.

"Knighthoods at the very least," Lewis agreed.

"But we cannot let their soldiers counter-attack or free them," Fawcett warned.

"Which is why we'll make them guests in your ship, good sir!" Lewis replied, reaching over to clap the young captain on the shoulder. He gave the other man a mock bow. "And tell me, good captain, how will you feel hosting royalty?"

"Honestly," Fawcett admitted, "the notion rather frightens me."

"You'll do fine!"

The guards were all clustered outside the double doors that led to mage Margen's classroom. They turned as the King Markel thumped down the hallway toward them. The captain of the guard told him, "The doors are shut, we can't open them, sire!"

"We'll see about that!" King Markel bellowed, motioning the guards to make room. He pounded on the door, shouting, "Open up in the name of the King!"

Nothing. He pounded again and then turned, eyes blazing, to the guard captain. "Get Mannevy." As the guard rushed off, he shouted after him, "And have someone get a battering ram!"

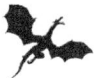

Skara Ningan held up a hand in warning as she, Thomas, and Bethany came to a corner. She peered around it for an instant then turned back to the others who were standing against the wall and shook her head firmly. Thomas gestured for them to move backwards and they retraced their steps until they were far enough away to not be heard.

"Guards," Skara said. "At least twenty. And they can't get the door open."

"Now what?" Thomas asked.

Bethany started to answer but turned at a noise behind her. Ellen and Tracker joined them. Skara repeated her news to them. Ellen frowned thoughtfully.

"Describe what I'll be seeing inside," Ellen said.

"It's our classroom," Bethany said. "We've got twenty desks and as many students."

"Margen will be there," Thomas vowed.

"And Vistos, probably more," Skara added.

Ellen turned to Bethany. "What's the best place to hide?"

Bethany gave her a surprised look, then said, "I know a place."

"Describe it," Ellen said. "Please."

"Let me," Tracker said, moving to grab Bethany's arm. "Think what you want and I can track it," she told the girl.

Bethany's eyes went wide and she drew a breath but nodded in agreement. She closed her eyes to concentrate.

"I see," Tracker said, releasing the girl's arm. She turned to Ellen. "I can show you but you would have to teleport to get there."

Ellen Annabelle smiled. "Show me."

"Before I do, what's your plan?"

"Go in, kill the bad mage, free the girl," Ellen said.

"Won't work, he'll have her hostage," Skara warned.

"And he may have more hostages, too," Thomas added. "Especially —" he glanced to Bethany "— did he have any sweets or candy?"

Bethany nodded.

"Cursed candy," Tracker said in a low voice. "Some mages use it for control."

"He controlled at least one mage," Thomas said. "He had a cursed tooth, like Skara."

"You can smell them," Skara said. She gave Ellen a pointed look. "At least, I can."

"So I take you," Ellen said.

"Take me, too," Bethany said. "I know where to hide, how the classroom is arranged."

"Make two trips, drop off the girl and the assassin first, come back for me and the horseman," Tracker said.

Ellen eyed her thoughtfully, then extended her hands to Skara and the girl. "Close your eyes."

"Why, are there going to be bright lights?" Tracker asked.

"Or nothing," Ellen said, closing her eyes and pulling forth magic.

The three disappeared. Thomas and Tracker waited nervously. Moments later Ellen Annabelle re-appeared, breathing heavily. "Grab on!" she ordered. "I can only do this once more!"

The horseman and the mechanical grabbed the little girl's hands. And they disappeared.

Mage Margen picked up the disturbance the first time, so he was ready when three people appeared at the back of the classroom, stepping furtively to join the other two behind the curtains.

Torvan Brookes narrowed his eyes at the mage but said nothing, keeping his attention on the other, aged mage and his sneering apprentice. *Vistos.*

"You're the steam maker," Vistos said, jerking his head at Brookes. "What are you doing here?"

"I have a writ from his majesty to select apprentices," Brookes replied. "What are you doing here?"

"I work for the king," Vistos replied haughtily. "And," he smiled nastily, "as it happens I'm in need of more apprentices." He shook Margiss' shoulder pointedly. The girl was caught in the crook of the taller man's arm, unable to escape.

"That, Vistos, is my granddaughter," Mage Margen said warningly.

"I know," Vistos said, his smile growing broader. He fished in the pockets of his robes and pulled out a lozenge. He stuffed the lozenge into the girl's mouth. "She'll make an excellent apprentice, don't you think?"

"Margiss, spit it out!" Bethany shouted, darting out from the curtains at the back of the room. "It's poisoned!"

"Tainted, cursed, but not poisoned," Vistos said agreeably. He waved his free hand in a strange gesture and beamed when Bethany found herself floating toward him. Vistos turned to Margen. "Perhaps I'll have two apprentices!"

He gestured to the lad standing beside him. "Halston, why don't you give this one a sweet?"

Halston took Bethany as she floated toward him and grabbed her, putting her neck in the crook of his arm and pulling a sweet from his pocket. He pushed it into Bethany's mouth but cried out and jerked his hand, bleeding back. "She bit me!"

"Feisty," Vistos said approvingly. He nodded toward the girl in his grasp, Margiss. "This one still hasn't swallowed her sweet." He smiled at Margen. "Doubtless she thinks that swallowing will complete the spell," he said. "She doesn't know that the candy itself —" he broke off as Margiss swallowed loudly and stopped resisting in his arms. "Oh, there you are? All ready, little girl?"

"That was good!" Margiss said, peering up at him, her eyes oddly bright. She turned her head back to the others. "It was very tasty," she told the class. "You should try it." She started giggling, stopped and started again.

Margen's face went ashen.

"You really should try it," Bethany added a moment later. She giggled. It was not a pleasant sound.

"What did you do?" Margen demanded.

"I only gave them sweets," Vistos said innocently. "I let them have what they really wanted."

*Boom!* The doors behind him shook and he turned his head idly, peering at them.

"They'll be good girls now," Vistos said. He peered down at Margiss. "Isn't that right, dear?"

"Yes," Margiss said with another giggle. This time she broke out into loud guffaws and bent over double, her expression pained as she panted for breath, all while still laughing.

"You may stop laughing now," Vistos told her. She stopped immediately. "Well," Vistos demanded, "where are your manners? What do you say?"

"Th-thank you," Margiss said immediately. Beside her, Bethany gestured wildly, crying between her bouts of laughter, "Master?"

"No," Vistos said. "You tried to thwart me. You can keep laughing. Until you understand."

Helplessly, Bethany continued laughing, doubling over, gasping for air, collapsing to the floor, tears streaming down her face even as she continued, uncontrollably to laugh.

*Boom!* The doors shook again and creaked, threatening to burst open.

Vistos glanced down at the stricken girl, thinking. "Perhaps I just need one, at that," Vistos said. He turned to Margen. "You think you're so powerful. But your magic won't save her." He turned to Halston. "Let's go."

The apprentice stepped back from the stricken girl and Vistos made a gesture. The three — mage, apprentice, girl — disappeared, leaving a gasping, red-faced, heaving Bethany sprawled on the floor curled in agony.

Ellen Annabelle rushed forward, turned to Margen and Torvan Brookes, asking, "Can you save her?"

"No," Margen said.

"I've never seen the like," Torvan Brookes agreed, face pale.

Ellen turned to Tracker. "Can you?"

"Her heart will stop in a minute," Tracker said, eyeing the purple-faced girl. She gave Ellen a hard look. "It will be a release."

"She's one of Ophidian's!" Ellen Annabelle swore, rushing forward and wrapping her arms around the still-squirming girl. She turned to Tracker. "Find him!"

And then she was gone.

"Where did she go?" Skara said, moving to Tracker.

"I would like to know that myself," Torvan Brookes said. He turned to Margen and raised an eyebrow. The mage shrugged.

"I cannot follow her," Tracker said, sounding surprised.

*Boom!* The doors crashed open and soldiers rushed in, swords drawn.

"What is the meaning of this?" Margen demanded.

"Exactly what I was going to ask *you!*" King Markel roared back.

Tracker pulled Skara and Thomas behind the curtains as the king's men rushed in. Skara and Thomas felt something and realized that, somehow, the mechanical had hidden them. At her touch, Thomas and Skara stilled their movements and slowed their breathing.

"Mage Margen, what is going on?" King Markel demanded as the soldiers fanned out protectively around him. He turned to the guard captain. "Someone send for Mannevy!"

"Mage Vistos decided he had the right to recruit my students," Margen replied, "sire."

"He said he was short-handed," Markel said with a wave of his hand. He glanced around the room at the youngsters and back to Margen. "Did he take anyone?"

"My granddaughter," Margen replied heavily.

"Really?" Markel replied. "I'm surprised you let her go."

"I had no choice," Margen said. He gestured toward Torvan Brookes. "The Steam Master is also here, apparently, searching for apprentices."

"Yes, well, we need to build rails," the king said. "Your students will find themselves well-employed, I'm certain."

"But, Your Majesty, I'm not of age!" Barbara Garrett protested, flouncing to her knees to bow to him. "And my parents!"

"Your parents," King Markel said, "and who would they be?" "My father is the Lord of Far Corner, sire," Barbara replied, glancing up to him from her kneeling position. "Duke of Far Corner, Lord Randall Garrett."

"Oh!" King Markel said, surprised. "So you come of good stock! That's surprising, seeing as you're learning magic!"

Barbara blushed but lowered her head to hide her anger.

"What is your ability, Miss Garrett?" Brookes asked in a no-nonsense tone.

"She is a mage of fire," Bree Emer replied from where she stood in a knot of students.

"Is she?" Brookes said in a pleased tone. He glanced at the king. "I've need of good fire mages," he said. "And earth mages, and air mages."

"No water mages?" Bree Emer asked, aghast.

"Water mages are not much use in my enterprises," Brookes said. He turned to the students. "Who is the best earth mage?"

"Freddie Fennimore!" the class roared. The lad flushed in surprise.

"And the best air mage?"

Hands pointed to Matt Evans who stepped forward.

"Why don't you three come with me and we'll see what you can do," Torvan Brookes said. He nodded toward Margen. "If they don't work out, I'll send them back."

"Tuh!" Margen said angrily. "And if they work out?"

"They'll be invaluable in building our new southern rail lines," King Markel said in a tone that discouraged argument. "I've promised the Duke of Southerland that we'll begin it immediately."

"I see," Margen said, sounding no less subdued. "And my granddaughter, sire?"

"If you cannot afford to lose her, see mage Vistos," King Markel said.

"But, sire!" Margen said. "Mage Vistos used some sort of spell —"

"I should hope!"

"A most foul spell, I believe," Margen said.

"I have learned that it is never wise to argue with my mages," King Markel said, nodding to his guards and turning toward the door. "I'll leave the matter with you."

"You three, come with me," Brookes said, moving to join the departing gaggle of guards. Over his shoulder he called to Margen, "I'm bringing them to the station."

Margen glared at the Steam Master but said nothing, turning his attention back to his much disordered and reduced classroom. With a wave of his hand, he caused the double doors to close. They wobbled as they turned and Margen glowered at them a moment before turning to the remaining students. "Take your seats."

"Sir, what about Bethany?" Bree Emer asked. "And Margiss?"

"You three, come out from where you're hiding," Margen said waving toward the pocket of silence that Tracker had created. He turned to his students. "I need your word on this."

"Sir?" Bree said, taking on the role of class speaker. "Our word on what?"

"Two things," Margen said, raising a hand. He extended one finger. "That you'll accept no sweets from anyone — even someone you think you know." There was a chorus of anguish over this. "Unless you want to get poisoned like Bethany," Margen told them heatedly. "You know people can take on disguises, you cannot trust anyone."

"How will we know you, then?" one of the youngest boys challenged.

"How *do* you know me, little Tim?" Mage Margen challenged. Margen waved his hand and a small smoky, purple ring appeared.

"Can anyone else make that, sir?" Tim Smith asked.

"No," Margen said, rapidly wafting away the smoky mark. He made a face. "Later today, I will teach all of you how to make your mark," he promised. "That way we will know each of you, truly."

A rustle of eager gasps swept through the room.

Margen gestured toward Tracker, urging her to come forward. "This immortal is Tracker."

"Tracker?" Bree asked. "And the other two?"

"You won't know their names," Margen said. "No one should know that they were here."

"Mage Vistos did," a girl piped up in challenge. "I think he'd seen them before."

"He tried to kill me," Skara Ningan said, moving up to the front of the class. "He fed me one of those sweets."

"How did you survive?" Bree asked.

"She had help of a sort that only happens once," Thomas Walpish said. "And together we gave our oaths."

"Oaths?" Tim Smith asked.

"To stop Mage Vistos from hurting anyone ever again," Skara Ningan replied.

"Miss, he hurt Bethany," Bree told her.

"And Margiss," Tim added.

"We're going to help them," Thomas Walpish promised.

"I shall track them," Tracker added emphatically.

"We shall need your help," Mage Margen told the class. He nodded toward Skara and Thomas. "I'm going to teach them magic."

"We'll help!" the class roared in unison.

# Chapter Five

"Ophidian!" Ellen Annabelle's voice pierced the high domed ceilings of the Dragon Palace. "Father!"

Krea Wymarc rushed toward the sound, followed by Jarin Reedis, and Nestor Pallas.

"He's not here!" Krea called, increasing her pace. "What is it?"

"She's dying!" Ellen shrieked. "She's dying and she can't stop laughing! It's killing her!"

Krea and the others found her on the circular balcony just outside the royal chambers, huddled over a small lifeless form.

Krea rushed to kneel beside her. Jarin Reedis stood further back, looking down appraisingly. Nestor stopped, eyes wide at the sight of a girl little older than Ellen.

"Who did this?" Nestor asked. He took a deep breath. "This is magic. It's foul, dark, poisoned."

"Poison!" Annabelle cried. "Ellen, your tears! Only your tears!"

"What?" Ellen asked in the same voice.

"She's been poisoned," Krea said in sudden understanding. "Use your tears to heal the poison."

"But — won't I make —" she raised a hand and cupped it to her chest "— another wyvern?"

"You have no choice," Annabelle answered for her.

"But without a twin soul —"

"I can hold her," Nestor Pallas offered, stepping back and turning into the snow serpent, frozen air wisping up from her nostrils.

"Her heart's stopped," Annabelle said, using Ellen's other hand to point to the still form below them. Ellen nodded, tears streaming. She raised her hand to her cheek, wet it with her tears and transferred them down to the cheek of the young girl. "Live."

For a moment nothing happened. And then the girl gasped, her lungs heaving. Her eyes opened and she stared up at the faces above her.

"Where —?" Bethany started.

"Stand back," Krea said, pulling Ellen and Jarin with her. She turned to the snow serpent. "Nestor."

The long, sinewy snow serpent stepped forward to the startled girl. Nestor Pallas breathed frozen, icy air over the recovered girl. Bethany had only a moment of panic before she froze completely, still.

"We must find her a twin soul," Ellen Annabelle said, reaching to grab Krea Wymarc's hand. "We can't leave her like this."

"Of course not," Krea agreed firmly. She leaned down over Ellen's shoulder and asked. "Any suggestions?"

"Well…"

"Don't you dare say *her* name!" Krea warned. The others took an involuntary step away from her, eyeing her anxiously.

"Actually, I was thinking of someone else," Ellen said. She moved away from the winter wyvern and turned to face her. Looking beyond her, she said to Nestor Pallas, "How long do we have before she comes to harm?"

"I've never done this before," Nestor said. "Not long."

Ellen nodded, unsurprised. She looked over to Jarin Reedis. "Would you like to learn a new trick?" Reedis cocked his head questioningly. "Something father hasn't taught us?"

"I'm all ears," Jarin said with Reedis' mouth.

"What are you planning?" Krea Wymarc demanded.

"I'm awfully tired," Ellen Annabelle confessed. She nodded to Jarin. "I need a ride."

"As a human?" Jarin Reedis asked. His face split in a huge grin. "Do you think a dragon can carry you as a human?"

"Of course," Wymarc snapped with Krea's voice. "It's done all the time."

"And we'll need to carry the girl," Annabelle said. She glanced to Nestor. "Jarin's flames can revive her, correct?"

"If he doesn't burn her to ash," Wymarc warned.

"Can a dragon burn a wyvern?" Ellen asked.

"It's not something to try," Wymarc said haughtily.

"I quite agree," Nestor said. He said to Ellen Annabelle, "You plan to find her a twin soul?"

"Yes," Ellen said. "I've got someone in mind." She gestured to Jarin Reedis. "We need to hurry, can you take us?"

"Are you going to teach us this new trick?" Jarin Reedis asked.

Ellen smiled. "Of course!"

They arrived over the castle at Kingsford moments later. Jarin Reedis bellowed in challenge as he spiralled down to the courtyard.

Ellen Annabelle scrambled down his side, carefully cradling Bethany's frozen corpse until both of them were safely on the ground. A moment later the dragon was gone, leaving Jarin Reedis in his place.

"That was amazing!" Reedis cried. "Why did father not tell us about this way?"

"I think he wanted to see if we could figure it out ourselves," Annabelle said, using Ellen's voice.

Reedis' eyebrows flew upwards momentarily. Then he nodded. "And I bet that Wymarc knows this way, too!" He made a face, stretching his arms behind his head. "It would have saved us an awful lot of work. It took me at least a solid week to recover from that flight before."

"Well, you look better for it," Annabelle admitted, causing Ellen's face to smile impishly.

"What are we doing here?" Reedis said, glancing around as the first smattering of guards poured out of the doors, their pikes at the ready.

"Looking for a suitable twin soul for Bethany," Annabelle said. She glanced up the stairs toward mage Margen's classroom. "I expect they'll —" she broke off, nodding as Margen and an eager group of children came boiling out and mingled through the unsuspecting guards.

"This is going to be too public, I fear," Reedis said, glancing around at the guards and the students.

"Yes," Annabelle agreed grimly. "We'll have to provide a distraction."

"Are you Reedis?" Mage Margen called as he passed through the guards. He approached Jarin Reedis with a hand outstretched. "You're that mage who made the airship fly, aren't you?"

Reedis nodded in agreement and, shyly, shook Margen's hand.

"That wasn't a bad bit of magic," Margen allowed, "flashy and not very difficult, but not bad."

Reedis flushed.

"Mage Margen, where are our friends?" Annabelle asked with Ellen's voice.

"You are more than you seem, aren't you?" Margen said eyeing Ellen's body warily. He glanced to Reedis. "Am I correct, sir, in surmising that you are a twin soul dragon?"

"I am," Reedis said, drawing himself up haughtily.

"Fascinating," Margen said. He glanced toward his students. "Children, this is mage Reedis who is sometimes a dragon."

The students, who'd heard of the dragon's arrival, all clustered around Reedis, eyeing him with a combination of curiosity and terror.

Margen looked past Reedis to Ellen Annabelle once more. "And do you, child, have a similar story to tell?"

"My story doesn't matter," Ellen Annabelle replied tartly. She nodded to the frozen form of Bethany, lying at her feet.

"So," Margen said sadly, "she could not be saved."

"Perhaps she can," Annabelle replied with Ellen's voice. She glanced around. "Where are the others?"

"Why do you ask?"

"We need a diversion, if we're to save this girl's life," Reedis spoke up, moving toward Margen. "Something that will keep everyone from learning what happens."

Margen eyed first Reedis and then Ellen Annabelle cautiously. He pursed his lips. "And if I do this, you will help me find and free my granddaughter?"

"I will," Ellen Annabelle said. She nodded toward Jarin Reedis. "I cannot speak for others."

"We are sworn to bring Vistos to justice," Thomas Walpish said as he strode forward with Skara Ningan and the mechanical just behind. "Skara Ningan has already tasted his poison."

"How did you survive?" Ellen asked. Annabelle continued, "His poison killed me."

Margen's eyes bulged as he caught Annabelle's words. She turned to him, eyes flashing, and said, "I will save your granddaughter; *your* life depends upon your honor."

"Also," Skara said to Margen, "I think your loyalty to the king does not serve you any better than mine did."

"I swore an oath to him!" Margen said.

"As did I," Skara replied. "He freed me of that oath when he ordered his mage to kill me." She gave him a cutting look. "Did he not break his oath to you when he refused to help your granddaughter?"

Margen's jaw tightened. He nodded — a tight, sharp jerk of his head.

"If you do what you're thinking, Annabelle, prepare for father's wrath," Reedis warned in a low tone.

Ellen Annabelle looked up at him. "I think father will be pleased that we're gaining allies."

"Something is happening," Tracker said. "Something big." The others looked at her in surprise, so she explained, "I track. I can track changes."

"I wish Rabel were here," Ellen said.

"You knew Rabel Zebala?" Mage Margen asked in surprise. When Ellen Annabelle nodded, he said, "He must be nearly dead by now!"

"He swore an oath to a god," Ellen said, her lips twitching upwards. "He's gotten *much* better!"

"You wouldn't recognize him," Jarin Reedis agreed. He turned to Ellen. "But your friend doesn't have much time."

"The guards —" Thomas said, turning to look at the knot of soldiers slowly marching down the stairs to surround them.

"They don't worry me," Ellen said. Thomas gave her an appalled look. She gestured to Bethany's frozen form. "If we do this, she'll need another."

"A twin soul!" Margen exclaimed. "You are going to make her a twin soul?"

"She'll be in pain for the rest of her life," Annabelle said with Ellen's voice.

"You're a twin soul," Margen said. "One of you said that Vistos had killed you with poison."

"Annabelle," Jarin Reedis said. He shook his head, sadly. "I wasn't there at the time."

"She will become a wyvern, like me," Annabelle said, turning Ellen's head up to meet the mage's eyes. "She'll be in pain from the poison."

"It got better, didn't it?" Ellen said, stealing her voice back from her twin soul.

"Yes," Annabelle said. "Having someone to share it with makes it manageable."

"I could work to find some way to neutralize the poison," Margen suggested tentatively, gesturing first to the frozen form of Bethany and then to Ellen Annabelle.

Annabelle snorted and shook Ellen's head. "We shall survive as we are, thank you."

"What do you need?" Margen said.

"You heard?" Ellen said, gazing down to students who were clustered around the mage. They eyed her warily. One girl nodded.

"I heard," Skara Ningan said forcefully. She eyed young Bethany's frozen form. "What do you want us to do?"

"A twin soul requires a choosing," Annabelle said. She used Ellen's arm to point at Bethany. "When we release the ice, she'll change. Someone needs to call her back, bind with her — it's different every time —"

"I won't tell you how I did it," Reedis said in a low voice.

"— but it must happen or the soul will go mad," Annabelle finished.

"And the distraction?"

"The guards must not see what we're doing, only see the wyvern when it appears," Annabelle said.

"Your dragon friend should be able to manage that admirably," Margen said.

"First we need his heat," Reedis said. "Actually... that might be enough." He glanced to Ellen Annabelle. "Wouldn't it?"

"It would," Annabelle agreed with a half-smile. She turned Ellen's head to the mage and, his students, and the two adults. "Are you ready?"

"I am," the group chorused.

"Reedis," Ellen Annabelle said, stepping back from Bethany's body and gesturing for the others to move away.

Reedis nodded and turned into his dragon. He bellowed at the guards warningly, shooting a gout of flame towards them. Then he turned back and shot flame at the body of the girl. An instant later, he was airborne, diving on the guards who fled in panic back inside the castle.

"Bethany," Ellen Annabelle called, "fly!"

Ellen Annabelle became her wyvern just as the form of Bethany distorted, melted, and drifted into smoke. A moment later, a silver form darted into the sky.

Ellen Annabelle screeched after it and took off, outflying the smaller form and herding it back toward the cluster on the ground.

"Mister Mayor, so kind of you to receive me on such short notice," Margaret Waters said when she arrived early that morning at Hamo Beck's office. She was always on her best manners when hatching plots, it was something of a hobby of hers.

"It is always a pleasure to receive you, Miss Waters," Hamo Beck said, rising from his seat and bending his head in a quick nod. He gestured her toward a seat. "I've taken the liberty of asking Nox to arrange —"

"That won't be necessary," Margaret broke in. Hamo's brows rose in surprise. "In fact, if you'd accompany me now, I think we can leave before the captain notices."

"Leave?"

"Let your Nox know that we will be looking at some caves," Margaret said, rising from her seat and waving him to the door. "I can't say quite how long we'll be gone."

"Caves?" Hamo Beck looked nonplussed. "I can't understand how a train —"

"I'll explain when we get there," Margaret said. As Hamo seemed to hesitate, she added in a more acerbic tone, "I *certainly* shan't explain where others might hear!"

"As you wish."

"That booming we heard last week," Granno said to Queen Diam as he entered her throne room. Diam nodded for him to continue. "It was the sky-touchers. They've got mages — three of them! — and they laid metal tracks through the pass."

"Yes," Diam said. "We knew about that. Why do you bring it up again?"

"Hamo sent word that they're planning on building a line to connect with the South Sea Pass."

"I'd guessed as much," the queen of the zwergs allowed.

"And they're going to build a line all the way north to the Sorian capital," Granno said.

"It would make sense," Diam allowed. "We've used trains here underground for time out of mind."

"But theirs are powered by *steam*," Granno protested.

"Yes, the same engines as are used on the airships," Diam agreed. "We wouldn't want to use them here where they'd stink up the air."

"With those iron rails, they can trap us, surround us," Granno said.

"They have to *find* us first to be a threat," Diam said.

"That crazy attack — two of them! — they are looking for us," Granno said.

"The humans have always been looking for us," Diam said. She gestured through the walls, toward the vast underground cavern that housed their captive airship. She grinned. "If they are not lucky, they even find us."

Granno grunted, unable to argue with the queen's logic.

"Besides, it hasn't always been a loss on our part," Diam said. "Rabel Zebala, Jarin Reedis, Ellen Annabelle —"

"Two of those three are twin souls!" Granno complained.

"And our own Abner," Diam continued, unfazed. "We zwerg have always had some commerce with humans. Often to our mutual advantage."

Granno accepted that with a grimace. "And, sometimes, to our loss."

Queen Diam agreed with a shrug. "So you are worried about the mages? Or these rail lines?"

"Both," Granno admitted. "With these trains of theirs crossing through our lands regularly, we run the danger of being discovered."

"But we're well into our new developments," Diam reminded him. "Another month or two and all the humans will find will be empty caves without any sign of habitation."

"And how many times can we move?"

"We move to our profit, Granno," Diam reminded him. "Always to our profit."

"And soon we'll have an airship," Granno said to himself. He raised his eyes to the queen's. "What plans do you have for that?"

Queen Diam smiled. "When the time comes, dear Granno, you'll be among the first to know."

"Minister Mannevy," Peter Hewlitt said as he entered the first minister's office. "Were you aware that there is a dragon outside?"

"Is there?" Mannevy replied. "And what does it want?"

Hewlitt shrugged. "I haven't a clue," he said. "Earlier, I'd heard that there was a disturbance in mage Margen's classroom, that our friend, Mister Brookes, had acquired some apprentices under the king's writ and that Margen and Vistos had exchanged some heated words."

"Did they?"

"And that the king had his guard break open the doors to the classroom before retiring to his quarters," Hewlitt continued, his eyes scanning the first minister's face carefully.

"The king was well?"

Hewlitt nodded.

"Then I see no harm in it," Mannevy said. "Brookes has his help, the kingdom will prosper."

"And Margen? And Vistos?"

"Is it not in the nature of mages to be contentious?" Mannevy countered. "It seems like nothing more than the usual exchange of insults." He raised an eyebrow to Hewlitt. "Unless there is more?"

"I have never thought it a good idea to encourage discord amongst the king's men," Hewlitt said.

"And yet it does happen," Mannevy replied with a shrug. "At the worst, one of the mages will decant and leave the other in power." He lifted one of the documents in a stack on his left, placed it in front of him, read it quickly, signed it and placed it to his right. "Is there anything else?"

Hewlitt's lips tightened for a moment. He shook his head and spun on his heels.

Mannevy watched until the spymaster shut his door, then turned his head down to his desk, grabbed another document and placed it in front of him.

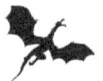

"There!" Tirpin said, clapping Jacques Martel on the arm and twisting him as he pointed. "That's an inn!"

"We've no money!" Martel said as he and the mage examined the small town in front of them. "How are we going to get a room?"

They had been trudging through the bitter cold for days, hiding when they had to, stealing when they could. Their last pair of stolen horses had collapsed the day before and they'd continued on foot.

"What is this place?" Martel asked. He frowned. "It looks like Korin's Pass."

"Do you know anyone there?" Tirpin demanded.

Martel shook his head. "I was a seaman, I didn't go inland."

Tirpin snorted. "So we go in, posing as travelers —"

"We *are* travelers," Martel said with a snort.

"— as travelers and we want a room for a night," Tirpin continued, ignoring the other man's outburst. "We'll see about getting — oh, damn! Are those soldiers?"

"Halt in the name of the king!" a voice shouted out from the distance.

"We've nothing to fear," Tirpin said in a low voice to Martel. "We're good Sorians —"

"Those are Kingsland soldiers!"

# Chapter Six

Two figures stood in front of the crowd waiting for the new wyvern's return — Skara Ningan and Bree Emer. The older woman smiled down at the young girl. Bree ignored her, keeping her eyes fixed on the rapidly approaching wyvern.

The new wyvern screeched in challenge… and pain.

*Come to me,* Skara thought to the pale figure racing toward her, *I know pain.* The wyvern seemed to hear her for it altered course directly toward her.

Little Bree, seeing the change, darted in front of Skara. "Take me!"

Following fast on the tail of the new wyvern, Ellen Annabelle heard the young girl's challenge and then saw something that turned her blood cold. With a screech of warning, she increased her dive and her speed, racing to get in front of the new wyvern. She could see Jarin Reedis in his awesome dragon form turn in surprise at her call, saw the old mage, Margen, and the others slowly raising their heads toward her in surprise. She strained every fiber of her being and folded her wings tight against her body in a desperate attempt to outpace the wyvern in front of her —

— but she was too late.

With a cry of triumph, a young girl rushed to the front of the group, held out outstretched arms, a leer on her face — Margiss, magic-tainted Margiss, stood ready to receive the new-made wyvern.

"Bethany, no!" Bree Emer cried, flailing to grab at Margiss' arm and pull her aside.

"My child!" Mage Margen cried in surprise and horror. "What are you doing?"

Margiss, her eyes filled with an evil gleam, turned back to her grandfather and said, "I'm doing what I'm told!"

But before she could turn back again to attain her victory, she gave a cry of surprise and was roughly tackled… by Thomas Walpish. "Skara, now!"

Skara Ningan leaped over the tangle of bodies and raised her head to the wyvern. "Come to me, Bethany! Together, we'll save Margiss!"

The new wyvern's eyes grew wide as the words registered and, with an anguished cry, she back-winged, her talons extended to rake Skara and tear her out of her way —

— but that didn't happen. Skara smiled as she reached up for the talons, taking one in each hand and deflecting them around her body, pulling downwards and bringing the new wyvern on top of her.

*Are you ready to fly?* Skara thought as the wyvern's flesh met her body. *Are you ready to show the world, child of Ophidian?*

*Yes!* And then there was only Skara standing, turning to face the melee behind her. "It is done."

"NO!" Margiss and Vistos cried in unison. Vistos waved his hands in a spell but found himself blocked. He turned to Margen with a snarl on his face but the other mage smiled at him and gestured with a hand back toward the pale wyvern.

"Her?" Vistos spat as he turned back to the wyvern. "What can *she* do?"

"This," the new wyvern said, grabbing the limp form of Margiss and pulling her upright. In a softer voice, she said to the limp form, "I'm sorry, this is going to hurt." And then her hand reached her hand into the girl's mouth. She turned to Margen so that the mage could see her eyes as she created her spell. Margiss woke with a cry and a wail of misery, squirming to get out of the wyvern's reach but she was no match for the new-made wyvern. The wyvern smiled at the mage and flexed her fingers on the cursed tooth in Margiss' mouth. With a wrenching yank she pulled it out.

Vistos gave a cry and clutched his chest.

The wyvern held the darkened molar between her fingers, raising it to display for all to see. To the sobbing girl in her grasp, she said, "I'm so sorry." Then she turned her eyes back to mage Vistos. "Your days are numbered."

Vistos hissed in surprise and vanished… just a moment before Jarin Reedis' flame landed on the spot where he'd been standing.

With a cry, Mage Margen rushed to grab his granddaughter. Skara released her to him.

"Are you all right?" Margen asked in spite of the blood pouring out of Margiss' mouth and the sobs of pain. He turned angrily to the new-made wyvern. "What did you do to her?"

"I did the best I could," the silver wyvern replied. "The tooth had to be cleansed." She nodded toward Margiss. "She'll take no more harm from it."

"'More?'" Margen repeated, his anger cooling.

"The longer the curse was in her, the more of her it would kill," the wyvern replied with Skara's mouth.

"How do you know this?" Margen demanded.

"I… felt it," Skara said. She made a face. "Something to do with your teaching, something with… Bethany's oath to Ophidian."

"We need to leave," Ellen Annabelle said, moving toward the new wyvern.

Jarin Reedis landed beside her, turned into his human form and nodded in agreement, saying, "We should go before more questions are asked."

"What should we call you?" Ellen asked the human form of the new wyvern. "I am Ellen Annabelle from both our first names." She pointed to Jarin. "He uses the name of his dragon first and the last name of his human." She made a face. "Krea Wymarc was most disdainful."

"So by this Wymarc's thinking, we should be named…?" Skara asked.

"You are something new," Annabelle admitted, "like me."

"So… Skara Bethany?" Skara asked.

"Perhaps Bethany Skara," Reedis suggested with an apologetic look to Ellen Annabelle. "Eldest name last."

"Huh," Ellen said, her brows furrowing. "I hadn't thought of that."

*Bethany?* Skara thought to her twin soul. She got a half-formed thought in response and realized that the young girl was still in shock and digesting her new life. *I'm here for you. I'll always be here for you.*

Skara felt Bethany's gratitude and also her fear, confusion, doubt.

*We'll get through this together,* Skara thought, mentally hugging the other twin soul tightly. She felt Bethany's resistance, then felt the tortured soul relax, release. Skara realized that tears were flowing down her cheeks and raised a hand to touch them in surprise.

"Are you all right?" Annabelle asked.

"I don't cry," Skara said in a shaky voice.

"Bethany does," Ellen said. She pursed her lips. "Let her cry, Skara. She can cry for the both of you."

Skara nodded jerkily, still amazed at the emotions that coursed through her body. She saw the way Thomas Walpish looked at her, half-fearful, half-speculative. She jerked when he moved forward to hold her and steadied only when his arms engulfed her.

"There is no shame in tears," Thomas told her... them. "Bethany, cry all you want. Skara will handle it."

Skara felt Bethany's sorrow well through her and let the tears flow, unchecked. Some of the tears, she realized, were her own. When she recovered enough to push away from Thomas, he smiled at her. "So," he said, "Bethany Skara?"

Skara felt Bethany's approval and nodded. "Bethany Skara."

She felt something inside her release. Bethany.

"Can we have some time to think about it? Maybe try it out?" Bethany asked with Skara's voice. Her eyes widened as she added, "I'm *tall!*"

"And you're an awfully small wyvern," Ellen Annabelle said.

"I think she'll grow as she ages," Reedis said. "Just like a normal person."

"I know *I'm* waiting for Ellen to get bigger," Annabelle said with Ellen's voice.

"Can you take us with you?" Thomas Walpish asked, gesturing to himself and Tracker.

"I think that would be wise," Annabelle said, nodding to Jarin. "Can you carry the immortal?"

Jarin nodded and turned to the metal immortal. "If you don't object."

"Where are we going?" Tracker asked.

"*That*," Jarin Reedis said, shaking his head sadly, "we cannot tell you."

"Someplace that will further your aims and ours," Annabelle told her.

"Can you take me, too?" Margiss asked, turning her head to peer over her grandfather's shoulder.

"You're hurt, you need a healer," Mage Margen told her.

"I know a healer," Ellen Annabelle told him. Beside her, Jarin Reedis chuckled, adding, "One of the best."

"I will send one of your father's *other* children to accompany you," Margen said.

"Oh, I think we won't have to worry about that," Walpish said with a grin, raising a hand up in invitation. A chirp in the distance echoed around the castle courtyard. It was joined by another chirp, more scolding.

"You'll take those two, then?" Margen said.

"I'll take mine, too," Margiss told him, raising a hand upwards. "She can keep you informed." The small form, nearly identical to Jarin Reedis in form but small enough to fit in Margiss' palm, dropped from the sky with a happy chirp.

"Very well," Margen said. He nodded toward Ellen Annabelle. "As you said, you should leave." He turned toward his students, moving toward the still sprawled Bree Emer. "Come along, Miss Emer! You've had more excitement today than is normal and doubtless it will take you some time to recover." He spread his gaze to the rest of the class. "No doubt the same is true of all of you." He made a sweeping gesture, motioning them back to the classroom. "We are going back to the classroom where there will be tea and biscuits — *not* sweets! — and we will talk over what we learned."

He turned and dropped Margiss onto the ground beside him, gesturing for her to join the gathering of wyverns. He gave an *oof* of surprise when Margiss turned and hugged him tightly. Gently he untangled her and sent her on her way. With a smile to her and the others, he whirled his hands in a spell and a multi-colored fog rose like a wall between them and the castle. He continued to hold the spell and urge his charges on until he heard the rustle of wings — three sets — and then he let the spell fade.

As the fog lifted, the palace guards rushed down the steps toward him and his students. Margen raised a hand and shouted, "Enough!"

The guards stumbled to a halt.

"Children, back to class now," he told his students. He turned to the officer of the guard, adding, "There's nothing more to see."

"There was a dragon!"

"Yes," Margen said. Keeping his lips from twitching, he added seriously, "As you can see, I got rid of it."

"The King will be pleased!"

"Yes," Margen said. "I'm sure he will."

The officer gave him a puzzled look, trying to match the mage's words to his tone and failing. With a tired wave, Margen gestured him back to his duty. As the officer collected his guards and they all moved back up the front stairs into the palace, mage Margen turned back to his students.

"We have a lot to learn today, let's be about it."

Bree Emer fell back until she came close enough to speak only to the mage. "Will your granddaughter be all right?"

"I have no doubt of it," Mage Margen lied. He put a steadying hand on her shoulder, guiding her forward and back to her education.

As they entered the corridor that led to the classroom, Margen glanced to the right — and the king's chambers. *Markel, you have much to answer for!*

"Are you not worried that we'll get lost in this blizzard?" Hamo Beck asked as he and Margaret Waters continued to walk away from the village of Korin's Pass and to the looming mountains that walled the village off from Kingsland in the south.

"Well, we might," Margaret agreed easily. "But I'm sure you know where I'm going."

"Pardon me?" Hamo said, stopping abruptly. "How is it that I could possibly know where I'm going?"

"Because you're half-zwerg," Margaret replied smoothly, "and I need to talk with the queen."

"The queen? What queen?"

"The queen of the zwerg," Margaret replied, her tone growing hot. "I think I can arrange a trade that would be beneficial to all."

"I have no idea what you're talking about and I haven't the slightest clue where to go," Hamo Beck said angrily.

"Well, if we don't get inside soon, you'll probably freeze to death," Margaret said unworriedly. "Besides, you are certain to profit from this." She glanced up to him and saw his expression. "There'll be gold involved."

Hamo Beck eyed her for a long moment, his expression hard. Finally, he said, "Close your eyes and don't open them."

Margaret did and was surprised when the taller man grabbed her arms, spun her around rapidly and then threw her over his shoulder.

"What are you doing?" Margaret demanded, putting a fierce tone in her words.

"Taking you to the queen," Beck said. "Keep your eyes closed. You will be killed if you try to discover the way into the realm."

Margaret, her head bouncing against his chest, kept her eyes closed. She didn't need eyes. A small breath of warm air tickled her left ear and she smiled. She had other ways of getting directions.

"All right men," Major Lewis said, "you know your orders. We have the plan." He pulled the leather gloves from his warm coat pockets and slipped them on. "Gloves on, grab your rope, jump over and slide down."

Below them was the dark form of a castle. They were aiming for a rooftop. Some of the men had done this same jump not all that long ago with Colonel Walpish as he captured the guard tower in South Sea Pass.

"Cast off your line as soon as you're down and draw your sabers."

Samuel Lewis waited until each of his picked squad were gloved and had grabbed their ropes. Then he pulled himself to the top of the railing. The squad joined him. "Ready, go!"

Sam Lewis felt the rush of air as he plummeted into the dark night and blizzard of snow. He tightened his grip on his line to slow his descent. A moment later, his boots thudded loudly on the roof of the Sorian castle. The other boots thudded beside him. He dropped his line, pulled his sword and cried, "Onwards, lads! For Kingsland!"

# King's Conquest
## Book 17
Twin Soul series

# Dedication

**In memory of**

**Grant Imahara**

# Chapter One

Alain Casman was not familiar with this part of the Jasram Plains. In truth, he was not familiar with much of the Plains beyond the city his father had ruled and its immediate environs.

The ground they trudged over was not promising: hard-packed dirt and scrub that seemed to offer neither food nor protection. And, in the distance… more of the same.

He was glad that the zwerg queen Alva had supplied him with water and food, although he was worried about his sister, the centaur. Lisette might eat human food but what about the horse part of her? Hay, oats, those would be the sort of food the horse half of the centaur needed. And water, lots of water. The two canteens were not enough to quench both their thirsts. And if Lisette Marie grew too thirsty or too hungry, what then?

"I'm taller than you, you know," Lisette said as she walked daintily beside him. Dainty for a horse, at least. "I can see farther."

"And what do you see?"

"Nothing," Lisette said. "An awful lot of nothing."

"The wyvern didn't want to get us too close," Alain said, suddenly wondering if perhaps the wyvern had more nefarious goals in mind.

"She has a name!"

"Two of them," Alain muttered curtly. His negativity was rewarded with a smack on his shoulder — reminding him once more that Lisette *was* taller than him. "Ow!" he cried, even though it didn't hurt. Usually his cry was all that was necessary to get Lisette to apologize profusely and promise to be better.

"That didn't hurt," Lisette said this time. "You know, sometimes I think you're a —"

"What?" Alain demanded heatedly.

Lisette dropped her voice. "We're being watched."

"Someone ahead?"

"Behind and to the side," Lisette said, glancing warily from side to side. She dropped her hand on Alain's shoulder, saying, "Don't do anything."

"I'm not sure what I —" his reply was cut off as something powerful and big smashed into him from behind.

"Murderer!" a gruff voice shouted into Alain's ears as he fell. His head was forced into the dirt and some of it got into his mouth. It did not taste good.

"What?"

"Leave him alone!" Lisette cried. A moment later there was a loud thud and she said, "I *said*, leave him alone!"

"You want to kill himself yourself?" the gruff voice guessed. Suddenly, Alain was released and pulled up harshly back to his feet. "Go ahead, I suppose you've earned the right."

Alain caught Lisette's fierce look, her teeth bared, eyes flashing, hands balled into fists and suddenly remembered how amazing his little sister could be when incensed.

Her hand flashed out and smacked someone across the face. "You idiot! He's my brother!"

"Brother! He's a human, anyone can smell it!" the gruff voice replied.

"A human and a centaur sister?" a different voice said in astonishment, it was a woman's voice — female, at least. "And she's a filly, hardly grown at all!"

"What are you thinking, Mayse?" the gruff voice asked.

"We need to get them out of sight," Mayse said. "*Now!*"

"All right, all right," the gruff voice said.

"Janzie, you don't understand," Mayse said. "If the Duke finds out…"

"She's a filly," Janzie said in sudden understanding. "He'll kill her."

"He'll have to get through me first!" Alain exclaimed, his hand going to his sword. Before he could do more, Janzie smacked him to the ground with one hand, his other grabbing his sword hilt.

"That won't be hard," the gruff man said. Alain glared up at him and swept one leg behind him and pushed against Janzie's knee with the other — the gruff man grunted in surprise and fell on his back. Alain was back on his feet, one hand going for the stiletto in his boot and the other coming up in guard position.

Janzie took in Alain's fierce look and shook his head, laughing. He raised his free hand in surrender. "I meant no harm, lad!"

"Alain!" Lisette called warningly. "They can help us!"

"I wouldn't go that far," Mayse said. "But the sooner we're out of sight, the better."

"How can we get out of sight?" Lisette asked, craning her head around. "There's nothing for miles."

"Nothing you can *see*," Janzie said, rising to his feet and passing back Alain's blade — hilt first. He glanced behind him and added, "Nice work, Mayse."

"Straight ahead and be quick," Mayse ordered. "We've been in the open for too long as it is."

"The only thing that could see us was that wyvern — and it's long gone," Janzie grumbled.

"The only thing *you* saw," Mayse said. "Who knows what lingers unseen?"

Janzie grunted at that but nodded. He gestured Alain ahead of him. "No talk," Janzie said. "Wait until we're safe."

*And how long will that be?* Alain wondered to himself.

"What is wrong with that child?" Wymarc demanded as Ellen Annabelle, Jarin Reedis and others returned to the small balcony of Ophidian's castle.

"She's bleeding," Annabelle said, stating the obvious. "She was assaulted by magic but Bethany Skara saved her."

"Bethany Skara?" Krea said, darting her eyes to the tall woman cradling the young girl with the bleeding mouth in her arms. Wymarc wrenched Krea's head toward Ellen Annabelle in alarm. "You made *another* wyvern?"

"You were there," Jarin Reedis said. "Nestor froze the wyvern until we could find her a twin soul."

"And so… Bethany Skara," Krea surmised for her astonished older twin soul, Wymarc. She waved a hand toward the other girl. "But who is she?"

"This is Margiss, the granddaughter of mage Margen," Ellen said. "She was cursed by mage Vistos and we saved her."

"And the others?" Wymarc demanded.

"The man is Skara's companion," Jarin Reedis said. "Apparently they've sworn an oath to a god — or gods — to have Vistos' head."

"That's one," Wymarc said.

"I am Tracker," the metal immortal said, nodding her head toward the twin soul.

"You brought a *mechanical* here?" Wymarc cried in surprise. "And a *Tracker?*"

"We didn't have much choice," Jarin Reedis said with a shrug. "We had to take the girl here so that Ellen Annabelle could do her magic without being seen."

"But — but — the girl will know!" Wymarc spluttered.

"Margiss, come here," Ellen Annabelle said. The taller girl eyed her dubiously but saw the way that Jarin Reedis — the dragon — nodded encouragingly. She took two steps and dropped to her knees. "I can heal you," Ellen told her. "But it has to remain our secret —"

"Why?"

"Because she's the only wyvern who can heal," a new voice, male, loud, and irritated said from under the arches leading out to the balcony.

"You are Ophidian," Tracker said. The immortal glanced at the dusky-skinned man moving toward them with smooth, flowing steps, and dropped to one knee. "I greet you."

Ophidian nodded to the mechanical quickly then turned his attention back to the rest of the group.

Ellen Annabelle ignored him, saying to Margiss. "Open your mouth, so I can close your wounds."

Margiss gave her a worried look but obliged. "Will it hurt?"

"It might," Ellen told her honestly. "Especially if you keep talking." She eyed the bleeding wound, frowned and moved one finger toward it.

"Think the skin whole and unblemished, if you wish to close the wound," Ophidian said with a sigh. He dropped to his knees and gave Ellen Annabelle an exasperated look.

"What about the tooth?" Ellen asked.

"I don't think you know enough for that," Ophidian told her. "Maybe in another ten years."

"I'm sorry," Ellen said to the girl.

"Wait!" Bethany Skara said, moving toward them. She glanced toward Thomas Walpish in inquiry.

"We made a deal that gave Skara back her tooth," Thomas said.

"That is not something I can do," Ophidian said, his smoky eyes looking thoughtful. He smiled. "Although I can guess who —"

"Aron!" Thomas Walpish cried, raising his head and turning in a long slow circle.

"You don't have to shout," a young boy's voice replied from the right of the lithe cavalryman. "I could hear you just fine."

"Ah, brother," Ophidian said with a nod toward Aron, the god of Judgement. "I might have guessed."

"Would have guessed," Aron agreed.

"If I cannot replace her tooth, I should heal her now," Annabelle said, nodding toward the boy god and glancing up toward Ophidian.

Aron grinned. "I like her! She's not afraid of you."

"I'm his daughter," Ellen Annabelle replied. "I owe him my life."

"Only one," Aron said, "and bought with the other."

Ellen nodded in agreement and returned her gaze to Margiss. "Don't listen to them," she said, pushing a finger against the gaping wound that had held Margiss' back molar.

Margiss felt a burning sensation then nothing. Ellen removed her finger and Margiss' tongue darted to the wound... only, it was gone. Her tongue, confused and intrigued, continued to probe the smooth jaw.

"Well," Wymarc said in a prickly tone, "now that that's all been settled — oh my gods, you didn't!"

She glared at a small form that chirped excitedly and darted down to land on Bethany Skara's shoulder.

"Don't you know —" she broke off as another small form landed on Thomas Walpish's shoulder. "Have you no sense?" she demanded. Another form streaked down from the sky and Wymarc jerked and squeaked in alarm. She glared at Ellen Annabelle. "Are you mad?"

"What?" Ellen Annabelle said in all innocence.

"Bringing *them* here!" Wymarc scolded.

Ellen frowned. "The humans?"

"No, the *drakes!*"

"It was bound to happen sooner or later," Ophidian said, raising a hand as a perch. One of the small creatures cried in delight and swooped down to land. He nodded toward it. "And what news have you, little one?"

Margiss looked from the drake on Ophidian's hand to Jarin Reedis and back. "Are... are they baby dragons?"

"No," Wymarc said reprovingly. "They're pests."

"Your daughter loves them," Jarin said to her.

"Her daughter?" Margiss asked, glancing toward Krea Wymarc. Krea Wymarc met her gaze. "Did you have a child when you were very young?"

"He doesn't mean me," Krea replied with a smile. "He means Wymarc."

"The twin soul wyvern," Ellen Annabelle explained. She saw the confusion in Margiss' eyes and continued, "Bethany Skara and I are not typical of wyverns."

"No," Wymarc said frostily, "not at all." Under her breath she muttered something more that could have been: *Thank the gods!*

"A twin soul is usually the union of a magical creature and a human," Jarin Reedis said, raising a hand to point to himself as an example. "Our Ellen decided to change the rules." His lips quirked as he nodded toward Ophidian. "Rather like our father."

"But the drakes?" Margiss asked. "They're not twin souls, are they?"

"No, thank the gods!" Wymarc growled, adding under her breath, "At least we have that much to be grateful for."

"The origin of the drakes is not something I will talk about," Ophidian said in a very firm voice. He swept his hand upwards and the drake perched on it flew back to Margiss. He turned toward Wymarc, adding, "But they are dear to me in their own way."

"They're terrible gossips," Wymarc said. "They're everywhere and eat everything and —"

"Daughter," Ophidian said quellingly.

Wymarc grimaced. A moment later, Krea said from the same mouth but in a very different tone and stance, "I think they're cute!"

"They are great at being unseen and hearing things," Jarin Reedis said.

"Mage Margen seemed to tolerate them and no more," Thomas Walpish said. "Skara and I thought that we could use them as messengers."

"Provided you can get them to go where they're meant," Wymarc muttered darkly.

Ophidian raised a hand, silencing the conversation. He turned to Aron, the young boy. "And what is your opinion on this?"

"They balance out," Aron said with a wave of his hand. "They are none of my concern." His eyes strayed toward the mechanical.

Ophidian followed his gaze and nodded. "Ah, yes." He turned to Tracker. "One of your kind is here already."

"Ibb," Tracker said, rising from her bent knee. "I felt him. He is not too close, however."

"He is working on something," Ophidian said evasively.

"For you?" Tracker sounded surprised and somewhat angry.

"To our mutual benefit," Ophidian said. "He is in my debt and helps another of my oathsworn."

"You are gathering a lot of them," Aron said with a frown.

"I am not the only one," Ophidian said, meeting the god of Judgement's gaze steadily.

"Take care," Aron cautioned before turning to smile at Walpish. "Some have other allegiances."

Ophidian nodded, turning to gaze at Walpish. "Is that so?"

"Can I tell him?" Walpish said to Aron.

"In private or only in the presence of the oathsworn," Aron said. He turned to Ophidian. "You do not want this knowledge shared."

"I see," Ophidian said with a jerk of his chin. He turned to Tracker. "Your presence here is your doom."

"Ibb is here," Tracker said, sounding serene.

Aron's brows narrowed and he turned to the mechanical, head cocked in surprise. "You seek her."

"Who?" Tracker asked.

"The one who destroyed the caravan," Aron said. His lips quirked. "You don't believe in us — how could you, being an immortal? — but you are beginning to have doubts."

"As is Ibb," Jarin Reedis said. He frowned.

"He said that a change is coming," Annabelle said with Ellen's young voice.

"More than one," a new voice spoke up. They all turned. Ibb the mechanical stood at the archway. Beside him stood a sturdy young lad, a girl, and a young man.

Jarin moved forward. He waved a hand toward the new group and turned back to the others. "Thomas Walpish, Bethany Skara, Tracker, and… uh, Margiss, may I make you known to Ibb the immortal, Angus Franck, Hana Renn, and Nestor Pallas?"

Margiss gasped in amazement and turned, dropping into a deep curtsy. "Your Highness, we thought you were dead!"

# Chapter Two

"See them below," Captain Fawcett shouted over the noise of the wind and the royal protests. "Secure them in the brig, but bring blankets and warm food."

His first mate saluted sharply and nodded to the soldiers who tugged the bound royals along with them.

When they were out of sight, Fawcett turned to Major Lewis and beamed. "Well done, well done! The king will be overjoyed at this news!"

"I certainly hope so," Major Lewis said, his emotions engulfing him as they always did after a combat action.

"You have them — the king, the queen, their son! What can the Sorians do now?" Fawcett said. He turned to his helmsman. "Turn about and set a course for the coastline!"

"Aye sir!"

Fawcett tuned out the helmsman's bellowed orders to his mates and turned back to the triumphant cavalryman. "We'll meet up with General Georgos and deliver our cargo." He waved a fist in the air. "Then let's see what happens!" He lowered his fist and waved it toward Major Lewis. "Just you wait, it will be *glorious!*"

"Yes," Lewis said glumly.

"It *will* be!" Fawcett declared. He eyed his companion and shook his head. "You're overtired, Samuel. Why don't you go below and take some wine in my cabin." He eyed his ship. "I'll join you presently."

Major Samuel Lewis pursed his lips tightly and nodded. "Aye, I suppose it's just the cold."

Fawcett clapped him on the arm. "Of course it is! Get below and get something to warm you!"

Sam Lewis nodded and turned toward the hatchway.

Inside the captain's cabin, he located the glasses and decanter, brought them to the table and poured himself a generous cup of wine.

Everything had gone well... except for the girl.

His men had been hangdog when they came to the roof with the prince. Lewis had eyed them in surprise. "Well?"

"This here's the prince, sir," the senior man had said, pushing the struggling prisoner toward him.

"Good, good," Lewis had said. But the two privates exchanged nervous looks, clearly there was more to their tale. "What?"

"He was in bed, he was," the other private said.

"With his doxie," the first private agreed.

"But you got him," Lewis said.

"Aye but the doxie — the girl — she put up a fight," the first private said.

"We had to stick her, sir, to get her to let go," the second private said, looking pale in the wintry night.

"Well, one life for a kingdom," Lewis said with a shrug. "I'm sorry that you had to do the deed but you've done your duty, no one will blame you."

"Yes, sir," the first private had agreed weakly.

*One casualty on their side and none on ours,* Lewis thought to himself as he took a sip, *that's a good mission.*

Still, the look on the prince's face, the heat of his gaze, had troubled Lewis. *There is a man who will not forget.*

Margaret Waters smelled the men — zwerg — as they approached. They smelled of earth and spice mixed. They smelled of worry… and anger.

"Are you mad?" a bass voice demanded from among the group, his attention focused on Hamo Beck. "What do you mean bringing a sky-toucher here? The queen will be livid!"

"I made him," Margaret spoke up, eyes still closed. A small breath of warm air brushed her neck beneath her ear. "I am Margaret Waters and I laid the tracks through Korin's Pass."

"Mage are you?" the bass voice guessed.

"I owe thanks to Hissia and Hanor for my powers," Margaret said. "I owe my father for my training, however."

"And who is your father?"

"My father is Torvan Brookes," Margaret replied. "But most know him as the Steam Master."

A hiss of surprise informed Margaret that her father's name had traveled even to the zwerg who lived underground.

Margaret forced herself not to smile. "The zwerg are well known for their great abilities with metal," Margaret said. "I know that my father would be most grateful to work with them."

"How grateful?" a voice, not the bass voice, asked from Margaret's right.

"Grateful enough to pay in gold," Margaret said. She heard the reaction of the zwerg: she *definitely* had their attention. "We're going to need a lot of steel, we plan to lay a lot of railroad tracks." She paused, gauging the moment. "But we'd pay twice for dragon steel."

"And who tells you that the zwerg know how to make dragon steel?" a different voice demanded. A woman's voice.

Margaret knelt to the ground. "No one," Margaret confessed, "not until you spoke. Your Majesty."

The gasps from around her confirmed Margaret's guess. Quickly Margaret continued, "My father knew Rabel Zebala. They worked together, along with Ibb the mechanical, to make the first steam engines and lay the first rail line." She paused, her ears straining to gauge their reaction. "Father knew that Rabel had worked with the zwerg from of old." She paused. "And when he heard that the fort at East Pass had shot down the airships, he guessed that Rabel was involved." Shrewdly, she added, "That somehow, Rabel had worked with others to make dragon steel and make the fort fly."

"It didn't fly, it floated," the queen corrected her. She added, "And how much, child, of what you are saying is your father and how much is you?"

Margaret smiled. "I guessed about the fort, the dragon steel, and the zwerg," Margaret admitted. "But father told me about you and Rabel." She paused, listening to the reaction. "And everyone knows that the zwerg love gold."

"Just as long as they don't know why," a voice spoke softly, not expecting Margaret's ears to catch it.

But Margaret had the wind to help her.

Alone in his chambers, mage Margen allowed himself a moment. A moment of fury, a moment of sorrow, a moment of anger, and a moment of calm. With each breath, he grew calmer, more thoughtful. Vistos had cursed his granddaughter. Vistos had cursed others, too. Vistos' apprentice was clearly under his control. That assassin, Skara Ningan, had been too.

*Where there is smoke, there is fire*, Margen thought to himself in a grumble. How many had Vistos ensorceled? And how many more would come under his control? And to what end? Would those cursed sweets doom them? Or would they merely become mindless pawns for the mage and his master?

*Sorcerer*, Margen thought to himself. *He's become a sorcerer.* Which made sense — Vistos was a pretty poor excuse for a mage.

"But the king does nothing!" Margen spat the words out aloud. *So where does that leave me? My allegiance?* In fact, the king was unconcerned about Vistos' attack on one of Margen's kin. King Markel had, in fact, approved the writ that allowed Torvan Brookes — the "Steam Master" — to steal Margen's students.

"I swore allegiance to him," Margen said out loud to himself, in reminder.

*"Did he not break his oath to you when he refused to help your granddaughter?"* the cavalryman — Thomas Walpish — had asked him that question.

"There are penalties for breaking an oath," Margen reminded himself.

"Indeed there are," a small voice agreed pleasantly. Margen looked around his room frantically, eyes wide. *Nothing* could enter his chambers when he'd spelled them! Nothing... except a god.

Margen looked down and found a pair of bright eyes staring back up at him.

"Aron, god of Judgement," Margen said, nodding to the young god.

"And friends," Aron said, waving a hand toward the air beside him. In an instant the space was occupied by a tall dusky-skinned man and...

"Margiss!" Margen cried in surprise and joy, rushing to engulf her in his arms. Margiss smiled and closed the gap just as quickly.

"You're safe!" Margen said, feeling the strength of her soul flowing in her body, feeling the wellness. He grabbed her by the shoulders and pushed her away so he could get a better view of her. "And your tooth?"

"Gone," Aron said.

Margen nodded to the young god and gave the taller man a nod. He motioned Margiss aside with his hands and went to one knee. "Great god Ophidian, I am in your debt."

"I know," Ophidian said with a smirk. "I've been waiting for this for a long time."

"I have other charges, students in my care," Margen said cautiously.

"You cannot speak for them," Aron warned. He turned to Ophidian. "And what do you plan?"

Ophidian glanced down at the small god. "I need allies. There is more going on here than we know."

"Agreed," Aron said. "But do not forget that allies can also become targets."

Ophidian grinned at him. "Which is why I need *smart* allies."

"What do you want of me?" Margen asked.

"Help," Aron said. "But nothing more than you can give."

"I work with all the gods," Margen said in warning. "I would lose abilities if I had to choose only one."

"I know," Ophidian said. He glanced toward the well-wrought wooden cabinet beyond Margen's desk, the one that held his figurines of the gods. "But I believe that some of the gods are not in your pantheon."

Margen's breath caught.

"You don't know everything," Aron warned Ophidian.

"And how boring the world would be if I did!" Ophidian agreed. He turned to mage Margen. "Ibb the immortal tells me that change is coming."

"Yes," Margen agreed.

"King Markel has decided that Vistos is his mage," Ophidian continued, "unless you can replace him."

"I wish to destroy him," Margen said fiercely. He pulled Margiss backwards against his chest and wrapped an arm around her. "He challenged me and threatened my kin."

"And progeny," Aron added, winking at Margiss. The girl's eyes bulged in confusion — a god winking at her?

"I swore allegiance to Markel because we agreed that knowledge needed to grow," Margen said. "That Kingsland would be richer if there were more mages, more educated tradespeople, more chances for learning."

"And," Ophidian said, "for a while that's what happened."

"Now the king thinks only of conquest, of grabbing territory, even at the expense of his people," Margen said.

"I need your oath if we're to continue any further," Ophidian said. "There are things that I will only share with my oathbound."

Margen released Margiss from his embrace and turned her around. He looked into her eyes.

"I would swear to him," Margiss said. "I would have sworn already but I owe you, grandfather."

"What would you have of me?" Margen said. "I will protect my charges, I will see that Vistos is destroyed, I will educate those who wish it."

"In exchange for what?" Aron asked. Margen glanced toward him in confusion.

"Rabel got thirty years," Margiss told her grandfather with a grin. She glanced toward Ophidian, saying, "You didn't tell me I couldn't say anything."

Ophidian chuckled.

"I would like more," Margen said. Ophidian closed his mouth with a snap. "I would like to consult with the immortals and with Rabel Zebala." Ophidian jerked his head in agreement. "And I would like to train Skara Ningan and Thomas Walpish — as I'd already agreed —"

"I can give you a few more to train," Ophidian murmured.

"They're Bethany Skara now," Margiss chirped.

"I shall need you to train Imay the zwerg princess, Angus Franck, Hana Renn, and Nestor Pallas," Ophidian said. Margen started to respond but Ophidian stopped him with a raised hand. "And a dozen more of my choosing at any time."

"Half a dozen or he'll get nothing done," Margiss said, stepping away from Margen's grasp to stand between the old mage and the smoldering eyes of the dragon god.

"Does she speak for you then?" Ophidian demanded.

"Usually she speaks far too much," Margen replied with a grin. "But, in this case let us say that I'll accept those you recommend if they meet my standards."

"We are being seen," Aron warned, glancing toward the cabinet of god figurines.

"I accept," Ophidian said, reaching his hand to Margen. The mage stepped forward to stand by his granddaughter and took the dragon god's offer.

Not many moments later, back in the Kingsland capital of Kingsford, in the king's castle, the doors to Margen's chambers flew open and mage Vistos sprang forward.

But the room was empty. The great desk was gone, the shelves were bare, and the cabinet of the gods was only a smoldering pile of ashes.

Vistos turned angrily and spied the boy who had led him here. "You were too slow!"

"Mr. Bastien!" Captain Fawcett called out when he was certain that all the Sorian royalty had been properly detained.

"Sir!"

"Are you ready with the signal rockets?" Fawcett called.

"Aye sir!" Bastien replied. Fawcett hid a grin: the midshipman had only just heard of their existence a scant hour ago.

"How many have we got?"

"Ten of each, sir: red, gold, blue, green," Bastien replied quickly, glancing toward one of the airmen standing at his side.

"Very well," Fawcett replied. "You are to take a detail to the crow's nest along with a lantern and you are to fire in this order: red, gold, blue."

"Red, gold, blue, aye sir," Bastien said, saluting sharply.

"You are to continue doing so every fifteen minutes," Fawcett continued.

"Aye sir," Bastien said.

"You will stop when you have used up six of each colored rocket or when you receive a reply."

"A reply, sir?"

"A green flare from the direction of South Sea Pass," Fawcett told him. "You will detail a lookout with a glass to watch."

"Aye sir," Bastien replied.

"Do you understand your orders?"

"Aye sir."

"Then carry on," Fawcett said. He moved over to the helmsman and nodded to the engineer. "Hold us steady over the capital." The helmsman nodded. "I'm going below. Call me if anything changes."

"Aye sir," the helmsman said.

It was cold in the highest turret of King Markel's castle. There was no light kept there, nor any fire — to preserve night vision. The man called Hewlitt's Eyes didn't mind. He'd grown inured to such hardest years back in a much harsher clime. Galvin Narvik's thick fur coat and thicker undergarments kept the worst of the night's cold from biting him. He'd grown up far north in Issia where the nights last all winter — this was but a warm day to him.

He scanned north and east, as ordered. Hanging from his neck by a leather strap was a pair of fine binoculars.

A light. There, north, in the distance. Galvin raised the glasses to his eyes for confirmation. Green. An acknowledgement. A moment later, in the same location, he spotted three flares high in the sky: red, gold, blue. That was the signal being repeated south. He lowered his glasses, went to the logbook resting on its stand, checked the time by glancing at the stars above and made a quick, accurate note. Replying to the message was not his responsibility.

The signal was repeated again. Galvin ignored it, turning his attention once more to the east.

There! Gold flare. He smiled to himself. He pulled out a piece of parchment from his pocket and marked it. He did not record the incident in his logbook.

He leaned over the parapet — gods, did he love this part! — and spied a guard on the walls below, nodding off over his spear. Sleeping again.

Galvin made a quick note with another bit of parchment, found a nice-sized rock, wrapped the note around the rock and took careful aim.

Far below, the sleeping guard yelped in surprise as a rock bounced off his metal helmet. He glanced up in the darkness but did not see Galvin. With a curse, the now-awake guard bent over and retrieved the parchment wrapped rock. Galvin smiled as the guard shook his fist up at him before turning his head and calling loudly, "Captain of the guard! A message from the tower!"

Message delivered, Galvin returned to scanning the horizon, looking. Being Hewlitt's Eyes.

Moments later, Galvin heard the expected sound of heavy feet rising up the long circular stairway that led to his tower.

"Any other news?" Captain Gufstafson said.

Wordlessly, Galvin handed him the strip of parchment with the note about the gold flare.

Gufstafson took it, read it, grunted, and pocketed the note. "Tell no one."

Galvin Narvik saluted and turned back to his watch.

# Chapter Three

"Sir, sir! Signal, sir, from the north!" the midshipman squeaked as he rapped on Commodore Evans' door.

"Enter!" Evans replied, rising from his bed and swinging his legs over to the floor. He pulled his night robe from its hook and fastened it about him, searching for his slippers absently with his toes.

The midshipman rushed through the door — it had been opened by Evans' marine guard — and came to a shambling halt as he caught sight of his commander.

Evans affected not to notice but coughed softly and nodded toward the lad's brow.

"Oh!" the midshipman squeaked, bracing to attention. "Sir, signals report a sighting from the northeast."

"Just the one?"

"Well, there was another from due east but…" the midshipman's voice trailed off. "I was told to tell you that they fired red, gold, blue, sir."

Evans stood and saluted the midshipman, showing him how it could be done even when *not* in uniform.

"Very good," Evans said as he lowered his salute. "And the other signal?"

"Just one gold flare, repeated twice on the half hour, sir."

"Where from?"

"The lookouts thought it was maybe not far from Korin's Pass, sir," the midshipman offered hesitantly.

"Hmm," Evans muttered to himself, "probably not meant for us." A moment later, he added, "Nor our eyes." He pursed his lips, then said, "My compliments to the first lieutenant, have him call the crew to quarters. Have the engineer and stokers report for duty and let Mage Firth know that we may have need of his crew presently."

"Aye sir," the midshipman said, knuckling a salute and turning to dash away.

"AND," Commodore Evans raised his voice to halt the midshipman who turned, ashen-faced back to his commander. "Signal to have all captains prepare for imminent departure and repair aboard the flag immediately."

"Aye, sir," the midshipman said. "Any further orders, sir?"

"No," Evans said, his lips twitching, "that will be all, midshipman."

The midshipman saluted again and turned to depart, moving more slowly.

"We haven't got all night, midshipman," Evans barked at his back. "And tell the cook to get us something warm!"

Peter Hewlitt was "relaxing" at the Inn of the Broken Sun when the messenger came to him. Hewlitt nudged his companion in apology then rose from his bed to gather the message.

"Very good," Hewlitt said, moving toward his clothes and dressing quickly. He nodded the messenger toward the bed. "It's a bitter night out, why don't you go warm yourself?"

Hewlitt's companion, wisely, said nothing of this change in the state of affairs. As the young messenger was enjoying the warm bed and the warmth of the bed warmer, Hewlitt went to the far side of the bed and kissed his companion gently on the cheeks.

Outside, he turned and walked down the hall, stopping to rap gently on one door. "Steam Master?" he called. "We've news of a signal that might interest you."

"Is that so?" Torvan Brookes, the Steam Master, called groggily. "What signal and where away?"

"Gold and Korin's Pass," Hewlitt replied.

Immediately there was a thump from inside the room as the Steam Master jumped out of his bed. "I'll be right there."

"So you have your orders," Commodore Evans said to the men gathered around his table. "Captain Wright, you and your brig, *Eagle*, will remain on station here. *Conqueror* will return to Kingsford for the King." He turned to the others. "The rest of you will follow *Victory* to join *Wasp* at Sarskar." He glanced around the table. "Any questions?"

"What of the other ships, sir?" Captain Malcolm of *Conqueror* asked.

"Fancy yourself flotilla, Terry?" Evans asked his junior with a grin. He shook his head. "Last I heard, the next batch won't be ready until the end of the week. I doubt his majesty will want to wait that long."

"Quite," Terence Malcolm agreed ruefully.

"Very well," Evans said, looking around the table once more. "If there are no more questions —" he rose "— you have your orders, gentlemen."

The others rose with him and made way for him to lead them out of the cabin and up to the deck.

First Lieutenant Melroy spotted the crowd and moved to intercept them, saluting Evans smartly.

"How are we, Michael?" Evans asked.

"About five more minutes, sir," Melroy replied. "I sent the hands to breakfast, figuring that we would want them to be in all respects ready."

"And it will take that long to get our guests —" Evans nodded to the cluster of captains "— back to their ships. Good thinking, Michael!"

"If you'd like, sir," Melroy offered, nodding toward the captains, "I can take over from here."

"No," Evans said, moving closer to his first lieutenant and lowering his voice, "if one of them has some last minute worry, they'll want to tell me themselves."

Melroy struggled to keep his expression blank as he absorbed the news. Evans clapped him on the back, "It's all part of command, Michael! You'll learn soon enough!"

"Aye sir," Lieutenant Melroy said, standing upright once more and sounding more cheerful. "I certainly hope so, sir!"

Commodore Evans laughed, gestured the lieutenant back to his station and genially followed the departing captains to the sally port.

His feet were killing him. Alain didn't complain. They must have walked *leagues* by now! It was almost full dark, the sun had set at least an hour ago and Alain was half-convinced that they'd been walking in circles.

Janzie, in the lead, held up a hand warning them to stop. Alain barely saw the gesture and nearly stumbled right into the man. Janzie turned to glare down at him. Alain glared right back. Janzie frowned then turned back, reaching an arm behind him to grab Alain by the sleeve.

Lisette, from her higher vantage point, had stopped just behind Alain. Mayse moved up beside her. Alain caught a satisfied look on her face. She caught the glint of Alain's eyes and nodded: they were here.

Janzie sniffed and muttered something that Alain couldn't catch. A moment later, the gruff man pulled on Alain's shirt, urging him forward.

There was something in front of them. It looked, in the dimness, like a solid wall of rock. But Janzie stepped through. Dimly, Alain spotted a light. He stepped forward and realized that they were passing through something that seemed like a curtain.

It was not. It was magic. Alain felt its weight upon him, felt a crackle of tension in his skin, felt the hairs on his arms and the back of his neck stand up in protest. And then they were through. Janzie pulled him to the side and nodded back toward the opening as Lisette and Mayse stepped hastily through.

Mayse smiled at Janzie, expanded it to include Alain and turned back to the magic "tear" that separated them from the outside. She raised her hands, frowned in concentration and spoke softly, running her hands along either side of the "tear" and pulling the sides together to form a seamless gap.

Alain felt the magic snap around him and turned to look wide-eyed at their surroundings. They were at the outskirts of a camp. It was not a permanent camp. Alain could see where wagons were circled, see a corral for huge — *six-legged!* — beasts.

"Those are hexine!" Alain exclaimed.

Janzie turned to him, surprised. "What do you know of them?"

"I thought they were myths!" Lisette said, trotting up to join them. Her eyes widened in awe. "They're beautiful!"

"They're all that's left," Mayse said with pain in her voice.

"What?" Alain said, turning sharply. "There can't be more than six!"

"Seven," Janzie said. "There's a foal you can't see."

"This secret is worth your lives," Mayse said, glaring at Alain, her hand going to her belt and the knife that hung from it.

"Why are there so few?" Lisette said.

"Because the Duke has vowed to destroy them all," Janzie said heatedly.

Mayse nodded and caught Lisette's eyes. "And all the centaurs."

Mage Vistos was smiling as he approached the door to Margen's classroom the next morning. First, he'd give all the children sweets, then he'd see how they behaved.

He turned the doorknob. Nothing. He frowned. Behind him he could hear Halston stop and wait expectantly.

Vistos stood back, raised himself to his full height and let loose a spell. The double doors remained closed. He cursed and tried another, stronger spell. It didn't work any better. With a hiss of anger, he called forth a blasting spell — he would blast the doors open.

The spell uncoiled with all the strength Vistos — and the power he pulled from Halston — could manage. The doors disappeared in a cloud of dust, vaporized along with a large part of the wall.

With a triumphant growl, Vistos started forward. He stopped abruptly as the dust settled and he had a clear view. He saw the green grass of the castle lawn and beyond that, the walls surrounding the castle. There was a ten foot drop from the hole he'd created in the castle to the ground below.

"Where's the classroom, Master?" Halston asked, coming to stand beside him. "I thought it was through the doors."

A small, winged creature flitted into view directly across from them and chirped.

Vistos, infuriated, blasted at it with a lightning bolt. The little drake dodged the bolt adroitly, turned to follow its path and screeched in excitement as the bolt burst against the castle walls. It turned back to Vistos, chirped once impishly, and disappeared.

"Where are the children?" Halston wondered as he examined the damage his master's thunderbolt had created and heard the alarmed cries of the castle guard.

"What, you didn't know about this?" Mage Margen said to Jarin Reedis. His eyes were twinkling in merriment as he took in the slack-jawed outrage of the former mage.

Jarin Reedis was staring at the large sign that adorned the front of the rather decrepit building before them. Children and teens were walking excitedly through the front doors and out of sight down the corridors and up the stairs of the three-story building. Jarin Reedis' eyes bulged and twitched from side to side as he continuously read the sign in disbelief.

"The Reedis Memorial Academy of Balloon Magic." Smaller print beneath added, "Established by his beloved friend and master mage, Air Mage Kendral."

"We could burn it down," Jarin offered to his human mate in silky tones. "It'd be quite justifiable."

"My students are there," Mage Margen noted reprovingly. "And your father wouldn't take kindly to the results."

"Or we could burn down this Kendral," Jarin added.

"Let's see who he is before we take action," Reedis replied with the same mouth.

Jarin took possession of their body long enough to sigh in bored acceptance. A day without flaming death was a day wasted, in Jarin's opinion.

Beside them, Margen sniggered. Jarin turned to give him an arch look. "Trouble with your human, dragon?"

"The other way around, I think," Reedis said. He shook himself and started up the steps. "We may as well get started."

"I've got to find my class," Margen said. "If you decide you must cause arson, I expect you'll give me sufficient warning."

"I was thinking larceny might be a better approach," Reedis said. He could feel Jarin's greedy acceptance of this new proposal. "But aren't you going to have trouble getting your students to recognize you?"

"That's why we're along," Margiss said, jerking a thumb at herself and then Bethany Skara. "They'll be certain to recognize us."

"Should I accompany you, Reedis, or go with the mage?" Thomas Walpish asked.

"Make sure he causes no harm," Mage Margen said, nodding to Jarin Reedis. "I rather expect that you'll find Reedis' teaching intriguing at the very least." With that, Margen — now a very young man with dark hair and a spring in his step — strode boldly up the stairs and into the building in search of his students.

# Chapter Four

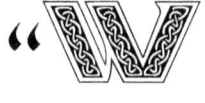"We are on a secret mission from the king and require all immediate assistance," Jacques Martel assured the Kingsland captain with a haughty disdain.

"Certainly," Captain Welless said with an easy air. "Just let me see your orders."

"Captain," Martel said frostily, "what part of 'secret' do you not understand?"

Welless blinked.

"The King," Martel said, "demanded that we carry out his orders with the greatest secrecy."

"And what were his orders?"

Martel looked at Tirpin in amazement and then back to the Kingsland captain. "Sir, I believe that I just said that I *cannot* tell you! They are secret."

Tirpin nudged Martel's shoulder and they exchanged looks. "Perhaps if the captain will swear himself to secrecy?" Tirpin asked.

"But the King —"

"I know, I know," Tirpin said, raising his hands. "He dispatched us from *Wasp* on this most secret mission and promised that all help would be provided by the army but… perhaps his orders were mislaid?" Tirpin turned hopefully to Welless.

"I haven't received any orders in days," Welless said, spreading his hands and sounding just as abandoned as he felt.

"There, you see!" Tirpin said. "The good captain was simply not informed!"

"But can we trust him?" Martel said in a low voice. He glanced back toward Welless with a thoughtful look.

"He was put in charge of the town and we all know how important that is," Tirpin said earnestly.

Martel frowned. "There is that," he allowed. He turned to Welless. "Sir, will you promise never to divulge this mission?"

"Of course," Welless said firmly. He cocked his head up at the two men standing before him. "I am an officer and a gentleman."

"As are we," Martel agreed. "Mage Tirpin and I have been dispatched on a most important mission."

"Which is?"

Martel glanced around the empty alcove and nodded firmly toward the door. He leaned down toward Captain Welless. "Is there anyone else here?"

"Mayor Beck is expected later," Welless allowed, nodding toward the door. "We are quite alone."

"Very well," Martel said, biting his lips. "What I now entrust to your ears cannot leave this room."

"You have my word," Welless said.

Martel glanced toward Tirpin, who nodded and gestured entreatingly. Martel leaned down so that his lips were just beside the captain's left ear. "We are on a mission to meet with the Emperor."

"The Emperor!" Welless exclaimed.

"Sh, sh!" Martel hissed. "No one can know!"

"I see," Welless said. "Well, your secret is safe with me."

"We risk our lives giving you this knowledge," Martel told him with a stiff expression. "But we need your help."

"What can I do to help?"

"We need two mounts and two spares — we must ride in haste — and provisions for a week's travel," Martel said. "The sooner we leave, the better it is for all."

"Very well," Welless said. "We don't have many horses, being infantry, but you're in luck — I have my string and some spares from the other companies." He pursed his lips. "How soon do you need them?"

"We cannot waste a moment," Tirpin replied. "Lives are riding on this mission!"

A dull *boom!* thudded through the air and King Markel looked up from this throne to over to his first minister, Mannevy. "What is it?"

"If I were to hazard a guess, your majesty, that was a signal cannon," Mannevy said. "If you'll permit, I suggest you send a page to check from the new landing."

"Page," Markel said, gesturing toward one of the languid court fops he had on hand, "go see what that noise was!"

"At once, your majesty," a young lad said, straightening himself, sketching a quick bow, and darting out of the throne room. As soon as he could turn his back on the king, he broke into a trot which could be heard from the throne room, fading in the distance.

"So, Mannevy, care to wager?" King Markel asked.

Mannevy chuckled and shook his head. "Your Majesty is too well known for his prowess in such manners. I should hate ever to bet against you."

Markel grunted, not entirely pleased.

"Your majesty," Mannevy began hesitantly, "if, while we're waiting, I might put another matter before you for your consideration?"

"What matter is that?" the king demanded with a pout.

"I am given to understand that a portion of the castle has disappeared and the part of your outer walls have been damaged," Mannevy said.

"What?" Markel shouted, sitting up in his plush throne. "What was that?"

"It appears that mage Margen's classroom is no longer part of the castle," Mannevy said. "And, further, that mage Vistos discovered this through the expedient of blasting a thunderbolt through the doors that previously adjoined said classroom."

"He did?"

"And that said thunderbolt went, unimpeded, straight to your walls, damaging, splintering, and blackening a section thereof."

"Huh," King Markel said, sitting back in his seat. "I'll bet Vistos was furious."

"I believe that could be safely conjectured," Mannevy agreed. "However, the issue still remains that you are not only missing a part of your castle but also that your castle walls are now in a previously unanticipated state of disrepair."

Markel waved a hand, dismissing the issue. "It won't matter, we'll soon be getting a better castle."

"We will?" Mannevy said. "Where, may I ask?"

"The castle in Sarskar," Markel replied. "I shall move the capital there."

"And what will become of this castle, your majesty?"

Markel laughed. "Why, fancy yourself as royalty?"

Mannevy brought a hand to his face in alarm. "I assure you, the thought has never entered my mind."

"Just as well," Markel said, "you don't have the money for this castle." He chortled. "The upkeep is ruinous, especially now that my mages have defiled it."

A pair of feet raced down the corridor, distracting them. The page had returned. He stopped at the entrance, breathless, and bowed low to the king on his throne. "Your Majesty, the airship *Conqueror* is approaching with dispatches."

"It is, is it?" King Markel said, glancing toward Mannevy. "I suppose we should greet them," he said, rising from his throne. He nodded toward Mannevy. "I presume our air dock is ready for us?"

In the course of the past week, King Markel had decided that the castle needed a special landing so that the king could walk from his castle onto any of his airships that docked. It had involved removing part of the battlements and building a new open landing but it had taken less effort than Mannevy had feared, being mostly made with magic. Vistos and his apprentice had not been involved. Instead, the new Steam Master had been invited to perform the duty, as part of his payment for his royal writ.

"It's down the corridor and up the stairs, am I right?" the king asked as he and his retinue left the throne room.

"Quite so, sire," Mannevy agreed.

"Then let's be about it," the king replied, increasing his pace. "I've been eager to try this dock out."

The page was dressed in fine clothes and courtly colors, as required. It had cost his parents dearly but his presence in the royal court was deemed to be worth the sacrifice. Mevin Kalenn, dressed in his fine purple doublet and gold stockings was not so certain now, having spent nearly a month in the royal court. He moved briskly to put himself in front of the throne and bowed deeply. "Your Highness."

"What?" Jenid Paulus, Prince of High Jasram, said in a slow drawl. He turned toward the woman serving him and nodded for her to place another peeled grape in his mouth. "Can't you see that I'm busy?"

"There's been a report," Mevin said, still deep in his bow. "From the plains, Your Highness."

Jenid Paulus lifted a finger, forestalling the servant, and straightened up in his chair. "From the plains?"

"Yes, Your Highness."

"What word?" Paulus demanded.

"The report says that a wyvern was seen —"

"A wyvern?" Paulus snapped, coming to his feet. "Where? And who sent this report? How old is this news?"

"The report was received just this minute," Mevin said. "I was sent by the commander of the watch."

"Stand up," Paulus demanded. "I want the full report."

"Yes, Your Highness," the page said, rising up from his bow. "The message was just received but it was sent by semaphore. It might be an hour or two old."

"And this wyvern, what did it do?"

"It was seen high in the sky then it descended and landed, Your Highness."

"Where?"

"In the Dry Plains, Your Highness," Mevin replied. "Just north and east of Vinjal."

"It landed?"

"It took off again, Your Highness, not long after," the page replied. "The sentry reported that it was on the ground only a moment."

"And where did it go afterwards?"

The page lips his lips, his eyes troubled. "It rose up and then disappeared, Your Highness."

"Disappeared?"

"It could be that the sentry lost sight of it in the haze, Your Highness," Mevin Kalenn guessed.

Grand Duke Jenid Paulus grunted, his expression sour. He waved a finger beckoning to a figure standing at the end of the royal chamber. "Gamden."

Gamden Ikar strutted forward, moving his arms as he moved his feet, like a person not used to them or a seaman fresh arrived on land. When he neared the Grand Duke he did not bow. Instead he gave Paulus a curt nod.

"How soon could you get there?" Paulus demanded.

"Two days," Gamden replied. "But I would have to rest afterwards."

"And your brethren?"

"There are only two of my moult here," Gamden replied. "Bax and Jaden are still young, they haven't reached their full growth."

"You should have the mother throw more out of the nest," Paulus said, his lips twisting wickedly.

"We threw out twenty and only those two survived," Gamden reminded him. He moved closer and said in a lower voice, "You are running out of guards."

Paulus gave him a sour look. "So these two, how fast?"

"It would take them three days and they'd be useless for another two," Gamden said.

"The wyvern would be long gone," Paulus said to himself. He fumed for a moment.

"I have not flown there before," Gamden said. Paulus raised his eyes and glared at him until Gamden gulped and hastily added, "Your Highness."

"You should go," Paulus said. "Take your two with you. Scout out the land, all the land and be back in…"

"Ten days, Your Highness?"

"Yes," Paulus allowed. "That will do." He waved the man away. "Go!"

"As Your Highness desires," Gamden Ikar said, moving away with the awkward gait of one unused to walking on two feet.

"I will go first, Colonel Walpish," Mage Reedis said in a low voice as they approached the closed door at the end of the hallway, the door marked "Principal."

"As you wish," Thomas Walpish said. He knew better than to argue with a flaming dragon and he wasn't at all certain that mage Reedis might not be even more alarming under the current circumstances. Certainly Reedis was not at all amused to discover someone running a school of mage under his name. And, whomever had arranged the travesty would shortly — and probably very pointedly — be made aware that the "Memorial" part of "The Reedis Memorial Academy of Balloon Magic" was grossly in error.

Reedis, much to Walpish's surprise, stopped at the door and knocked politely.

"Enter!" A muffled voice called in response.

Reedis turned the knob, pushed the door open but did not enter. Walpish nodded to himself: a wise precaution, certainly.

The room was tidy if hardly furnished. There was a large desk behind which was a chair which was turned away from them. A small bookshelf was visible on the wall to the right, notable mostly for the very few books that occupied its shelves. The windows were bare, no curtains or other flourishes visible. There were no other chairs in the room. The desk was a work desk and was surprisingly clear and uncluttered.

Reedis paused just long enough to be certain there were no magical traps about to spring and thumped boldly into the room.

"What is the meaning of this?" he bellowed — and stopped, surprised to find the same question being shot back at him.

"I demand to know —" he began again, but the *same* words were being thrown at him at precisely the same moment. He broke off, flustered. "Show yourself!"

The person in the principal's chair turned to face them.

"It can't be!" Reedis and the principal said once again in unison.

"If you're just going to talk to yourselves," Thomas muttered tartly, moving into the room, "clearly you're going to get nothing done."

Reedis and the principal turned to gape at him.

Walpish took their lack of action to take his own. He moved forward, past Reedis and held out his hand. "Thomas Walpish," he said to the principal. "And you are… ?"

"Nelly," Reedis said.

"They said you were dead," the principal, apparently 'Nelly', said in a small, shocked voice.

"I told you I'd be back," Reedis said.

"But they said you were dead and father —" Principal 'Nelly' stopped short. She was a short woman, compactly built. Her most noticeable feature was a huge bloom of curly red hair radiating around her head.

"You're Kendral?" Reedis said.

"Really?" Thomas spoke up, giving Reedis a judging look. "Nelly Kendral," Thomas said as he recovered, "delighted to make your acquaintance." With a twitch of his lips and a nod toward Reedis, he added, "However long that lasts."

"You never asked my last name," Nelly Kendral complained. She looked to Walpish, adding, "We'd only just met — he sold my father a magical icebox and that was the last we saw of him."

"Your father put a price on my head," Reedis said sourly.

"The icebox exploded," Nelly said by way of explanation.

"Oh," Jarin said with Reedis' mouth in a dry tone, "*that* ice box."

Nelly gave Reedis a worried look.

"Nelly Kendral," Walpish said, moving to Jarin Reedis' side, "permit me to make you known to Jarin Reedis, the twin soul dragon."

"Dragon!?" Nelly squeaked. "Twin soul?"

"He was going to eat a girl," Reedis said in his defense. "Maybe two."

"And so he ate you *instead?*" Nelly said, her hands clenching into fists at her side.

"It was mutually beneficial," Walpish said, moving in readiness to interpose himself between the incredibly *un*-defenseless fire-breathing dragon and the irate girl.

"He was lonely, he'd lost his human half and he was going crazy with the pain," Reedis said in Jarin's defense. Jarin, to Thomas' surprise, was silent. Then, to Jarin, in anger, Reedis said, "You destroyed my icebox?"

Jarin took over his body and shrugged. "I was mad at you, you'd killed my friend."

"You killed his friend?" Nelly repeated. "Oh, Reedis, how could you!"

"I didn't do it directly," Reedis replied, raising his hands defensively.

"No," Jarin agreed, lowering Reedis' hands, "he just built the airship that fired on the wyvern."

"Your friend is a wyvern?" Nelly asked. Her brows creased. "Not that wyvern at the docks?"

"Krea Wymarc has agreed not to eat me," Reedis said, "and I've agreed to serve her."

"That was before you joined with me," Jarin said with Reedis' voice.

"I see that you're having no trouble following the change in souls from one to the other," Walpish observed to Nelly.

"I only met him the once," Nelly said in her defense, "but it was a memorable meeting."

Reedis smiled at her just before Jarin took over their body and said, "Most memorable indeed, from what I can see in Reedis' memories."

"Do you mind?" Reedis demanded.

"Not at all," Jarin said. To Nelly he explained, "We share a body but it takes us effort to share memories."

"What do you look like when you're a dragon?" Nelly asked Jarin shyly.

"Much handsomer," Jarin told her grandly.

"He's huge, mostly black with some red," Thomas Walpish explained.

"You were the dragon at the castle yesterday?"

Jarin nodded.

"This is all quite a shock," Nelly said, moving back to take her chair. Seated, she looked up to Jarin Reedis and seemed to recall her situation. "I named the academy in honor of your memory." Her voice broke when she continued, "I never thought to see you again."

"But now that I'm here…" Reedis prompted gently.

"You'll be giving us a royalty, right?" Jarin prompted, not so gently.

"My father still has a price on your head," Nelly told them. "If he knows you're here…"

"Miss Kendral, do you really think your father would try to match his hand against a fire-breathing dragon-mage?" Thomas Walpish asked. Nelly glanced over to him. "He runs a tavern, doesn't he?"

Nelly nodded.

"Well, then he must be a rather practical man," Thomas continued, "so I doubt he'd be very interested in —"

"Nelly," Reedis broke in, dropping to one knee, "will you marry me?"

Nelly flushed bright red and nodded hastily, her eyes suddenly leaking tears and a look of absolute joy on her face. Then her expression changed. "And the dragon, too?"

"I'm given to understand that with twin souls, it's rather difficult to separate the one from the other," Thomas said drolly, thoroughly enjoying himself.

"Would that be a problem?" Jarin asked in a small voice. "I... I promise I would respect your privacy and — well, Reedis loves you much more than he has ever said —"

"I think those should be my words, thank you very much!" Reedis said, harshly reclaiming his mouth.

"Whatever happens, Miss, it won't be boring," Thomas promised.

"Of *course* I'll marry you!" Nelly declared, rising from her chair and leaping into Reedis' arms. "I'll marry you both!"

Reedis uttered a cry of joy but before he could even finish his embrace of his new fiancée a scream rose from the far end of the school.

All three bodies rushed out of the room immediately, with Nelly in the lead.

# Chapter Six

It was an undignified way to ascend and General Armand could see the disgust in his officers' expressions as they spied the rope chair rising slowly toward the high tower on the city wall. But Ingam Oliver — mage, formerly general — was too old to climb the stairs by himself. And Armand needed his advice. The Kingsland airship hovered tauntingly not a mile from the city walls.

Oliver cackled gleefully as he caught sight of the officers standing glumly beside the Sorian Army's commander. "You'll get old one day, if you're lucky!"

The soldiers working the chair hoist stopped lifting and an enterprising office hooked the line to drag the chair to the side of the wall. Oliver's aide — younger and spritely enough to climb the stairs to the tower unaided, helped the old man out of the chair and onto the battlements.

General Armand contained his impatience long enough for mage Oliver to recover his breath and move toward the nearest crenellation. Wordlessly, Oliver stretched out a hand and Armand placed his telescope in it. Oliver gazed at the sight brought closer by the magnification of the lenses for a long moment before passing the glass back.

"We could bring up one of our catapults," General Armand suggested, "it *might* reach."

Oliver snorted and shook his head. "How long has it been there?"

"Our sentries spotted it at first light," Armand replied.

Oliver reached out again for the telescope. Armand dutifully handed it over. While the mage grunted and wrestled with the long tube, Armand continued, "Of course, we'll have to tell the King but I wanted —"

"You won't have to tell the king a thing," Oliver said, straightening up from his perch against the outer wall and passing the telescope back once more. He cocked his head up at the general, adding, "And when did you last see His Majesty?"

"Well," Armand replied slowly, "last night as he retired with his queen."

"And you haven't heard from him since?" Oliver asked, his expression gleeful.

"No…"

Oliver waved toward the floating ship in the distance. "Well, feast your eyes."

"What?"

As if in answer, smoke billowed from the side of the airship and, a moment later, the *boom* of the gun could be heard. A pennant broke out from above the balloon.

"There's our king!" Oliver cackled. With a pitying look, he added, "You might want to send some guards to see about the queen and her son."

Armand fumbled for the telescope and steadied the enlarged image it presented to his eye. He growled as he identified the flying pennant: it was the royal pennant of Soria.

"What is he doing?" Armand muttered. "Is he trying to —" he broke off as he caught sight of people moving toward the front — the bow, as sailors would call it — of the airship. He gasped and lowered the telescope slowly. "No need," he said to his nearest officer. "I know where the queen and her son are."

"Where, sir?" a younger, less intelligent subaltern asked in surprise.

Mage Oliver cackled and pointed to the airship. "They're keeping His Majesty company aboard our enemy's vessel."

"Keep up!" Gamden Ikar shouted as he found another thermal and flapped higher in the sky.

"I'm trying, I'm trying!" Ostan Jaden cried back, banking to catch the thermal and grinning with glee as it lofted him higher. "This is fun!"

"We're on a mission," Gamden shouted down to the other eagleman, "we're not here to have fun!"

"Pity Toras didn't make it!" Ostan added wistfully.

"Pity!" Gamden scoffed. "The fool panicked when I pushed him off the wall!"

Ostan said nothing. Gamden Ikar had barreled into the two birdmen and shoved them over the wall. Ostan had managed to change into a bird on the way down. Toras Bax had not.

Such was the way of the eaglemen of Hinoma.

Gamden eyed the terrain below them, comparing it with the map he'd seen at Paulus' castle. They'd made good progress. If they were lucky, before night fell — and the thermals died — they'd be halfway to their destination. The problem was finding a good eyrie, one high enough that they could just fall back onto their path. Gamden eyed the mountains to their right, searching for a good peak in the distance. Perhaps they would do better to climb even higher, to find thermals over the mountains — even at the risk of getting too little air.

Gamden banked to his right, toward the mountains. "We're going higher!"

Beneath him, Ostan Jaden cried in dismay.

"We'll find better air over the mountains, go faster!" Gamden promised. He beat his mighty wings hard in example. He thrilled at the surge of power that he created, the burst of thrust that propelled him ever upwards. He found the edge of the thermal, banked back into it and continued his climb. The ground beneath dwindled, faded as the haze in the day's air obscured it. Gamden was untroubled — he knew their course — he didn't need to see the ground below. He was an eagleman, lord of the skies.

"You would trade gold for dragon steel?" Queen Diam asked Margaret Waters. "How much?"

"As much as we can get," Margaret replied. "Oh, you mean the gold?" She shrugged. "I am sure we can arrange a fair trade."

"And how soon do you need it?"

"We want to lay our tracks west from here to South Sea Pass," Margaret said, adding, "And from here north to Sarskar."

"And east to the Pinch, I'd imagine," Queen Diam guessed shrewdly.

Margaret shrugged and, realizing they were still in darkness, said aloud, "Yes, I imagine that will be so, presently."

"Your King wars with Soria," the bass voice said. "What is to stop him from warring with us?"

Margaret giggled. "Oh, I've heard about that fool that tried to get your gold!"

"Which one?" Diam asked tartly. "The general or the airships?"

"Airships?" Margaret said. "I thought they were destroyed by the fort."

"The first pair, yes," Diam agreed mildly. "But not the second pair."

Margaret frowned. "I have been busy, I have not heard of this second set of airships."

"It is of no matter," Diam allowed. "Your gold, where is it?"

"It's on its way," Margaret assured her. "Your dragon steel, where is it?" She paused. "And, forgive me, but do you always negotiate in the dark?"

Queen Diam chuckled. "Only with those we don't want to see."

"It will be hard to assess the dragon steel, or the gold, without being able to at least weigh it," Margaret replied.

"We have still not decided whether we want to trade with you, sky-toucher," the deep bass voice said threateningly.

"Does he speak for you?" Margaret asked the queen.

"He is one of my trusted counselors," Queen Diam replied. She turned to address the bass voice, "We have not always been hurt by humans."

"This one does magic," the bass voice replied.

"As did Reedis, if you'll recall," Queen Diam said in a low voice.

"Uncle Reedis?" Margaret cried joyfully. "When? Did you see him?" Her voice faltered as she added, "He went north in his airship… they say he is dead."

The bass voice snorted and the queen shushed him.

"'Uncle' Reedis?" Queen Diam repeated. "How is it that you know him?"

"My father worked with him when they made the first steam engines," Margaret replied. "Reedis claimed rights to the airships while father claimed rights to the locomotives." She sniffed. "It was Reedis who showed me how to ask the air."

"Ask the air?" Diam repeated.

"Hissia and Hanor, the gods of air, really," Margaret chattered on. "Reedis isn't really my uncle — I'm an orphan — but as the Steam Master took me as his apprentice and daughter, Reedis became my honorary uncle." She sniffed again. "Or he was. I miss him."

"You were the one who laid those tracks through the pass," Queen Diam said. "You called on the gods for that?"

"They loved doing it, we all did," Margaret said with a giggle. "It was so much fun to lift the timbers and the rail into the air, to lay them out in the sky and then place them back on the ground."

"Timbers?" the bass voice repeated. "What about the weight?"

"When the gods want, nothing stands in the way of their winds," Margaret said solemnly. "For them it is but a game to lift the timbers."

"But they do it through you," Diam said.

Margaret nodded. "Yes, I am proud to help them and grateful for their kindness."

"Not all gods are kind," the bass voice muttered.

"None of the gods are kind all of the time," Margaret said in agreement. "But they are not mean all the time, either."

"True," Diam murmured. Margaret could hear the queen's clothing rustle as she turned from one guard to another in inquiry. Finally, she said, "Enough of this! Let there be light."

A dim glow grew all around them, the luminescence of night glows. Margaret's eyes adjusted slowly. When she could make out the form of the queen, she knelt courteously. "Your Majesty."

"Come along, Margaret Waters, air mage, come and see our kingdom," Queen Diam said, gesturing for Margaret to rise.

"She must swear, first, majesty," the bass voice warned. Margaret identified it as belonging to a sturdy well-muscled zwerg standing close by the queen.

"As you wish, Granno," Diam said. "But if she is a friend of Reedis' —"

"You know Reedis?" Margaret said. "How?"

Granno gave her a smirk but nodded toward his queen.

"Jarin Reedis did us a favor just recently," the queen said. She smiled as she added, "Rumors of his death in the north were wrong."

"He's alive!" Margaret said. "Oh, where is he? I'd love to see him!"

"He left a while back, on a mission which was secret from us," Queen Diam said.

"Imay went with them," a young girl's voice piped up. Margaret turned toward the voice and lowered her gaze to a young zwerg, dressed in finery. The girl smiled up at Margaret.

"Princess Lissy!" Granno said chidingly.

"What?" Lissy said, shrugging off the older zwerg's frown. "She was going to find out soon enough." She waved a hand toward her mother, the queen. "Besides, mother's going to want a favor from her, you can just tell."

Margaret stiffened at the words. *A favor?*

"Shut the door, shut the door!" Madame Aubrey screamed at the urchin who raced inside. Chastised, the young… girl… although it was hard to tell from the grime and the shapeless tunic that she wore, closed the door and curtsied in a misguided attempt at an apology. "It's too bitter cold outside to let the wind in here!"

Madame Aubrey spent a moment wondering how the little bunch of sticks that was the urchin had survived in such cold — she would not survive long, that was certain.

"What do you want?" Madame Aubrey demanded, her tone harsh to cover her fleeting sympathy for the urchin girl.

"Do you have any news?" the girl said in a thin, piping voice.

Madame Aubrey recoiled as she recognized the child's voice. She turned her head toward the kitchen. "Maurice! A bowl of gruel, immediately!" She gestured the girl to a seat. "Sit, sit, Babette! Sit and warm yourself by the fire!"

Babette Collet nodded in thanks and sat nervously at the proffered seat. Maurice, the cook, came out with a bowl of steaming gruel and, at Madame Aubrey's insistence, set it in front of the small child. Madame Aubrey knew that Babette was ten years old, not the starving six that she looked.

Babette lowered her head and closed her eyes in a quick prayer which ended with a much louder, "And thank the gods for the kindness of Madame Aubrey and her chef."

After that she dug into the gruel, downing it in short order. When she was done, she looked up to Madame Aubrey, "Thank you, madame, for your kindness."

"Think nothing of it, child," Madame Aubrey replied. She sat back. "Now, tell me about your mother."

"My mother is dead," Babette said in a very small voice. "She died this morning or maybe last night." She glanced up to Madame Aubrey. "You know they threw us out of our apartments."

"I'd heard," Madame Aubrey said. "No word of your father?"

"No," Babette said. "He was taken prisoner with the other soldiers but no one can find him." Her lower lip quivered. "He was a captain, they should know where he is!"

"Yes," Madame Aubrey agreed softly. She patted the girl's hand. "Press on, my dear! I'm sure you'll find him if you keep looking!"

"You haven't heard anything?" Babette asked, her eyes wide and pleading.

"Nothing more than you know," Madame Aubrey replied.

Babette lowered her head and half-whispered, "They talk of the queen."

Madame Aubrey shuddered. She'd heard the rumors.

"The queen and the mages," Babette said. "I heard someone say that some of the new King's men are sick, they will not stand to arms."

"Then they are fools!" Madame Aubrey declared. "The South Sea Pass is part of Kingsland, conquered and subdued."

"They say that the soldiers were killed because of the murder of their queen," Babette whispered. She turned her eyes up to Madame Aubrey. "Do you think it's true?"

Madame Aubrey's jaw dropped. She'd heard the rumors but now she was hearing them from the mouth of a young girl — the news was spreading. Babette's pleading eyes begged for a response. Slowly, almost imperceptibly, Madame Aubrey nodded.

"But they'd surrendered!" Babette cried in shock. "My father, the others — they had no weapons. No weapons and he killed them!"

"Come!" Mayor Pierre Juin of the South Sea Pass said in response to the knock on his door. The door opened and a man entered quickly, closing the door behind him. The mayor controlled his surprise at the sudden entrance, instead smiling at the intruder. "Have a seat, Monsieur Rafkin. To what do I owe the pleasure?"

Henry Rafkin looked nothing like a spy. And, in truth, though he worked for Peter Hewlitt — the Spymaster — his normal duties included bookkeeping and writing letters.

He took his seat quickly. He seemed to grope for words before he finally managed, "I've been hearing some rumors."

"Ah? Of what, may I ask?"

"There are people talking," Rafkin said. Mayor Juin motioned for him to continue. "They are saying that soldiers are missing."

"About a thousand," Mayor Juin said in a dead voice. He caught Rafkin's reaction. "This is news to you?"

Rafkin nodded glumly. He raised his head slowly. "What do you know?"

"Rumors only," the mayor said, spreading his hands wide. "Your king — our king — ordered them in reprisal for the murder of his queen."

"A thousand men?" Rafkin said incredulously. "Where are the bodies?"

"I believe they were placed under your queen," the mayor said.

"Does anyone else know?" Rafkin asked.

"People are talking, the dead are missing," the mayor said. "It won't take long before the rumors become more."

"More?"

"If I were you, I'd be certain to tell my master as soon as possible," the mayor warned. He gestured toward the door. "Now would be a good time."

Rafkin nodded jerkily and left, closing the door behind him quietly, almost apologetically.

They left the village of Korin's Pass at a gallop and continued east until the village was lost in the blizzard behind them. Only then did Jacques Martel signal to mage Tirpin that they should slow to a trot. He glanced back again over his shoulder. "I don't believe our luck!"

"The gods are watching over us," Tirpin said. Martel gave him a startled look and snorted. "Well," Tirpin said, "they *could* be."

"The gods watch after those who watch after themselves," Martel replied. He waved forward, "Come my friend! A week's hard ride and we'll be at the Pinch."

"And then?"

"Then, with just a bit of your magic, we'll cross the border unseen and introduce ourselves to the Emperor."

"I'm sure he'll be glad to see us," Tirpin said doubtfully.

"He'll be glad to hear our news and see your plans," the former airship captain told him.

"Will he be interested, really?"

"He will if he wishes to survive," Martel said. "And, if he doesn't, he's got a brother."

"Break's over, back to your classes!" Jarin Reedis shouted to the throng of students loitering outside the Reedis Memorial Academy of Balloon Magic.

"Reedis! What are you doing?" Nelly hissed at him.

Reedis gave her a confused look. "Aren't they supposed to be in class?" he asked. "Isn't that how we make money?"

"But they don't know you," Nelly said. "They might not understand."

Despite her words, the students were rushing to get back inside the building, casting glances nervously toward Jarin Reedis.

"It seems to be working," mage Margen said as he turned to follow his students back inside the building. He glanced to Bethany Margiss. "Do you need anything?"

The young girl shook her head but then, impulsively, dashed to her grandfather and hugged him tightly. Margen patted her awkwardly and she pulled away, turning to Jarin Reedis. "What do I do now?"

Reedis pointed to Ophidian. "You might ask him."

Ophidian heard him and accepted his words with a nod, moving to stand close to Bethany Margiss.

"I could take you home," Ophidian offered.

"My home is here," Margiss said, glancing toward mage Margen.

"And so it will be," Ophidian agreed. "But *my* home is where Krea Wymarc is and she is the best one to help you through your grief."

"Grandfather?" Margiss called.

Margen turned back to her, saw the worry in her eyes and nodded toward Ophidian. "He called you daughter," Margen told her. "Aren't you curious about that?"

Margiss nodded, a slight jerk of her chin.

"You'll let her back if she asks," Margen said to Ophidian. The dragon-god nodded. "Good."

"Come," Ophidian said, raising a hand toward Bethany Margiss. "There is much to discover."

The twin souled girl took the dragon-god's hand and they vanished.

"And that," Margen said, raising his voice to carry and shooing the students back to their classrooms, "is why you should be very careful when dealing with gods."

"Where are we?" Margiss asked as they emerged upon the balcony outside Ophidian's palace.

"What?" A girl's voice demanded. "You were here just a minute…" she trailed off as she took in Margiss' expression and glanced toward Ophidian.

"Oh, my poor dear!" another girl's voice called out. Margiss found herself folded into the strong embrace of the albino girl, Krea. Rather, she realized, she was being comforted by the twin soul, Wymarc, using Krea's body. "Come! This is quite an ordeal, I know! There's a tea that helps with the transition, and we have some ready."

Margiss allowed herself to be hauled off by Kea Wymarc, followed by the other young girl, Ellen Annabelle. She was surprised when the tall form of Prince Nestor fell in beside her and asked, consolingly, "How are you doing?"

"That god," Bethany said with a sob in Margiss' voice, "he killed Skara."

"He does not like change," Ophidian's voice carried from where he stood on the balcony. "He fights for the past."

# Chapter Seven

"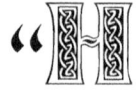ow are you feeling?" a woman's voice spoke close to Alain's ear and he startled awake. The woman — Mayse — chuckled. "You seemed half-past dead."

Alain rolled and stretched. His muscles complained and he ached all over. He rose to his knees and stood up slowly, stretching. "I'm thirsty, is there anything to drink?"

"And what would you like, little human?" a deep voice came to him, speaking over his head. Alain turned in surprise and then stepped back in shock as he looked up — and up — to see the face of Janzie peering down at him. Alain gasped in shock as he saw Janzie's feet — no, hooves.

"You're a centaur!" Alain exclaimed. A young girl laughed from behind him and Alain twirled once more. "Lisette?"

Lisette rushed up and hugged him tight. "Janzie showed me how to change!"

"Change?"

"From human form to centaur form," Mayse said, handing Alain a flask. "Have some water."

Alain took the flask with a nod of thanks and drank heartily. When he was done, the flask was empty.

Mayse glanced and gestured over her shoulder. "The stream's there," she said. When Alain made ready to move off and refill the flask, Mayse stopped him with an upraised hand. "You can do it later."

"I can't change into a horse yet," Lisette said.

"A horse?" Alain repeated, his attention now on his sister.

"Of course," Lisette said with a giggle. "And I'll bet that I'll be the best horse you ever saw!"

"A centaur has three forms," Janzie told him. "Horse, human, centaur." He shifted once more into a human, smiling at Alain.

"You'll be able to do it, too," Mayse said to him.

"Me?" Alain cried, jerking his head back in surprise. "I'm just a human!"

"No," Janzie said. Before Alain could respond, the older man said, "At first I thought it was just your sister but when you slept — and we taught her how to change — we caught your scent."

"Scent?"

"A horse smells better than a human," Lisette said. "Even a centaur can smell better."

"And you smell of centaur," Mayse said. She cocked her head. "Only something has a hold on you." She waved her hand at him. "You are trapped in this form."

"We'll figure it out," Janzie said confidently, "and free you. We need more centaurs."

"My father was human!" Alain declared hotly. He pointed to Lisette. "She's a centaur only because —" he cut himself off. He could not explain how Lisette became a centaur.

"Yes," Mayse said. "Your father was a human." She smiled at him. "But what of your mother?"

"Hah! There they are!" King Markel bellowed as he spied *Wasp* floating triumphantly just out of range of the Sorian guns. "Now we have them!"

"Indeed, sire," first minister Mannevy agreed. "But now that we have them, what next?"

"We'll get that ass Wendel to surrender the throne to me," Markel said. "I'll let him keep his head."

"Your Majesty, what if he refuses?"

"Then, Minister, you'd best hope that your plan works," Markel told him coldly. "I've no wish to spill my blood."

"As you say, sire," Mannevy replied with a half bow.

"Sound the challenge," Markel said to Commodore Evans. "Have all ships fire, let them hear our guns!"

"As you wish, sire," Commodore Evans replied. He turned and raised his voice to call, "Signal the challenge!"

One by one, the guns of the six airships fired off, filling the air above Sarskar with smoke and thunder.

King Markel had come triumphantly to his new capital.

# Epilog

"ou are dead," Terric said.

Mage Vistos looked up at him, affronted. "I can't be!"

"How is that?" Terric asked mildly.

"My god, Quenkorian —" Vistos cut himself off. The memories came back to him. He was in a white room, sitting in a white chair. Beside him, dressed in black, was the god of Death. "They got all the teeth?"

Terric smiled and twisted his hand, palm up. A small black bag appeared in it, bulged open, showing many teeth — all molars — and then disappeared again when Terric closed his fist. He smiled. "All of them."

"Oh," Vistos said, sounding deflated.

"Some days I love my job," Terric said with a cherubic smile. He nodded to Vistos. "This is one of them."

"Because I'm dead?" the mage asked in a soft but bitter voice.

"Because you're no longer killing others," Terric corrected.

"I thought you liked that."

"You thought many things," Terric told him. "All were wrong." He shifted his stance, as though releasing a humor. "Now, then, if you'll just give me the gold, I'll get you on your way?"

"Gold?" Vistos repeated dully.

"Two gold pieces, one for each eye, to pay the Ferryman," Terric told him.

"I'm the Ferryman," a younger, cheerful version of Terric spoke from where he suddenly appeared beside Death. He held out his hand expectantly.

"I don't have any gold," Vistos said. He licked his lips. "You don't suppose I could borrow some, do you?"

The Ferryman snickered and smiled evilly.

"If you can't pay your way, you'll have to earn it," Terric told Vistos with a sigh. "How are you at gardening?"

"Gardening?" Vistos sneered. He drew himself back in disgust. "You mean sully my hands with dirt and worms? Never!"

"That can be arranged," the Ferryman said with a smile, nodding toward Death.

"Hang on," Terric said. He waved his hand and suddenly two more people were in the white room. They were holding hands.

"I know you!" Vistos cried in recognition. "You're my assassin!" he pointed to the woman. Then he pointed to the man. "And you're that cavalryman!" he glared at the woman. "The one you were supposed to kill!"

"Didn't work out, did it?" Thomas Walpish replied, smiling at the sneering mage.

"Magic isn't everything, is it?" Skara Ningan added.

"He hasn't any coins for Bryan," Terric said, pointing at Vistos.

"Bryan?" Vistos said.

"Hi," the Ferryman replied, waving a hand.

"And you know," Terric said in a voice that carried a particular tone, "if you can't pay Bryan, he can't take you beyond."

"And father will make you work your way," Bryan added cheerfully, nodding toward Vistos. "This one is afraid of dirt and worms."

"I like worms," Skara allowed.

"Worms are okay," Thomas agreed with somewhat less enthusiasm. He glanced to Terric, reaching a hand into his trousers. "How long?"

"It depends on my mood, honestly," Terric said, his lips twitching.

Thomas Walpish glanced at Skara Ningan. Their eyes met. She nodded slowly, squeezing his free hand. Thomas nodded and pulled his other hand out of his pocket.

"Here," he said, passing the coins to Bryan the Ferryman. "That's good for one person, right?"

"Yes," Bryan said, taking the coins with a dubious look. "You wish to go?"

Thomas Walpish shook his head and pointed at Vistos. "No," he said, "take him."

Bryan smiled and vanished, along with Vistos.

"Huh!" Terric exclaimed, taking in a deep invigorating breath. "The air smells fresher already!" He glanced at the two remaining figures, still holding hands. "How about a bite to eat and then I show you the gardens?"

"We'd be delighted!"

# King's Treasure

### Book 18

Twin Soul series

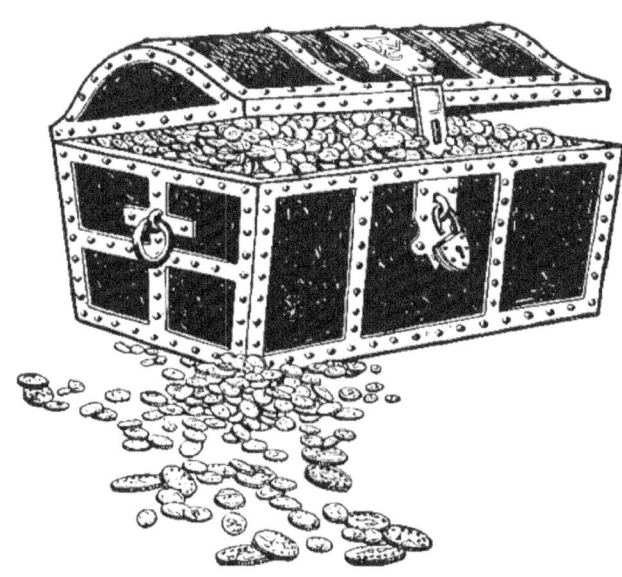

# Dedication

**In memory of**

**Zadie John E. Silver**

# Chapter One

"I am sorry, Your Majesty," Captain Fawcett declared once more, bowing deeply. His face was pale, his expression frightened.

"He just *jumped?*" King Markel said again, looking toward the bow of the airship *Wasp*.

"One moment he was there, the next he was gone," Queen Rassa, still weeping, said in agreement.

"I'm *certain* it was the sight of your ships which drove him to such despair," Crown Prince Sarsal added. He shifted from one foot to the other. "He was just standing there and then… he was gone!"

King Markel looked at each of them in turn then nodded. He spoke to Mannevy, his first minister, "Have the body recovered. We shall bury him with all due honors."

"Of course, Your Majesty," Mannevy replied smoothly. He nodded his condolences to the dowager Queen and her son, turning to wave for his attendants and issue orders.

"Captain Lewis!" Mannevy called.

"It's Colonel Lewis now, first minister. Acting-Colonel," Lewis corrected mildly, bringing himself to attention. "Would you like me to arrange a party to retrieve the body?"

"Perhaps you could send your cavalry instead," Captain Fawcett said, waving toward a distant motion on the horizon.

Lewis grinned as he moved to the side and saw that, indeed, the rest of his squadron had arrived. Behind them, he could see the darker smudge of moving infantry — the Kingsland division had arrived.

"Captain Fawcett, may I borrow your signalman?"

"Of course, Colonel," Fawcett replied formally. He snapped his fingers toward his signals ensign. "Have at it."

"And you're certain it was the king?" General Armand repeated to the officer.

"You saw it, too, Michael," Ingam Oliver, formerly commanding General of the Sorian Army, now a practicing mage, reminded the distraught general.

"Was he pushed, did you see?" Armand demanded, ignoring his former commander.

"There were two people close by, it was hard to get a good look," the officer temporized.

"Except that one was the queen and the other the crown prince," Oliver muttered.

"Neither would seem to be too inclined to remove the royal head," Armand said in reluctant agreement. He waved a hand to the view beyond the city's walls. "Not that it matters at the moment."

"The gates are still closed," Oliver said.

Armand waved a hand at the ten airships floating above them. "And what does that matter?"

Oliver sighed. "Yes, I suppose there is *that*."

"And that's how they captured the king," Armand said. "They may have used magic —" he cast a glance to the mage but Oliver shook his head firmly. "So they had their airship come in the cover of dark, land a party, and abducted the entire royal family without anyone being alarmed."

"Well… except the ones killed," Oliver allowed. He gave Armand a thoughtful look. "As a military operation, it was exemplary."

Armand snorted. "Except that it was not *our* military which operated."

"True," Oliver said. He tapped the Sorian commanding general on the shoulder. "Stop stalling Michael."

Michael Armand stood silent for a long moment. Finally, he nodded. He raised his head again and told the watch officer, "Open the gates! Lower the royal banner. Raise the Kingsland flag!"

The officer gave him a shocked look. "Sir?"

"Do you see anything else we can do?" Armand roared at the officer. He glared at his staff which had slunk away as far as they could. He waved at them. "Go on! Do it! You're still soldiers, act like it!"

"Sir! Yes sir!" the officers called back, saluting and moving off quickly.

Satisfied that they were following orders, General Armand turned back to mage Oliver. "Now what?"

Mage Oliver searched in his robes, patting them until something clinked. He smiled and pulled it out. It was a silver flask. "I don't know about you, but I'm having a drink."

Angus Franck reeled from all the commotion that sounded from the balcony at Ophidian's palace. He cast an imploring look toward Hana which she returned in full measure.

"What are you doing for the dragon-god?" the metal immortal, Tracker demanded of Ibb.

Ibb creaked as he turned his red eyes toward her thin metal frame.

"I am in his debt," Ibb said. "I was crushed when the East Pass Fort collapsed and it was because of him — and his get — that I was rescued and repaired."

"Fixer must have helped," Tracker said.

"That debt has been paid," Ibb replied. He turned to Angus and Hana. "Perhaps we would be best returning to our project."

Angus nodded gratefully, glanced toward Hana who smiled in agreement, and held out his hand to the girl. Hana took it.

Ibb paused. To Tracker, he said, "I cannot take you unless you give your oath."

"Oath?" Tracker repeated.

"To me," Ophidian said, suddenly appearing before them. He waved a hand to the continued commotion on the balcony. "It will be some time before they need me again."

"I am an immortal," Tracker said. She turned her glowing blue eyes to Ibb. "I am not accustomed to swearing oaths to gods."

"Oaths go both ways," Angus offered.

Tracker turned her glowing eyes on him. "I am also not accustomed to listening to mortals."

"Forgive me," Ibb said to Angus with a nod to Hana. "Tracker is single-minded and I have done her the discourtesy of not introducing you yet." His head creaked as it moved downwards in a jerk of apology to the other metal immortal. "Tracker, I wish to make known to you Angus Franck, formerly apprentice to Rabel Zebala, and Hana Renn, formerly twin soul to the first *kitsune*."

"Kitsune!" Tracker exclaimed, awed. She nodded to Hana. "That is the first time I have heard of such a pairing."

Ibb rumbled deep within his chest — his way of laughing. "You are wondering, I am sure, how the bond was broken and by whom."

Tracker squeaked as she moved her head rapidly from side to side in disagreement. "It is of no matter to me."

"Ah, but it is," Ophidian said. The immortal woman turned her glowing eyes to meet his dark ones. Her joints squeaked as she cocked her metal head slightly to one side in curiosity. "The one who broke the bond is of interest to you."

"How is that?" Tracker said.

Ibb turned his red eyes to Ophidian and raised a hand. "If I may…?" Ophidian nodded. Ibb turned to Tracker. "The person who broke the bond is the one known as Lyric."

"I am tasked with finding her," Tracker allowed, clenching her metal jaw tightly. She turned to Ophidian. "Am I correct, Lord Ophidian, in guessing that you have information I would find useful?"

"*Lord* Ophidian," Hana murmured, shocked.

"The immortals generally do not believe in the powers of the gods," Ophidian told her with a glint of amusement in his eyes. "But they are wise enough to know not to push their luck."

Tracker bent in a half-bow. "Indeed, as an immortal, one learns discretion."

"Which is good," Ibb said in a warning tone. Tracker turned to look at him. "Because one must remember, above all, the knowledge that we share."

Tracker's blue eyes flared — just slightly — and then she nodded, a tiny jerk of agreement.

"You have seen and learned things that must not be shared with others," Ophidian told her.

"I keep counsel with my own," Tracker replied immediately. She waved a hand toward Ibb. "As does he."

"I cannot let you share what you've learned with others," Ophidian said, his voice growing heated. "There are —"

"If I may," Ibb said, raising a hand toward Ophidian but turning to Tracker. "There are forces at work, forces we are just beginning to understand —"

"'We?'" Tracker said.

"We immortals," Ibb replied. "I have reported this already. We are seeing signs —"

"What you reported, I know," Tracker said. "I see no reason —"

"Immortal," Ophidian interjected, "I must have your word on this —"

"Or what?"

"He was prepared to destroy us all to keep this secret," Ibb told her. "Including his children. You are tempting your destruction."

"What oath must I swear?" Tracker said to Ophidian.

"The others are under *geas*," Ophidian said, waving toward Angus and Hana. "But you are metal and cannot be so compelled."

"What oath, Ibb?" Tracker said.

"Nestor could freeze her," Angus suggested, "that way you wouldn't have to worry about her for a while."

"No!" Ibb said. "Her mission is important, her powers essential to our task."

A noise from the balcony startled them and Tracker turned toward it. When she turned back, her eyes dimmed. She looked at Ophidian. "Our memories say that the last new dragon was created thousands of years ago," she said slowly, her voice shaky. "We think —" she nodded toward Ibb "— that something happened to you, something that ended your power to make new children..." she broke off, turning back to the balcony and the piping voice of Ellen Annabelle offered comfort to the other girl.

"No one must know," Ophidian told her. "Even your Memories."

"Because they might trade the knowledge," Ibb added in warning.

"What you ask," Tracker said slowly, "goes against my oaths."

"For your life," Ibb said in a slow, deep voice, "I will vouch this unto you." He glanced toward Ophidian. "This knowledge is as dangerous to me as the knowledge you wish to guard."

"You're a Memory," Ophidian said. Ibb took a step back in surprise. The dragon-god chuckled. "I will keep your secret." He turned to Tracker. "Will you?"

"You are a Memory?" Tracker said to Ibb. "But I thought —" she broke off. For a long while she was silent and then she started squeaking — chirping really — and the others realized that she was laughing. "Well, that explains so much!"

"You did not hear it from me," Ibb said, nodding toward Ophidian, "so my oaths are not broken." He gave the dragon-god a grateful look. "But knowing part of my function —"

"Part?" Tracker interjected. Angus gave Ibb a thoughtful look and nodded to himself.

"Part," Ibb repeated. "Knowing that I am a Memory for our people, you know also that you have not forsaken your vow to tell us what you learn."

"And you'd make such a mess on the floor if I have to melt you," Ophidian added in a tone that caused both Angus and Hana to jerk their heads toward him in surprise.

"You can make new children," Tracker said to the dragon-god. The edges of her lips rose in a metal smile. "I am glad of that." Ophidian accepted that with a nod and then raised an eyebrow questioningly. "I shall keep this knowledge safe with the Memory known as Ibb."

"And?" Ophidian prompted.

"I shall tell none other, save by your leave," Tracker said.

"Unless others discover it themselves," Ibb added.

Tracker nodded acceptance of that amendment and continued, "And I shall not act in such a way as to hint or otherwise reveal this secret until you, Lord Ophidian, give me leave."

"And I, god Ophidian," Ophidian replied, "shall give you my protection as you might require and offer you the freedom of my realm and the protection of my children, for as long as you honor this oath."

"Agreed," Tracker said, extending her hand to the dragon god. Ophidian cocked his head like a bird at the proffered hand and then, with a sigh, took it and shook it firmly.

"And now that that's out of the way —" Ibb began.

"And we don't have a mess to clean up," Hana muttered.

"Let me show you what we are devising," Ophidian concluded, opening a portal to another part of his castle and gesturing for the others to precede him through it.

Tracker was the first to go through.

"Here come the barbarians," General Armand muttered acidly under his breath as the trim little airship floated down toward the city walls.

"Our new lord and master, too," Ingam Oliver reminded him.

Armand snorted derisively.

"You know, Michael," Oliver said quietly, careful to keep his voice pitched only for the general's ears, "this wouldn't have happened if you'd listened to me."

"Would it not?" General Armand said, his jaw taut with anger. "And what would you have done?"

"If you had acknowledged the threat and planned accordingly…"

"You expected me to take your 'word' that Kingsland would attack in winter," Armand reminded him angrily. "That they would use their cavalry through the snow, that they would use these —" he waved a hand at the docking airship "— *things* to launch an attack —"

"Yes," Oliver replied, his tone mild. "I did." He waved toward the city gates which were wide open, greeting the head of the Kingsland cavalry. The city's inhabitants watched the horsemen ride through with wonder and not a little fear. Oliver could imagine their surprise: What had happened? Where was the King?

It would only be when they saw the body slung over the horse's back, lying face down, led by a Kingsland cavalryman, that they would begin to wonder — was that the king? What had happened to good King Wendel? Wasn't he asleep in his bed just the night before?

"It is time," Armand said, moving forward to the front of the crowd that waited as the gangplank was thrust across from the airship to the wall.

"At least they're sending the queen across first," Oliver muttered as he moved to keep pace.

"Wise," Armand agreed. "Unless she tells us, firmly, that there was no foul play…"

"If there was, what of it?" Oliver replied. He gestured toward the cavalry heading up the wide boulevard toward the castle proper. "We have no king, our gates are open, and their troops are here, arrayed, and in force."

"And if their soldiers are still a mile away?" Armand muttered. "Could we not overwhelm their cavalry, close our gates, and deny them the capital?"

"General Armand!" Queen Rassa cried, her face warming with recognition.

"My Queen," Armand replied, bowing low. "I am so sorry for your loss. All Soria will grieve."

"I don't know what came over him," Rassa said, her voice quivering theatrically. "One moment he was… and then…" she raised a hand to her mouth and closed her eyes in pain.

"Interesting," Oliver murmured to himself. Armand made a pleading gesture with the fingers of the hand trailing behind him, out of sight. "She's lying. She did know what happened to him."

"Here is my good son, the Crown Prince, devastated at the loss of his step-father and so soon after the loss of the king of his blood," Rassa said, reaching back to grab Crown Prince Sarsal's hand and leading him safely from the gangplank to the stone walls of the city. She turned back to the gangplank and pulled her son down into a bow to match hers. "And here is our new king, Markel!"

"King Markel," Armand said, moving forward to stand beside the queen and Crown Prince. He went to one knee. "I greet you."

# Chapter Two

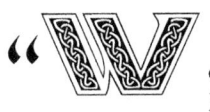"Well, I must say, I don't think all that much of your general," King Markel said as he and Queen Rassa were finally left alone in the royal bedchamber.

"*I'd* get rid of him, if that's what you're wondering," Queen Rassa agreed, divesting herself of her fluffy outer dress and peeling off her petticoats with obvious relish. She turned back to Markel and rushed to embrace him. "Armand was no better a general than Wendel was a lover," she said. She buried her head against his neck and added lasciviously, "It will be so good to finally sleep with a *proper* man!"

Markel allowed himself a smile even as he explored the soft flesh of the Sorian queen.

"Mind you," he said as he took a step back and pulled his shirt over his head, "I can't say that any of *mine* are that much better."

"Well, they did beat ours, so that's something," Rassa allowed, taking a seat on the side of her bed and peeling off the last of her clothes. She patted the spot beside her imploringly. "But now, darling…!"

King Markel did not need to be asked twice.

"You there!" a sharp voice rang out down the corridor. Colonel Samuel Lewis turned toward the caller and was surprised to find the Crown Prince — Sarsal — storming toward him.

"Your Highness?" Lewis asked.

Sarsal stopped just in front of him, fuming. He raised his hand and pressed it against Lewis' chest. "You're the one who abducted us."

"My men and I had that assignment, yes," Lewis agreed, his tone neutral.

"Your men killed my woman," Sarsal said, his nostrils flaring with rage. He dug his finger into Lewis' chest. "She died because of you."

"I am sorry, Your Highness," Lewis replied. "I was following orders." He allowed his expression to soften. "I had no ill-will toward your lady."

"Her blood is on your hands," Sarsal growled. He dropped his finger. "When the time comes, I'll remember." He turned and stormed back down the corridor.

Samuel Lewis stared after him for a long while then turned back to his duties.

"Father." Margaret Waters ducked her head as she met Torvan Brookes, the Steam Master. They were in the new station room, the headquarters for the Korin's Pass train station.

"You sent a signal," Torvan Brookes said without preamble.

"I believe we can get the rest of our track from the zwerg," Margaret said. "Made of dragon steel, no less."

"How much?"

"A chest of gold and they'll make enough rail to run west to South Sea Pass," Margaret said.

"And to get north to Sarsal?" Brookes demanded.

"Another chest and a favor," Margaret said. The Steam Master's eyebrow rose. He was not fond of favors. Margaret's lips twitched. "They want to learn more about steam engines."

"Harumph," Brookes grunted. "Why?"

"Apparently they want to build them," Margaret said. Her jaw tightened as she added, "Or repair one."

"And where would they get a steam engine?" Torvan Brookes demanded.

"From what I can tell, Reedis gave them one."

"Reedis? Before he died?"

"He's not dead," Margaret said. She paused. "He's the twin-souled dragon, the one that captured the airships *Pace* and *Harbinger*."

"Oh, really?" Torvan Brookes said. He rubbed his chin in thought, looking down to the floor of the trim room. He was silent for a long time. When he looked up, he gave her a grudging look of approval. "Do they want me?"

"No," Margaret said, smiling. She pointed to her chest. "Me."

Tracker turned once they'd stepped into the huge dimly lit cavern to look behind her. There was no door, only a solid wall. She turned back, noting the way that Ophidian grinned at her. She decided that he wanted her to say something so she didn't. Instead, she scanned their location.

"Is that —?" she cried as she spied a large shape in the distance. She turned to Ibb. "Is that *yours?*"

"Yes," Ibb replied. He gestured above them even as he started walking forward into the widening space.

Tracker looked up. And up. And up. "Is this open to the sky?" she asked Ophidian.

"Not at the moment," the dragon god replied smugly.

"Is there a Fixer here?" Tracker asked, looking around for signs of another person moving in the distance.

"Well… in a sense," Ophidian replied, grinning and pointing at himself.

"I am tempted to believe that the Fixers learned from him, actually," Ibb rumbled deep in his chest.

As they moved further in, the ceiling above them disappeared. Ophidian nodded toward Tracker in warning, waving a hand and suddenly the whole area was filled with lights.

The lights were tiny in the distance and Tracker realized that they were in a space far larger than any she'd ever seen before.

"Are those... books?" Tracker asked, pointing to tiny shapes climbing up on a far wall in the distance.

"Part of my library, yes," Ophidian allowed.

"You are enjoying this," Ibb observed. He turned to Tracker. "He did the same with me."

"And me," Angus said. He jerked a thumb toward Hana. "And her."

"He might be a bit vain," Hana said before adding excitedly, "but this is only a *small* part of his library!"

"So it's just a library?"

"It is a library, a workshop, laboratory, observatory —"

"Observatory?" Tracker broke in. "What do you observe?"

Ophidian stopped and leaned his head point, raised a hand to point to a spot far up above them and away in the distance. "The sun, the stars, whatever can be seen with a good telescope."

"You observe the heavens?" Tracker asked in awe.

"Well, it's not as if I don't have a lot of *time*," Ophidian allowed.

They crossed closer toward Ibb's caravan. Tracker swiveled her head slowly in a complete circle, stopping once in a while to investigate some new amazement. Finally, she stopped and pointed. "There is something *wrong* in that."

"Yes," Ibb agreed blandly. She looked at him, her metal brows lowering in agitation.

"Can you guess?" Ophidian asked.

Tracker turned toward the object and strode quickly toward it, stopping a body length away. The others joined her.

"This is *wrong*," Tracker said again, this time with more vehemence. "It is twisted, a blight..." she stopped and turned toward Ibb, her metal brows going straight up. "This is a *caravan?*"

"The one I gave Lyric," Ibb agreed.

"It is all *twisted*, warped," Tracker said. She turned to Ophidian. "Your doing?"

The dragon good shook his head once, quickly.

"Is it safe to touch?" Tracker asked, cautiously moving forward.

"I would not," Ophidian said.

Ibb went further and grabbed her arm, pulling her back. "As you say, there is something wrong with it."

"*Lyric* did this?" Tracker asked, still eyeing the crushed shape in front of her.

"Or she had help," Ophidian said.

"If so, we are in great danger," Tracker said.

"Yes," Ibb agreed. "Will you help us?"

Silently, the metal immortal nodded, her glowing blue eyes never leaving the wrecked caravan.

The blood drained from Margaret Waters' face as she saw the Steam Master's expression harden. A muscle jumped in his jaw.

"You were supposed to arrange it that *I* made the deal," the Steam Master told her coldly.

"I tried, but —"

"I do not accept 'buts'," Torvan told her. He nodded curtly toward the door. "Go to my room, pick out two belts and prepare yourself for instruction."

Margaret's eyes widened but she knew better than to complain. She left. Outside the room, Drake gave her a hopeful look. She waved a hand at him and shook her head sharply, biting back any sound that might further inflame the Steam Master.

Drake saw her look, took in the silence, and trailed after her. He stopped outside the door to Torvan Brooke's room but peered in while Margaret carefully cleared the bed of the Steam Master's bags, placed them neatly in the corner of the room nearest the windows, and opened one bag. He gasped as he saw her pull out the Steam Master's horde of belts. His eyes went wide with worry as he saw her sort through them, picking two — one very thin, the other only slightly thicker.

Margaret laid the belts on the bed and moved to the door, closing it slowly in Drake's face, shaking her head to forestall any protests or words of sympathy.

Drake knew the drill, having done it many times himself. For a moment he thought he caught a half-sob coming out of Margaret's throat but he couldn't be sure.

Torvan Brookes' feet resounded heavily on the floor as he approached his room. Drake stepped back from the door, drew a breath to speak but was silenced by the Steam Master's upraised hand, and simple: "Don't."

"I can stay, so when you're done —"

"I'll call you," Brookes told him coldly.

Drake Fisher, mage of fire, adopted child of the Steam Master, mutely stepped away, not turning his back until the Steam Master had entered his room and closed the door behind him. He increased his pace hoping not to hear the first — *thwack!* — as a thin belt hit flesh but he was not fast enough. He winced at the sound, imagined the clenched jaw, the suppressed wail, and walked to his room.

Just outside, another door opened and the slimmer form of Chandra Evening peered around the edge. Her dark eyes met Drake's — and then she flinched as another *thwack!* escaped the muffling of the door. Drake's face burned hot and he glowered at her even as he opened his door and stepped inside, helpless at the power of the Steam Master.

"General Gergen," the man in Sorian garb guessed as he approached the commander of the Kingsland Army. Gergen nodded and the man extended his hand. "General Armand, sir."

"General," Gergen said, taking the proffered hand and shaking it firmly.

"May I say," Armand continued as he pivoted and gestured Gergen toward the staff room, "congratulations on a well-run campaign."

"Even though it was in winter?" Gergen asked drolly.

Armand waved a hand. "The season was part of the strategy, was it not?"

Gergen nodded. "And may I say, general, that I am sorry for the loss of your king."

"I have served many kings," Armand replied, "and hope to serve many more."

General Gergen raised an eyebrow in surprise.

"I was given to understand that King Markel has appointed Crown Prince Sarsal as his heir," Armand explained hastily.

"In the event that Queen Rassa does not provide another," Gergen allowed. He cocked his head at Armand. "I found it very surprising how quickly your queen and my king found their affections swayed."

"As did I," Armand agreed. He pushed open the doors to the formal meeting room and waved at the assembled officers, who rose immediately in response. "If you would, permit me to introduce my staff."

"Yes," Gergen said, entering the room. He swept the assembly with an encompassing look. "We have much to discuss and much to plan."

"We are at your pleasure," General Armand allowed, ducking his head subserviently.

"Well, that was far more excitement than I'd desired," Nelly Kendral said expansively as she sat at her desk, a pot of tea brewing beside her. The sun was setting and, already, Jarin Reedis had grandly lit all the lamps in the building, much to mage Margen's amusement.

The older mage nodded now in agreement with Principal Kendral.

"Even I, accustomed to life in the courts, found today a bit more exciting than I'd desired," Margen allowed.

"And your students?"

"Those that survived are more than eager to renew their efforts to learn the craft," Margen said with a thankful nod in her direction. He sat in one of the two chairs arranged opposite the desk, facing the open windows. "I suppose I could move them back to the castle, if you're pressed for space."

"No, no," Nelly said hastily, her dimples flashing. "I mean, I'm sure we can come to an arrangement, if you'd like."

Mage Margen snorted. "My dear, if you don't mind honesty —"

"No, never!" Nelly allowed hastily.

"— you are a bit young for this, aren't you?"

"I'll teach her," Reedis told the older mage testily from the other chair. "After all, this academy is named in *my* honor."

"So it is," Margen agreed equably, "and I doubt that I am your equal in matters pertaining to airships."

"But —?" Nelly prompted.

"I have more than fifty years' worth of knowledge in the magic arts," Margen said with a nod toward her. "And I am… obliged… to provide teaching to students in my agreement with the god Ophidian." He paused and spread his hands, palms down to either side of him.

With a quick glance to Jarin Reedis, he said to Nelly, "I would be honored if you would consider accepting my humble aid."

Nelly gasped in surprise but looked immediately toward Reedis to gage the other's reaction.

"All my life," Reedis said, his voice radiant with emotion, "I have looked for someone to teach me." He held out his hand to Margen. "I would be honored."

Margen took it solemnly. They shook once and then, almost awkwardly, let go. Margen turned his attention back to the Principal.

"When Vistos and I first came to this city, it was with the desire to create a center of learning," Margen said, his tone reminiscent. He leaned forward in his chair and said to Nelly, "And never once did we consider reaching out to everyone, setting up an academy in the very middle of the city." He nodded firmly to Nelly. "I am flattered that you would have me."

"Good!" Nelly said, reaching for the pot. "And with that, gentlemen, who's for tea?"

"Actually," Margen said, rising from his chair, a hand raised out in front of him, "I feel the need for something more substantial." He added hastily, "No offense, dear lady, but this day has been rather… strenuous, if you'd permit me to say."

"Hmm," Nelly replied, putting the pot back down. "I suppose a good meal is in order." Her eyes brightened. "And I know just the place!"

"No, not your father's tavern!" Reedis said, jumping out of his chair. "He threatened to kill me the last time I was there!"

"Well, he *had* suffered quite a loss," Nelly allowed somberly. "And mother was most put out — some of our best meats were in that cooler."

Jarin laughed and Nelly gave Reedis' body an alarmed look.

"I'm sorry, Miss Nelly," Jarin said with Reedis' voice. "The failure of that 'cooler' was not the good mage Reedis' but rather the result of my ire."

"Ire?" Margen repeated.

Jarin Reedis turned to him and nodded. "The airship had just shot down my friend," Jarin said, his voice going cold. He pointed a finger at his chest. "The airship that this body helped create."

"And I've apologized already, Jarin," Reedis said, taking control of his voice. "And Wymarc has accepted my apology —"

"And your service," Jarin added snidely.

"— *and* my service," Reedis agreed with a dismissive wave of his hand. He turned back to Nelly. "But I would rather, my love, not break our news to your parents while at the same time we arrive on their doorstep looking for sustenance and hospitality."

Nelly looked hurt.

"My dear," Mage Margen interceded, "if I may, I must agree with Reedis. We've had enough excitement for the moment."

"Then where would you suggest?" Nelly asked stiffly.

"I know just the place!" Jarin replied cheerfully. "And it's not twenty minutes away!"

"Very well, good dragon, we'll follow your lead," Nelly said, waving Jarin Reedis to the fore of their small party.

As Jarin Reedis passed in front of mage Margen, the mage shot him a worried I-hope-you-know-what-you-are-doing look.

Jarin, being Jarin, failed to notice.

Peter Hewlitt was just sitting down to a fine meal of prime rib smothered in mushrooms with potatoes and nearly fresh peas on the side — aided by a good strong red wine when a commotion startled him.

"Here!" A young woman's voice shrieked. "You can't mean here! Don't you *know* what this place is?"

"It's an inn for weary travellers," a voice replied, desperately trying to soothe the irritated woman. "I've been here many times."

"Not me," the voice added in a slightly different tone and emphasis — like two people were vying for the same tongue.

Hewlitt leapt from his chair and moved out of his secluded alcove toward the front door with silent speed.

His motion was spotted by a person standing at the side of the confrontation, someone who looked vaguely familiar but Hewlitt couldn't place him immediately. There was something different about the man, like —

"Mage Margen?" Hewlitt cried out in surprise.

Margen and the other two turned at the sound of his voice.

"What are you doing here?" Hewlitt asked.

"Looking for a quiet place to eat," Margen replied, casting a glance toward his companions that made it clear that he feared they would *not* provide such.

"This — this — *place!*" the young woman growled, shock and anger written all over her face. She turned to her companion again. "And you *came* here?"

"Just me," Jarin replied, "I was on the run at the time. Looking for someone."

"If you would," Hewlitt stepped forward, "I would be delighted to entertain you as my guests." He waved a hand toward his alcove. "I was just sitting to eat but I'm sure the cook could make whatever you require in short order." He gave Margen a thoughtful look. "And I would be very interested to talk with you Margen. I've heard only rumors."

"That must cause you no end of pain," Jarin said in a low voice. Nelly glared at him.

Hewlitt gave him a sharp look. "You are wearing the shape of Reedis, who was thought lost in the bitter north."

"I am Reedis," Reedis replied with a half-bow. "Rumors of my demise are —" and here he took the woman's hand in his, affectionately "— fortunately rather premature."

Hewlitt's eyes narrowed as he examined the woman. Suddenly, he recognized her, "You are the Kendrals' girl."

"Nelly Kendral," Nelly replied frostily with a quick curtsy. She turned to Reedis, adding, "And my father would *kill* me if he knew I was —"

"Nelly!" a gruff voice cried from the far end of the room.

Nelly Kendral's face drained white as she finished faintly, "— here."

The knock, when it came, was not unexpected. Torvan Brookes thrust open the door long enough to look inside. A pale, frightened Chandra was by his side.

"Your sister needs you," Brookes said, tossing two bags into the room. "Take your stuff, I'm staying here tonight."

"Yes, father," Drake Fisher said, grabbing his bag and hefting it to his shoulder. He stood aside as the Steam Master swaggered into the room, seeming thrilled, almost drunk. Drake kept his eyes on the ground as he made his way out the door. Chandra pulled it closed quietly after him.

"It must be bad," Chandra said in a whisper. "I've never seen him look so happy."

Drake could only trust himself to make a grim nod in reply. He strode forcefully up the hall to the other room. The door was open which surprised Drake — usually father would keep his punishments private.

The red slab of meat lying motionless on the bed pulsed blood with each heartbeat. Chandra sobbed when she saw it.

"We must get help," Drake said, throwing his bag to the ground. "Find some sheets or something to… cover her."

"She's bleeding too much," Chandra said. "He whipped her too hard, too long!"

Drake knelt at the nearest side of the bed, his right hand raised but not touching the tortured skin that housed Margaret Waters. He turned to Chandra. "We've got to do something, we've got to get help."

"Who?" Chandra said, turning toward the door. "Who would —?"

"I smell blood," a man's voice spoke from the end of the hallway. "What has happened?"

"My sister," Chandra began, licking her lips nervously.

"No!" Drake hissed from his place at the side of the bed. "If father —"

"What in the name of the gods is —?" the man had moved even as he spoke and rounded the corner of the doorway. His words cut off abruptly and his eyes narrowed with a look of death. "Who did this?"

"If he finds out you know, he'll kill you," Chandra told the man — a Kingsland soldier by his dress — in a worried whisper.

"Not if I kill him first," the man replied coldly.

A snort from Drake at the bedside caught the man's attention and he turned angrily toward the brown-skinned man. "Not likely," Drake said, glancing to meet the man's angry look.

"Why?" the man replied, his hand going to the sword at his side.

"He's the Steam Master," Chandra told him in a whisper. She grabbed the man's hand and dragged him into the room, closing the door hastily. "And if he hears you, not only will he kill you but he'll punish us."

"Punish?" the man repeated. He glanced toward the slab of meat that was once a young girl and gestured. "Like that?"

Grimly, Chandra nodded.

# Chapter Three

"Soooo," First minister Mannevy dragged out the word to hide his disbelief, "you're telling me that Soria *has* no first minister?" Heads shook. "No prime minister?" Heads shook again.

"There might have been one, once," Grekken Jallir allowed hesitantly, glancing to the others in the king's chambers, who all nodded eagerly, "but, if so, it was before my time."

"Mine too," chorused the other nobles in the room. The half-dozen men in the room constituted the most powerful and responsible men that could be mustered for a meeting of this importance on such short notice. Mannevy had been informed that several others were out of the capital, wintering in their own fiefs. Doubtless, Mannevy was told, they'd come as soon as they heard word to bend knee to the new king.

"Who sees to the treasury?" Mannevy asked. "Who pays the army, who levies taxes, who rules your kingdom?"

"The king," Jallir replied with a shrug.

"Did he not have councillors?" Mannevy asked, trying to hide his desperation.

"He would ask for advice, sometimes," Jallir said agreeably. "But mostly he would talk to the generals or… I suppose you want to talk with the treasurer."

"Yes, that would be a good idea," Mannevy said. He glanced around at the assembly. "Is he here?"

"No," Jallir said, shaking his head. "He's out on his farm. Won't be back until spring."

"And when *he's* not here, who pays the gold?" Mannevy asked.

"Well..," Jallir began slowly, "if there's an emergency, the king throws me the keys and tells me to get him so much gold."

"So *you* have the keys?" Mannevy persisted.

Jallir shrugged. "No." Mannevy sighed. "I expect they're still around his neck."

"Then," Mannevy said, rising in exasperation, "let us pay our respects." *And acquire the keys to the treasury!*

"What is *he* doing here?" Kenid Kendral said, sneering at Jarin Reedis. "I thought he was dead!"

"No, thankfully not at all," Reedis said.

"You owe me for that 'cooler' of yours — and expenses!"

"Come, let us sit and eat together," Peter Hewlitt said, gesturing the crowd toward the alcove. In an aside to Margen, Hewlitt added, "Kenid and I were just discussing business."

"Old client?" Jarin asked slyly. Using Reedis' mouth, of course.

Nelly slapped his arm, hard.

"What's that for?" Reedis asked.

"It was for *him*," Nelly said firmly. She reached over and rubbed his arm, full of sympathy. "As for you, I'm sorry."

"I don't owe you anything," Reedis said to the older Kendral.

"But *I* do," Jarin added in the same voice. "I destroyed the cooler out of pique. It was childish of me."

"Well," Reedis continued in the same voice, "you are only… four, isn't it?"

"What," master Kendral demanded of his daughter, "is going on with him?"

"He is a twin soul," Mage Margen replied. "They are newly joined and still learning how to cooperate together."

"A twin soul?" Kenid asked, his eyebrows rising in alarm. He turned to Reedis. "Are you half-dragon now, boy?"

"Yes," Reedis replied smoothly. "I am twinned with a dragon." He nodded to Kenid agreeably. "I am also the air mage who led the royal airship *Spite* to the bitter north, met with the god Arolan, and helped free him." He spied the table in the alcove, saw Hewlitt's meat sitting, cold and lifeless, and said to him, "Oh, I'm sorry! We've kept you from your meal! How about I warm it for you?"

And, keeping his eyes on his future father-in-law, Reedis sent a wave of flame to hover gently over the meat until it sizzled with renewed flavor. He added as he sat near the now warm plate, "And the cooler worked. Perfectly. Until it was tampered with."

"For a price," Jarin added, grabbing a roll from the breadbasket and placing it on his side-plate, "we could make a better one. Tamper-proof."

"Please," Hewlitt said, gesturing to master Kendral, his daughter, and the mage, "be seated." He gave Jarin Reedis a grin. "Perhaps our friend here will aid the chef in preparing some special meals."

"I'll help!" Nelly squeaked, grabbing Jarin Reedis and pulling him up out of his chair. "Come on, Reedis, let's go to the kitchen!"

"I'm not sure I want my daughter —" Kenid began anxiously.

"Oh, I wouldn't worry about that," Reedis told him. Jarin, piqued, spoiled it by adding, "After all, we're betrothed!"

"Jarin!" Nelly cried, dragging the twin-soul body away forcefully.

"Betrothed?" Hewlitt said to Margen while dragging master Kendral into a chair and softly patting the rage-spluttering man on the back with one hand.

"Happened today," Margen said. "At the end of a rather long and eventful day."

"I'd heard rumors," Hewlitt said. He gestured to the table. "I'm willing to pay to hear more." He reached for the bottle of wine and waved it questioningly toward the mage. "It's got quite a bouquet, well worth the effort."

"Well, in that case, please pour," Margen said. He glanced around the dining room appreciatively. "I've always wondered what this place looked like."

Hewlitt stifled a snort and converted it into a surprised, "Really?"

"And," Margen said, his tone rising and his head swivelling toward Kenid, "I am so glad that I'll be able to tell Mrs. Kendral how gracious her husband was in allowing me to *prevail* upon him to provide me with his keen hospitality insights."

"Ah!" Hewlitt replied with a knowing look. "Yes, I imagine Mrs. Kendral might take it amiss to hear that her husband had been a guest at this establishment without good cause."

Kenid Kendral looked from one to the other and threw up his hands in surrender. "Very well!" he said grudgingly. He glanced to Hewlitt. "What's the price?"

"Nothing you won't mind paying," Hewlitt assured him. Kendral gave him a neutral, if slightly doubtful, look. "You may have heard that we are expanding our rail lines." Kenid nodded. "Which means that I'm going to be looking at expanding our hospitality —"

"No!" Kenid Kendral swore, half-rising out of his chair. "You've got a good business here but there's no way that I'm going to take on *your* sort of customers at *my* establishment!"

"Sit down," Hewlitt said, waving the offended man back to his seat. "I'll be expanding here, too." Kendral, still flushed with anger, sat back down. "I would not dream of asking you to change the nature of your business."

"That's good," Kenid replied. "People deserve a good place to sleep, a chance to eat out, and a friendly place to speak freely."

"All of which I appreciate and wish to reward," Hewlitt assured him. Kenid's brows rose. "There must be a place where people can speak freely —"

"Without the king knowing!"

"Without anyone knowing," Hewlitt agreed. "A place of safety, of rest. And with the rail lines there will be more people coming into our city. More will need places to stay, places to do business —" he glanced toward Margen "— places to learn."

"What are you proposing?" Kenid asked, still looking as though he smelled something foul.

"I wish to invest in your business," Hewlitt said. Kenid began to reply hotly but Hewlitt waved him down. "*Strictly* as a business, sir, nothing else."

"I'm a commoner, not a sir," Kenid said.

"Nor am I," Hewlitt replied, his lips twitching. "I meant it as a recognition of your good nature, not a mark of nobility."

"The two should be the same," Margen muttered to himself.

They were interrupted by the sound of shrieks from the kitchen and the smell of charred beef.

"There you are!" King Markel's voice boomed as he tromped down the hallway toward the open door of the room where Mannevy was crouched, looking busy and perplexed.. "I've been looking all over for you!" He glanced around the Sorian palace possessively and beamed. "Quite a place, isn't it?" When Markel reached the door, he peered inside. "What is this place?"

"It's the royal treasury, sire," First Minister Mannevy replied without glancing up from his counting. He gestured to the person crouched beside him. "This is Grekken Jallir."

"He is?" Markel said, his eyes going narrow. "And does he not know to bow before a king?"

"Please, sire," Mannevy replied in a pressed tone, "we're right in the middle of our accounts and we can't lose a moment."

Markel drew his head back in affront. He drew breath for a royal bellow but stopped as he looked around the bare walls of the room. "Where's all the money?"

"That's what we're trying to determine, sire," Mannevy said without looking up. He waved his hand around, gesturing toward the few forlorn piles of gold and silver coins. "At the moment, however, *this* is all that we know of."

"What?" Markel cried in surprise. "There can't be more than — than —"

"About two hundred in gold, sire," Mannevy told him with a heavy sigh. "We've more gold in our treasury back in Kingsland."

"Someone stole it?" Markel said, groping for any solution.

"The keys were on King Wendel's body when he was recovered," Mannevy said, shaking his head. "They were brought here immediately by our master Jallir. I inspected the lock before opening the door." He waved his hand around the room again, his expression grim. "This is what we found."

"Magic?"

"The walls are spell-proofed," Mannevy replied with a shake of his head, "the spells are fresh. I can tell that much."

"Been breaking into treasuries, have you?" Markel asked darkly.

"No, sire," Mannevy replied, "I've been protecting them. As you might have reason to recall."

King Markel's shoulders fell in dejection. He peered around, still dismayed. "So this is all there is?"

"It appears so," Mannevy replied grimly. "Apparently the late King — and perhaps others of the royal court — made free with the royal treasury."

"We could raise taxes," Markel suggested.

"I thought it best to first ascertain the depth of the treasury," Mannevy replied. He stood up and brushed off his knees. "Having done that, I think my next action should be to come to grips with our current expenditures."

"Well, don't let me keep you!" King Markel said, turning and abruptly leaving them to their own devices. "I'll expect a full report in the morning!"

"Of course, sire," Mannevy said in a long-suffering voice.

Markel turned back, his brows creased. "How is the larder? Don't tell me we've nothing to eat!"

"I have no idea," Mannevy said, moving toward the doors and gesturing for Jallir to follow him.

"King Wendel set a good table, sire," Grekken Jallir offered. "And, it being winter, I'd be surprised if he didn't lay in a good larder against the cold."

"I doubt he expected to feed —" Markel paused thoughtfully "— what is it? About ten thousand troops?"

"Fortunately the number is near half that," Mannevy said. He looked up. "But I take your point, sire. Shall I send someone to examine the state of the larder, sire?"

"When you can," King Markel said nobly. He turned back down the corridor and added, as he stomped away, "I realize you have your limits, after all."

Mannevy stared after him for a long moment. Then he blinked and turned to Jallir. "Perhaps a foray to the larder — and the kitchen — before we seek out the royal accounts."

"Mr. Brookes," Captain Welless called loudly outside the closed door — for he was the man who had found Drake, Chandra, and the bloody ruins of Margaret Waters earlier, "This is Captain Welless of his Majesty's Infantry. I have placed a guard on your room, sir."

He nodded to the two privates what braced to attention, one on either side of the doorway.

Chandra, who had accompanied him out the door, whispered worriedly, "I don't think that's a good idea —"

*BOOM!* There was a huge explosion on the other side of the door and the sound of ruins falling to the street below. Captain Welless jerked in surprise.

"He's a mage himself, you see," Chandra finished lamely.

"You two," Welless snapped at the soldiers, "guard *this* room." He jerked his finger toward the open room in which Drake knelt grimly beside the shivering form of the young girl. He glanced at Chandra. "You do magic?"

"Earth magic," Chandra admitted with a small curtsy.

"Please come with me, I might need your aid," Welless replied. Chandra cast a worried look at the open door. "She needs more help than we can provide," Welless explained gently. "I'm going to see if I can find it."

Chandra darted to his side and dogged his heels as he took off, went outside and down the street.

"Well, I must say, whatever your faults, there's no doubting your skill in the kitchen," Kenid — "call me Nid" — Kendral roared as he slapped Jarin Reedis' shoulder with rough affection.

"Nelly helped," Reedis said honestly.

'Nid' Kendral beamed and nodded his head. "'Course she did! She learned from the best!"

The red wine had been followed by white, then by a sweet dessert wine, then by port, and was now joined with a stronger whisky, all courtesy of the ever-kind Peter Hewlitt, the king's spymaster.

Mage Margen, who had drunk little and said less, grew more and more grim with each new toast or loud guffaw. He gave Hewlitt a sour look which the man shrugged off with a pleasant look but Margen wasn't fooled — he was *up* to something.

"Did you know," Jarin said, smiling at the spymaster, "that dragons don't get drunk?"

Hewlitt's smile slipped. "I haven't had the occasion to meet many dragons."

Nelly turned her attention to them, placing her silverware carefully on her plate.

"You have been ever so kind," Nelly said now, hoping to defuse any tension.

"And you've got my hand on that bargain," Nid Kendral said, proffering his hand in evidence. "Together, we'll *be* the hoteliers of Kingsford."

"And beyond," Hewlitt agreed, not taking his eyes off of the twin-souled Jarin Reedis. He turned to Nelly. "Actually, miss, your father's words are perhaps more to the mark than most here know."

Nelly gave him an attentive look, encouraging him to continue.

Hewlitt returned her look with a smile then swept his gaze over to Margen and, finally, back to Jarin Reedis.

"While it is true that I am honored to work for the king — may the gods bless his soul — some forget that I have other enterprises which require management," Hewlitt said. "And tonight —" he nodded to master Kendral "— I have been so engaged." He nodded to Margen and Jarin Reedis. "Your unanticipated presence has allowed me the chance to get to know you both more personally." He turned to Nelly. "And, I must add, to make the acquaintance of the Principal of the Reedis Memorial Academy."

"Here it comes," Margen muttered under his breath.

"Indeed," Hewlitt, whose ears were better than the mage had credited, agreed. "Miss Kendral, I hope your academy prospers. I hope it grows." He nodded toward Margen. "It is in the interest of the kingdom to have a large and growing supply of well-trained mages to protect our borders and our interests."

"I quite agree," Margen said, his expression puzzled.

"And today," Hewlitt pressed out a thin smile, "I'm given to learn that the academy — and its teachers — have proven themselves capable of protecting themselves against the untoward incursions of a god."

"Not without help!" Margen growled. "No one goes against a god without help."

Hewlitt nodded in acknowledgement.

"Even so," he continued, "you were able to attract such help."

"At the cost of two lives," Reedis added solemnly.

"My point is," Hewlitt persisted, "that your establishment has shown to all that it is ready to take care of its own."

Nelly nodded, reaching for Reedis' hand under the table. He took it firmly in his and squeezed it supportively. She beamed at him.

"Which means, all things being equal," Hewlitt continued, "that as of today, the Reedis Memorial Academy of Balloon Magic is the premier school of magic in the kingdom."

Nelly took a deep breath and blushed with pride. Hewlitt acknowledged her reaction with a congratulatory nod.

"So, thinking ahead," Hewlitt pressed on rapidly, "I imagine that the school will be inundated with applicants." Nelly's eyes got bigger and she exchanged hopeful looks with Reedis and Margen who both nodded in agreement. "And that, of course, means that your premises will shortly become overburdened with eager students."

"We'll expand, of course," Nelly said. She turned to Reedis. "I always knew that the academy would grow. It had to, because of you."

Hewlitt smiled at her, and continued, "Of course. And, as with such things, the academy will be beseeched to provide education to those from outside the capital. And that will mean —"

"I had always planned on making it a combined day and boarding school," Nelly said firmly. "I have plans —"

"No doubt, mistress, no doubt," Hewlitt continued smoothly, raising his hands palms down and spreading them wide. "And it will be to the profit of all."

"Hear it comes," Margen said, catching Hewlitt's slight emphasis on the word 'profit'.

"There's nothing wrong with a decent profit," Reedis said, coming to Nelly's aid. Under the table, she patted his hand.

"What I propose," Hewlitt said, realizing that prolonging the discussion would be to his detriment, "is that I underwrite your expansion and the construction of a proper campus."

"In return for what, sir?" Nelly asked, her tone all business now.

"I would like a place on your management board and a decent return on my loan, nothing more," Hewlitt assured her.

"And first chance at our students," Margen guessed.

"I would be more than happy to get to know your students," Hewlitt agreed. "I will be honored to follow their exploits."

"What with airships, rail lines, and goodness knows what else, it's a fair venture," Nid Kendral spoke up, his expression surprisingly sober given the amount of liquor he'd consumed. He nodded across the table to his daughter. "A good bargain benefits all."

Nelly smiled at him. He was quoting a phrase she'd coined years back.

"The details will need to be determined," Nelly said to Hewlitt. The spymaster nodded but there was a slight caution in his expression — as though he was coming to recognize the business acumen in the young woman's eyes. Before he could backtrack, Nelly stretched out her hand. "But, that being so, Mr. Hewlitt, I believe you have a deal."

Hewlitt took her hand and shook it once, firmly.

Gamden kicked the heel of Jaden Ostan's boot, hard, startling the other rudely awake. "Get up!"

Jaden grunted and turned over. Gamden kicked his other boot, harder. Jaden pulled his feet up.

"Dawn's coming, we've got a ways to go," Gamden growled. Jaden opened up an eye and winked blearily. "You don't get up now, I leave you."

"Ugh," Jaden grunted, turning over and coming to his knees. "I'm up."

"You're still on the ground," Gamden said. "Up is on two feet and ready to soar."

"Food?" Jaden asked, rising to his feet and stretching.

"We'll find something when it's light," Gamden promised.

"I'd like to eat more than a bird," Jaden muttered.

"Have two," Gamden offered grandly. "By the gods, have three!"

"I'd be happier with a side of roast beef," Jaden said.

"That in your gullet and you'd fall straight to the valley below," Gamden said with a snort, pointing toward the darkness looming to their left. He'd guided them up to a high plateau well above the valley, knowing that it'd make their first flight easier in the morning — they'd nearly need to drop over the cliff and glide until they found a suitable thermal.

"Is there any air moving?" Jaden asked, sniffing the darkness dubiously. "Didn't you say that the hot air comes with the sun?"

"I did," Gamden allowed. "And the sun's coming soon enough. If we catch it when the ground's just heating, we'll get lift enough the whole day."

"Just as long as we don't go too high."

"Air gets thin when you're too high," Gamden said by way of agreement. He shot the other eagle man a dirty look which was unseen in the darkness. "I'd warned you about that."

"But you didn't say how high was too high," Jaden sniffed.

"It's different for every body," Gamden said. He stabbed a finger in the other's direction. "You're out of shape, haven't learned to breathe like a bird. You'll get better in time." He turned to survey the darkness below them. In the far distance, to the east, he saw the beginnings of a lightening. South, he could just barely make out the whiteness of breakers on the shoreline, fifty leagues distant. "Come on," he said, grabbing the other man's hand and pulling him over the cliff.

"Wait!" Jaden wailed as they plummeted. Gamden pushed him aside and Jaden fell, terror-stricken into the darkness.

A moment later, Gamden's eagle cry pierced the morning sky.

For one terrible instant, Jaden feared that he couldn't find his feathers and then — with an echoing screech — he was flying.

"Well, what are we to do?" King Markel asked first minister Mannevy imploringly. They were in the royal audience chamber. Queen Rassa was there, holding Markel's hand and looking at Mannevy with a mixture of disgust and fear. Crown Prince Sarsal sat next to them. They had just finished breakfast and had strolled leisurely into the audience chamber, only to have their stomach curdle with the news Mannevy brought them.

Markel glanced to his queen. "And you didn't know anything about this?"

"Wendel…" Queen Rassa began slowly. "Well, I thought he was better with his numbers."

Markel turned to the prince. "And you?"

"Not a whisper," Sarsal said, shaking his head in quick denial. He turned to his royal mother. "You know how much he loved the army. He was always buying them things, raising troops, paying for new swords."

"And now —" Markel turned to Mannevy. "How bad is it?"

"I had hoped, sire," Mannevy said with a deep sigh, "to combine our treasuries at a profit." He shook his head slowly and spread his hands out beside him, palms down. "But with *this* news…"

"Well, we don't need the army any more," Markel said. "We can let them go —" he broke off as he caught Mannevy's pained expression. "What?"

"It is the middle of winter, sire," Mannevy reminded him. "Even to disperse our army back south will take time, require food, and money." He shook his head. "Dispersing will cost as much, in the near term, as keeping them where they are."

"We could put them up here," Markel said, glancing to Rassa and the Crown Prince for confirmation.

"Five thousand infantry, sire?" Mannevy asked, shaking his head. "I doubt there is room enough in the city for less than half that number. And if we insisted on forcing our troops —"

"They're *Sorian* troops now!" King Markel exclaimed.

"— but they would be seen as lately enemy soldiers, sire," Mannevy said. "And forcing them into people's homes would not make them seem less so."

"Surely, first minister," Queen Rassa said with an attempt at a winning smile, "you have *some* plans."

"Obviously, we will have to reduce expenses, starting immediately," Mannevy said. "We should send word to the capital — to Kingsford — to cease construction on our airships —"

"Good!"

"But that will cause almost as many problems as it solves," Mannevy continued. "For instance, we have begun levying taxes on the earnings of those building our ships and we'll lose that income when we let those workers go." Mannevy pursed his lips thoughtfully. "And then there'll be a lot of unemployed workers in the capital, in the middle of winter."

"So?" Crown Prince Sarsal demanded. "What concern is that of ours?"

"Your Royal Highness, it is sometimes wise to look beyond the immediate and to the future," Mannevy said with a deferential nod to the young princeling. "Without money coming in, the men will not be able to pay for food, lodging, or clothes."

"And?" Sarsal demanded with a sniff.

"If they aren't making money, who will buy the food that comes in? Who will pay for lodging?" Mannevy said. "If there's no one to buy the food, what of the farmers? They'll have to drop their prices, and they'll lose money. The innkeepers will lose money, too. With everyone losing money, the Crown will be making less money as well." Mannevy frowned. "This losing of income by the airship builders will cause a drop of income throughout the capital."

"Kingsford," Queen Rassa corrected. She nodded toward Markel. "The capital is *here*."

"Of course," Markel agreed readily.

"The loss of income in Kingsford will be felt in the royal coffers, wherever they may be," Mannevy said.

"But you have a *plan*, don't you?" Queen Rassa demanded testily.

"As I say, we will have to stop construction," Mannevy said.

"But you made that sound bad," Markel observed.

"Well, we could perhaps change the nature of our construction," Mannevy said. King Markel urged him on with a brusque gesture. "If we chose to make the new ships *cargo* ships and sent them out to seek out trade and commerce —"

"In winter?" Queen Rassa barked.

"We have no choice, Your Majesty," Mannevy said. "We could slow down our construction, divert more efforts into building rail lines and —" he stopped, his eyes suddenly going wide. He turned to his king. "Do you recall, sire, that we gave Torvan Brookes — the Steam Master — an advance against future work?"

King Markel blinked and nodded dumbly.

"Two large chests and one small chest," Mannevy continued, rubbing his hands together.

"Chests?" Crown Prince Sarsal asked.

"Of gold," Mannevy explained. He gave his king a scheming look. "Enough to run the capital for at least a month, perhaps more."

"And get him crowned?" Queen Rassa asked, pointing to the king.

Mannevy's expression grew more glum. Finally, he said with a small nod, "If we keep a strict eye on our expenses."

"Then by all means, first minister, let us retrieve them," King Markel said with all pomp. He beamed at the dark man. "I *knew* you'd find a way to save us!"

# Chapter Four

"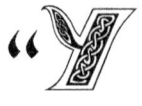our orders are clear, are they not?" First Minister Mannevy demanded of Colonel Lewis when the other presented himself later that day.

"I'm to take the same detachment I used to capture the Sorian royal family, take ship with Captain Fawcett's *Wasp*, and proceed to the capital —"

"No, Colonel, to Kingsford," Mannevy corrected. "Sarskar is now the capital of the kingdom. Of *both* kingdoms."

"Proceed to Kingsford and relieve Torvan Brookes, also known as the Steam Master, of the gold entrusted to him by the king," Lewis continued, accepting the correction with the merest jerk of his chin. "Once we have retrieved the gold — measuring two large and one small chests, the larger chests weighing one hundredweight and the smaller chest weighing half that — I am to return here in all haste to deliver the chests to the treasury."

Mannevy lowered his chin in agreement. "Good, Colonel," he said, "I'll let you go about your affairs at once."

"And the rest of my men, sir?" Colonel Lewis asked in a choked voice. He really *was* trying to hide his outrage, his anger, his sense of betrayal but 'choked' was the best he could do.

"I'm sure that General Gergen and the others will see to their needs," Mannevy said with a dismissive wave.

Lewis hesitated. Mannevy looked up, surprised.

"If I may, sir?" Lewis said. He pressed on before getting a response. "I should like to brevet ensign Falco — Berry Falco — to lieutenant. He's been outstanding and it would be good for the troops' morale —"

Mannevy cut him off, "I think that should be left to the new commander."

Lewis took a deep breath, preparing to argue his cause, met the minister's brown eyes, and gave in.

"Very well," Lewis said, "May I make my report to General Gergen?"

"No," Mannevy replied coldly. "You are to leave immediately, Colonel. At the King's orders."

Defeated, Samuel Lewis snapped to attention and performed a perfect about-face, marching away from the minister's small office briskly.

"Ah, General Armand!" General Gergen said as he approached the Sorian commanding general.

"General Gergen," Armand replied with a stiff nod.

"I am told by my king that we are to consider our two militaries united into one greater whole," Gergen pressed on.

"Am I then, sir, to be your subordinate?" General Armand asked in a careful tone.

"At His Majesty's wishes," Gergen replied.

"Until the official coronation," General Armand said tentatively, "I should find myself in a most difficult position."

"Does it help that the King has already agreed that Crown Prince Sarsal shall be his heir," General Gergen said, adding in a lower tone, "His first son being, as we all believe, lost in the bitter north."

"Indeed."

"And Queen Rassa has — to the surprise of many — agreed to join our king in matrimony, permanently aligning the two realms," Gergen added. "So I think that the coronation is merely a formality."

"An important formality —"

"To be sure," Gergen agreed testily. "However, General, I went looking for you to offer something you might find enjoyable —"

"And what might that be?" General Armand asked, trying to look like he hadn't sucked on a lemon.

"Colonel Lewis of the cavalry — the man who captured your royal family —" Gergen added the dig because Armand needed to be reminded of his place "— has been assigned a special mission by the king and must, regrettably, leave the bulk of his cavalry squadron behind."

Armand nodded and raised an eyebrow in question.

"Well," Gergen continued, "I thought that nothing could be better in cementing our new united relationship than in asking you to appoint a cavalry officer to take charge of this illustrious unit."

"Really?"

"Yes, this cavalry not only caught your king but it was responsible for the surprise liberation of the South Sea Pass," Gergen said. "So you see it is, in effect, one of the best units in our combined armies."

"And you want *me* to appoint the next commander?" Armand asked, genuinely surprised.

"If you would, yes," Gergen replied.

Armand drew himself up to attention. "General, it would be an honor."

Captain Fawcett looked thoughtful as he said, "I suppose we *could* go straight for the capital —"

"Kingsford," Colonel Lewis interjected.

"Yes," Fawcett said, giving the colonel a surprised look.

"The *capital*," Lewis said with emphasis, "is no longer Kingsford."

"It isn't?" Fawcett's brows rose in surprise.

Lewis pointed to the ground below them. "It is Sarskar."

"Oh," Fawcett blinked as he absorbed that change in nomenclature. "Well, regardless, we could head straight to Kingsford. We'd get there in about three days but we'd have to cross the Silver Mountains… about mid-way, at a guess and that's a danger."

"Silver Mountains, it is," Lewis told him.

"But, colonel, we'd be running on scraps," Fawcett said in warning. "And if we met any adverse winds…" he shook his head "… that could be *very* worrying." He glanced around the deck to steady his thoughts. Brightening, he added, "Although, if the winds *are* bad, they'll probably blow us inland and we could make for Korin's Pass."

"The fort's been destroyed," Lewis reminded him.

"Not the fort," Fawcett said, waving a hand in negation, "the village. They've got the rails there so they're certain to have a supply of coal."

"Good," Lewis said, nodding in agreement. He looked up at the young airship captain and smiled. "Very good! How soon can we depart?"

"Hamo, Hamo!" Captain Welless shouted as he barged into the front room that was his office — and the ante-room for Hamo Beck's office.

Hamo opened the door to his office and looked out in surprise. "What is it?"

"This is Chandra, she's Margaret's sister," Welless said by way of introduction. Chandra eyed Hamo curiously — they were the same height although he was clearly much older.

"Glad to meet you, Chandra," Hamo said absently. "How may I help you, captain?"

"We need a healer," Welless said without preamble. "My man in the company can't handle this."

"Handle what?"

"Father beat her," Chandra said, lowering her eyes to the ground. She raised them again long enough to meet Hamo's eyes as she confessed, "She's bleeding terribly."

"He beat her?" Hamo's voice rose. He glanced to Welless. "Where is she?" Immediately, he added, "Where is he? *Who* is he?"

"He is Torvan Brookes, the Steam Master," Chandra said. She bit her lip. "Margaret was making a deal with you and… some others."

"She told you?" Hamo asked, his brows rising.

"No," Chandra said. "But she wouldn't have sent a gold signal unless it meant trade. And father came, so it must be important."

"So you're wondering if we've got a healer in the village?" Hamo asked.

"No," Captain Welless replied, "I doubt your village healer is any better than my man." He took a breath. "I was wondering if perhaps you knew a way to get the zwerg healer here."

"The zwerg?" Hamo said, sounding surprised. "I don't know why you would think that *I*—"

Welless stopped him with an upraised hand and a small smile. "Who else would Miss Waters want to see for a trade?" He said. "And you must remember that my late commander assaulted the zwerg entrance on the other side of the pass."

Hamo cocked his head to one side in challenge.

Welless snorted. "I am not the sharpest knife in the armory, old bean, but when I get time to think… well, usually I catch up with the rest of the team." He smiled as he saw the other man absorb his meaning. "But now," he continued brusquely, "a young girl's life is at stake and I fear if we can't get her help immediately, we'll lose her." He hesitated just a moment before adding, "And I don't think your *friends* will like that one bit."

"Please, take me to them," Chandra said. "My magic is earth magic, they'll listen to me."

Hamo frowned. He looked at Welless. "No time to waste?"

"Her father beat her backside raw — and I mean *raw* — and he didn't spare one part more than another," Welless said grimly. He made a face. "Frankly, I've never seen a person beat so bad, even in the military."

"Very well," Hamo said, turning to Chandra. "If you'll follow me." He motioned to Welless. "You'll need to stay here."

"I'm going back to the tavern, to keep an eye on Margaret," Welless said. "Her father burst out of his room — I'm afraid you'll have to replace the wall — and I don't know if he plans her any further harm."

"Go, then," Hamo said, grabbing Chandra by the arm, "we'll be back as fast as we can."

"I just hope it's not too late," Welless said, turning the other way as they left the building.

The man known as the Steam Master for his creation of the great locomotive engines and rail lines that had propelled small Kingsland to victory over the much larger Soria raced into the night.

*She had* no *right!* Torvan Brookes swore to himself as he found a cluster of snow-covered trees far enough from the small village of Korin's Pass that he felt safe to look back for pursuit. *I was supposed to deal with the zwerg! Setting herself up before* me! *Who does she think she is? I should have beat her* harder!

"Yes, you should," a man's voice agreed smoothly from the darkness. Torvan twirled trying to find the voice's owner.

"It was most disrespectful of her," an old woman agreed with a cackle.

"After all you did for her," the man added. "Took her in, fed her — and I'm sure she *did* eat —"

"Stuffed herself silly, more like," the old hag cackled. "Children these days!"

"Try to teach them, instill respect and —" the man added.

"Show yourselves!" Torvan shouted into the night, raising a hand, palm up, and conjuring a ball of fire.

"Do you really want to see us?" the man asked.

"And us, see you?" the hag added.

Torvan growled and threw his strength into his fireball. It blossomed into a huge ball and rose into the night, illuminating all around him.

"Well, I guess he does," the man said, stepping out of the shadows into the light. He was smiling.

"Poor ducks," the hag said, stepping into view. Beside her, a hooded figure stepped forward, nodding in agreement. "All that hard work and none of his brood are willing to give him the *least* respect!"

"You trained them, fed them, made them yours," the man added. "Of course, when they were wilful, when they paid you no heed, you owed it to them to show them the error of their ways."

"You used a firm hand," the old woman said.

Torvan turned his attention from the woman, back to the smiling man, and then to the silent hooded one. "I've seen you before."

"More often than you know, ducks," the old woman cackled agreeable. "When you doubted yourself, we kept your faith."

"When you taught, we were in the shadows," the smiling man said.

"And when you —" the old woman broke off and turned angrily on the hooded man. "You know, for once — just *once* — Kor, I wish you'd speak up! Here we are, doing all the talking, all the work, and you just stand there and nod knowingly! It gets old, you know?"

The hooded one stepped closer to the hag, put an arm on hers and nodded in silent agreement.

"We've been over this," the smiling man said. "Kor gets to do the silent brooding part."

"Well, you know how hard it is on my throat to do all this cackling," the woman swore. "I'll have to bathe my throat in syrup and warm tea for the rest of the week, I tell you!"

Torvan Brookes glanced at the three in hurt surprise.

The smiling man noticed. "Oh, Quen, look! You've hurt his feelings!"

The hooded man turned toward Torvan Brookes, his eyes gleaming at the back of his hood and opened his mouth to reveal large, gleaming fangs. Involuntarily, Torvan took a step backwards, pulling his fireball back to his palm.

"Oh, now, Kor, look what you've done!" Quen snarled. "He was just about ours and you've scared him, poor ducks!"

"This is why we never get the good things," the smiling man said, nodding angrily at the hooded man.

Quen, the crone, turned back to Torvan. "But never mind Kor, dear. He's just reminding us that the time is at hand."

"Time?"

"We offers you a choice," the smiling man said.

Torvan Brookes' eyes widened in surprise. "My gods!"

"Well, three in one, really," the smiling man allowed with a small nod.

"Quite the package: order, tradition, obedience," the crone, Quen, agreed. The silent hooded one closed his mouth and tried to look non-threatening.

"The three-headed god," Torvan whispered in awe.

"Well, I wish they wouldn't say that," Ian said.

"It's not right, not right at all — we're three bodies in our own right," Quen agreed. Kor nodded silently.

"But enough of that," Ian said. "As my sister said, you've a choice."

"Choice?"

"Well… maybe a decision is the better way of putting it," Quen allowed. She jerked her thumb back to the village and the tavern whence Torvan had fled. "There's no going back there."

"And they'll take your magic," Ian told him with a grin.

"No one can take magic!" Torvan declared hotly. After a moment's thought, he added diplomatically, "No one, that is, except the —"

"Gods," Quen finished amiably. "Yes, that's the ones. Hissia and Hanor, for certain."

"Don't forget Vorg and Veva," Ian warned.

"Really?" Quen gave him a quizzical look. "They'd get involved? She didn't *do* fire, did she?"

"But her 'brother' —" Ian shot a look at Torvan "— nice move there, by the way — he'll have his say."

"Well, if so, I imagine that Geros and Granna will just *have* to chime in," Quen allowed with a shrug. "Not to mention Ophidian —"

"He's getting *quite* full of himself these days," Ian agreed.

"So that's — what? — *seven* gods?" Quen surmised. She shook her head. "Oh, dear, oh dear! I imagine you'll be powerless before the sun rises tomorrow."

"And dead, not long after," Ian added looking at his sister, "wouldn't you say?"

"Certainly, certainly!" Quen agreed. She turned to Torvan and smiled, showing her one scraggly tooth. "So what's it to be, ducks? Dead before noon or —?"

"Or what?"

"You know," Ian said, moving closer. "You know the way of things. You understand power, teaching, faith — the right way of doing things."

"And we can help you," Quen said, moving up to stand beside Ian. "We can protect you, give you power you only imagined."

"Power to beat the gods," Ian said.

"No one can beat the gods!" Torvan Brookes exclaimed. "No man —"

"Precisely," Quen agreed. "No, a man against the gods is without hope."

"But, with a god?" Ian said temptingly.

"Against us, few dare raise their hands," the silent hooded one spoke up. His words were like dry leaves, dead men talking.

"Nice of you to join in," Quen said sarcastically.

Kor shrugged and nodded silently at Torvan.

"We can give you power that you could not imagine," Ian said. He raised a hand and a branch flew into it, growing larger, stronger, taller — powerful. He smiled at Torvan as he passed the staff to Quen.

"Good choice," she said approvingly. Another bit of wood flew to her hand and she bent it around the first piece, causing it to grow and expand until the two pieces were joined together into a twisting spiral staff taller than a man.

Kor took the staff and nodded at it. The two pieces writhed and glowed with power, flaring brightly with a light and heat that caused Torvan Brookes to flinch away, eyes closed. When the light dimmed, where the twin spiral staff had been there was now a staff made of four spirals, each a different color.

"We control fire," Ian said, waving a hand at one spiral which flared with heat and light.

"— water," Quen said, pointing to another strand which turned a liquid blue, like ice. She turned to Kor but the hooded one merely nodded. "Still won't do it, will you?" she snarled. She passed the staff back to Ian with a snarl.

"Air," Ian said, and another spiral turned misty white and seemed to write from top to bottom in an endless shimmer of bound motion.

"Earth," Quen said, taking the staff for a final time. The fourth spiral turned a rust brown color, grew more knobby, strong, stiff as it took on the form of the very iron of the earth below. She passed the staff to Kor, the hooded one who took it, twirled it swiftly, and waved a hand over one end. Where his hand moved, a large glowing pearlescent sphere formed, forcing its way inside the four spirals which tightened around it to bind it tightly. He paused, his dark eyes glowing as he stared at Torvan Brookes.

"Take this," Quen and Ian said in unison, "take our staff and be our servant with the power over all."

Torvan Brookes stepped forward, his eyes bright with desire, and grabbed the four-wood staff. He knelt in front of the three, dropped his head to the ground. "I accept your offer, Quenkorian."

"Done!" the three gods cried, even ghost-voiced Kor.

"Come," Quen said, moving forward and gesturing to him to stand up.

"We have much work to do," Ian added.

"But first," Quen said, her gap-toothed mouth opening in a parody of a smile, "you must be punished."

"Why?" Torvan asked.

"You're ours now, best you know what that means," Quen said with a gleeful chortle. The three bodies of the one god surrounded him, crushed together, then crushed him until all that could be seen was the staff and all that could be heard was Torvan's tormented wail.

And then they were gone, leaving only the sounds of torture in their wake.

# Chapter Five

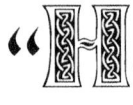ow much longer?" Chandra demanded as Hamo Beck led them into the cold blowing snow of the night's blizzard.

"Minutes," Hamo told her. He veered toward the right, westwards.

A cold wind kissed Chandra's cheek on the right. She reached up, felt her fingers chill.

"You are not leading us the straight way," Chandra said, her tone growing dark with menace.

"I —" Hamo started.

*BOOM!* The ground shook and the air rumbled as the earth moved. Hamo turned toward the young girl with wide eyes.

"Granna, Geros!" Chandra shouted, her voice carried by the ground beneath them. "I call upon you, beg your mercy!"

"We're going —" Hamo began but Chandra felt the cold breeze brush against her right cheek once more.

"Show me," Chandra said to the small air sprite at her side. "Mark the ground —"

"What are you —?" Hamo began but stopped as a small blast of air dug into the snow in front of them, marking a straight line. A line that led to the left of the path Hamo had indicated.

"I have *no time* for foolishness!" Chandra roared, her voice echoed once more by the rumbling of the ground.

"If we don't take the right path," Hamo explained, "they won't let us in."

"They'll let us in," Chandra said firmly, moving in front of Hamo and stomped off along the line indicated by the air sprite. "If they don't, *I'll* get us in."

Hamo hurried after the dark-skinned girl.

"Your majesty," Granno called, "there's a disturbance at the north entrance!" He made to guide her toward safety.

"What is it?" Diam, queen of the zwerg, asked. Her expression brightened. "Is it Margaret?"

As if in answer, the ground, the walls, all their caverns shook with a distance *boom*.

"That's not Margaret!" Lissy exclaimed. "She does air magic."

"That was earth magic," Diam agreed, her eyes going wide. She turned to Granno. "Powerful earth magic."

"Let me get you away, your majesty," Granno implored. "I always feared that the girl would sell you out, lead others to steal our treasures."

"No!" Lissy cried in horror.

"No," Diam echoed a moment later. "She is many things but she holds her honor dear."

"She is not her own master," Granno warned. "Recall that Rabel warned about this so-called Steam Master and she is his servant."

*Boom!* The quakes were getting stronger, closer.

"Get the others to safety," Diam ordered, gesturing for Granno to take Lissy. The little zwerg girl squeaked in surprise as the burly zwerg guard lifted her off her feet.

"Put me down!" Lissy shrieked. "Granno, put me down or so help me —!"

"I am following your majesty's orders," Granno told the girl firmly. "You might consider doing the same, princess."

Lissy turned her eyes on her mother. "Mother! Mother, I should be with you! I know about dragons, and I have Annabelle's elemental, I can... can..." she spluttered off, furiously trying to think of more to aid her cause.

"Granno, put the princess down," Diam said with a sigh. Granno gave her a surprised look but, at her insistent gesture, lowered the princess back to the ground. "After all, as she said, she is a princess." Diam smiled at her youngest. "And I've a spare safely in Ophidian's realm, so we can easily afford her loss."

"See, Granno?" Lissy said, giving their bodyguard and friend a triumphant look.

"Get the others away, leave a squad with me," Diam said. "We'll go to the gate and parley with whomever seems so excited to make our acquaintance."

"After, we'll seal that entrance," Granno growled. "It's too close to that dratted town anyway."

"Let's wait until 'afterwards' before we make our decision," Queen Diam declared. She reached down and grabbed her daughter's hand. "And now, my young princess, let's earn our crowns!"

With that she took off at a trot which she soon increased to a full gallop. Crying in joy and amazement, Lissy kept pace with her, waving at all the zwerg heading toward safety and laughing at their appalled expressions.

At the gate they halted, winded from their sprint. Abner Crippens, the human from the airship, and three of his men were there, carrying swords and spears. At the sight of the queen, Abner and his men bowed deeply. "Your majesty, we are ready to defend your life with ours."

Queen Diam's eyes lit with pleasure. "Arise, Sir Crippens. You and your men are most welcome this day." She moved close enough to whisper up to the midshipman's ear. "And I hope we don't need you."

Abner Crippens smiled back down at the diminutive zwerg queen. "Neither do I, your maj—"

The earth shook, the gates groaned in unison and dust fell from the ceiling.

"Stand ready, men!" Abner Crippens, newly knighted in the kingdom of the Silver Mountains, cried, rising to his full height, drawing his sword, and standing ready to defend his queen with his life. The three picked men arranged themselves around the two royals, their weapons raised, their eyes steady, their expressions fierce.

"No one has the strength to break these gates," Diam said assuringly to the men around her. "This is zwerg steel, and the stone is our —"

*CRACK!* A long line ripped through the floor, sending everyone tumbling to their knees.

Light, dim in the night and snow, burst in from the outside.

"I *said*, Hamo Beck, that I have *NO TIME!*" a young woman's voice roared over the sound of the earthquake. "Margaret is dying, we need a healer *now* and not when protocol *allows!*"

"Margaret is dying?" Lissy cried, rushing through the gap of the men's arms and leaping over the crevice in the ground in front of her. "Where is she? What can we do?" She turned back to the stunned assembly behind her. "Mother, send for the healer!" She turned to the source of the voice. "How bad?"

"She's dying, her back is cut to shreds," the woman — no, girl — replied, her voice filling with grief. "I came as quick as I could." A sob escaped her throat. "But it may be too late."

"She bled a lot," Hamo Beck added, moving carefully to avoid cracks, fallen rubble and the remains of the impervious zwerg steel, "she's nothing but meat on her backside." He stood beside the girl and rested a hand on her shoulder. "Chandra is right, if she doesn't get help soon —"

"She'll die," Chandra finished in a grim voice.

"I can send for the healer," Queen Diam said, stepping forward, gently pushing Abner Crippen's sword down, "but if the damage is as bad as you say…"

"There is only one person who can heal her," Lissy said, reaching into her vest and pulling out a bright light. She bent down over the glowing form and begged it, "Go! Go find Annabelle! Tell her we need them!" And with that, she threw the glowing elemental into the night sky.

"I'll have my healer come, to do what we can," Diam said, reaching to grab Lissy's hand.

"Thank you," Chandra said with a sob. "That's all I ask." She seemed to realize the destruction she'd created around them and gave the queen of the zwerg an apologetic look. "I'm sorry about all this," she said, "I'll clean it up."

"No," Diam said, "we'll seal this entrance up. It's not secure."

"I can help," Chandra said. "But please, we have to help my sister!"

The dinner was winding down, everyone was replete, the last of the port offered and politely rejected. The obvious next thing was to say thanks and head off to a well-earned slumber. But mage Margen was still nervous.

Spymaster Hewlitt had struck deals with Nelly Kendral regarding her school for mages, and with her father, Kenid "call me Nid" Kendral for expanded lodgings of the less dodgy sort — they all currently being seated in an alcove of the dining hall of the House of the Broken Sun — but he had yet to make a proposal or settle a deal with Margen himself. The mage was torn between being relieved and insulted.

Jarin Reedis glanced at Nelly, who stifled a yawn and turned to Hewlitt, saying, "Well, this has been a most enjoyable evening and —" he nodded toward Nelly who answered him with a game smile "— profitable for many, but I believe my dear betrothed and I should seek our rest."

"And just where, dragon-man, do you propose to do *that?*" Nid Kendral asked with a fierce expression.

"I have my quarters at the school," Nelly said quietly, glancing between her father and her betrothed. Shyly, she added to Reedis, "The bed's small."

"We'll manage," he assured her with a comforting look, patting her hand. He stretched his arms and yawned theatrically. "I am *quite* ready for slumber."

"Hmph!" Nid grunted. "If you think that *you're* going to spend the night with *my* daughter —"

"I do," Reedis told him firmly. Jarin added, "And I support him in this."

Nid turned to Margen. "You're a mage, what do you have to say to this?"

Margen blinked in surprise at being brought into this dispute. "Me?" Margen said. "Well, sir, I think that your daughter is well past the age where she needs permission." He smiled at Nelly. "She has shown herself to be resourceful, forceful, and well able to fend for herself."

"But he's *half* dragon!" Nid protested, waving a hand toward Jarin Reedis in emphasis.

"Today, your daughter faced down a god," Jarin said. "And, speaking from personal association — and full access to his memories — I will add that my good friend Reedis is not the sort to take advantage of any lady, let alone the love of his life."

"Well said," Hewlitt agreed quietly. He turned to Nid Kendral. "I'm more worried about you, to be honest."

"Me?" Nid barked in surprise.

"It's late enough that the walk home will not be well lighted," the spymaster warned. "However I think it might not be wise for you to seek to stay here the night."

"Mother would kill you," Nelly agreed.

"If you wish, I could escort you back," Margen offered.

"Aren't you staying at the school?" Nid asked. When the mage nodded, he continued, "Well, it seems to me that you'd have to go out of your way for that." He turned to Jarin Reedis. "I think the lad here can escort me and you can keep an eye on my daughter."

Reedis and Nelly started to protest but Margen spoke over them. "I think that's a perfect idea!"

Nid rose from the table, wobbling only a little. He glared down challengingly at Jarin Reedis. "Come on, lad, you can tell me about your prospects on the way."

Peter Hewlitt rose with the others, barely concealing a smile at the solution proposed by the senior Kendral.

Margen shot him a look and said, "I wondered if you wanted to speak with me this evening?"

"It's no great matter," Hewlitt replied, spreading his hands in a wide arc. "I was merely curious if you'd heard any word from your late students."

"You mean the ones Torvan Brookes stole?" Margen replied, his jaw clenched. He shook his head. "No, and I am concerned. Especially that you would ask the question. Does that mean you know something?"

"Actually," Hewlitt replied heavily, "it does not."

"And you should," Margen guessed. He nodded to himself. "If you haven't heard and I haven't heard, perhaps we should arrange to check on them."

"In the morning?" Hewlitt asked.

"Well," Margen temporized, "I have my classes."

"And more students," Nelly reminded him.

"Perhaps a field trip?" Hewlitt suggested.

"That," Margen said with feeling, "is quite an excellent idea!" He glanced to Nelly, and proffered an arm. "And now, my dear, shall we?"

Nelly took the arm and waved gaily to Hewlitt as she left on the arm of the last royal mage.

Jarin Reedis grabbed at Nid Kendral as the latter stumbled over a cobblestone, propping him upright.

"That's it lad, gotta keep an eye on the old man," Kenid muttered. "Don't want anything to happen to him 'fore the wedding!" He took a ragged, drunken breath, and added, "And when's that?"

"We hadn't set a date," Reedis told him in a quiet voice. "I only just asked her today."

"Well, you need my permission," Kenid warned, stumbling once more. "What are your plans, anyway?"

"We haven't had a chance to talk about plans yet," Reedis told him.

"So you're just hoping to marry her and stumble on through life?"

"I am too busy being amazed that she agreed to wed me, to be honest," Reedis told him.

"And why's that?"

"Well… until very recently I had little prospects," Reedis admitted. "Of course, now I'm twinned with a dragon. That's changed things a bit."

"I can bloody well imagine!"

"But I loved Nelly when I left for the north," Reedis said. "I'd never hoped that — but when I found about the academy —"

"And when was that?"

"When mage Margen told me," Reedis said. "I was quite affronted, thinking that someone would take my name for their profit."

"Hah!"

"Until I learned that it was Nelly," Reedis said. "And then…"

"What, boy?"

"Then I realized how much I meant to her," Reedis told him with feeling. "I hadn't even *hoped* — but she was going to remember me even if I was gone!"

"That's a woman for you," Kenid agreed. "Once they make up their minds, they won't let go." He stopped, pushed Reedis' hands off him and stood up straight, turning to stare at the other man. "That's the way with my wife, too," he said in a different tone. "If my Nelly wants you, there's nothing you can say otherwise."

"So I hope!"

Kenid Kendral snorted. He struck out a hand. "Well, you're part of the family now. It's best to get used to it because that's the way it'll be."

"For the rest of my life," Reedis said with feeling, taking the proffered hand.

"You be good to her, you hear," Kenid said, dropping their hands and turning back toward his tavern. "'Cuz if you don't, I'll skin you alive, dragon or no."

# Chapter Six

*Shh! Lie still or you'll break the moment!* The words came to Alain at the edge of his dream. *Don't move, just breathe steady, lad.*

Alain forced himself to relax. He was awake and yet not. Dreaming and still thinking, remembering. The voice spoke with a warm, deep tone. It reminded Alain of something… of —

*Lie still or you'll wake!* The voice warned him. It felt like he was being cradled in something soft and warm, like the cradle he was in as a baby. Alain forced himself to relax once more, adding a tendril of thought, *Like that?*

*Softer, easier. Just breathe, feel. Let yourself drift. You are safe. No one can harm you. Mother moon looks down on you, guards you with her soft light.*

Mother moon. Alain had heard that phrase before, when he was little. *Mother?*

*No,* the voice replied softly, *I fear she is long gone. She was only a little thing, poor foal! She met a human and — well, such things never end well.*

*My father,* Alain thought.

*They loved,* the voice replied, *and thought it was enough.* Alain felt a deep sadness, a sigh of tears shed long ago.

*Why wasn't it?* Alain wondered. Enough? Isn't love supposed to overcome all obstacles?

*To break the Way, one needs more than love,* the voice replied softly. *You, little one, you will come to know this yourself.*

Alain felt that the voice was crying for him. The thought made him angry. With a start, he woke up. He jerked up out of the blankets that covered him, moved harshly away, looking for the source of the words, the voice. There was no one around. Lisette Marie was sleeping as a horse far away. Mayse and Janzie were on guard duty, somewhere in the distance. Alain had settled himself near the hexine, far away from humans and centaurs alike. The hexine were standing on their six feet, sleeping upright. Only the little filly was lying on her side, near her mother.

After three angry circuits around his bedding, Alain settled back down, angrily. He'd lost half a night's sleep. *Dreams!*

The light woke her. Of course it would, moving closer and further, becoming impossibly bright and then faint. Ellen was a prudent sleeper, waking up easily, sleeping when she could. And — with the light — she couldn't.

"What is it?" she asked, her eyes still closed. She — and Annabelle, of course — were sleeping at the edge of one of Ophidian's impossibly large and impossibly comfortable beds, covered with just enough blanket to keep her from freezing. She managed to snag Bethany Margiss as a sleepmate — Ellen didn't like sleeping alone, wyvern twin soul or no. In truth, Bethany Margiss was all too happy to sleep with Ellen, being just so new that it helped to have the soft sounds of someone nearby. Imay had crawled in later, after they were asleep from whatever strange work Ophidian had enticed her into — something to do with Ibb, that new metal immortal, Tracker, Hana, Angus, and Ophidian himself. That group was tight as thieves. Ellen had been surprised to learn that the zwerg princess Imay was nearly fifty years old — hardly a *child!* — but the zwerg girl had assured her that zwerg were considered young for far longer than humans. *Fifty!* Ellen could hardly imagine such a number! Annabelle had kept silent when Ellen had expressed her amazement.

But now, here was this light. And no one answered her. Ellen put a hand over her eyes to protect them, then opened them.

"I know that light!" Annabelle exclaimed with Ellen's lips.

"You made it, and Captain Ford gave it to me!" Ellen said in agreement. She looked to the other side of the bed, where Imay was sleeping — snoring in that soft way of hers that she completely denied when awake. "Imay?"

Bethany Margiss, in the middle, snorted and turned in her sleep. She was bigger than Ellen — *everyone* was bigger than Ellen, even Annabelle — but the two souls were each only a few years older — well, three! — than her.

Imay grunted and turned toward Ellen. "Mprh? It's late, I'm tired. Can it wait until morning?"

Ellen sat bolt upright, twisting as she did so that she was looking across the bed and down at the zwerg princess. "That's not your light."

"Light?" Imay repeated woozily. And then she, too, shot upright, glancing toward Ellen, eyes wide with surprise. "The elemental?"

"Yes," Annabelle said. "I can feel it. It's not yours, though." She made Ellen's eyes grow wide with worry and surprise but before she could speak, Imay was out of the bed. "It's Lissy's!"

And then — Annabelle could not quite figure out how, later — everyone was out of bed, awake, alarmed, and shouting.

"What is it?" Krea's voice called from the doorway with Wymarc's fierce tones. "What are you all doing awake?"

"The light!" Ellen said, dropping her feet to the carpeted floor and pointing toward the bobbing elemental.

"Imay!" Wymarc began immediately, "How many times have we —" she broke off as Imay brought her elemental to life beside her and there were two lights — two elementals. "That's not your light."

"It's Lissy's," Imay said. "She sent it. Something must have happened." She turned to Ellen even as Bethany Margiss sat up, rubbing her eyes and stretching in the middle of the bed. "Can you take me to her?" She begged. "Now?"

"I've got to get some clothes on," Annabelle said, moving Ellen's body toward the dresser that she'd been given on her arrival. Ellen didn't have the nerve to ask if Ophidian had meant that the marvelous wooden armoire was really *hers* or just a loan. She'd never seen anything so pretty before. The clothes in it were just as amazing, silken undergarments, sturdy but richly-woven woollens and cottons — and the socks!

"Can I — we — come?" Bethany Margiss asked. Rather, Margiss asked for the both of them.

"I think you should," Wymarc said, her tone going firm and formal. "I'll let Ophidian know —"

"He knows," Ophidian said, moving to stand beside her in the doorway. He glanced toward Imay, his expression unreadable. "Your sister?"

"That's her light," Imay confirmed, pointing toward the light that was bobbing around Annabelle.

"I made it," Annabelle said. "Captain Ford gave three to Ellen here."

"Take a drake," Ophidian ordered. He glanced at Imay. "Do you want me to come?"

"Only if you wish it," Imay said, seeming suddenly all shy.

"They'll get dressed quicker if they don't have to worry about decorum," Wymarc told her great sire in droll tones.

Ophidian ignored her long enough to pull something out of his pocket — whether it had been there when he'd reached for it was of no matter — and toss it toward Imay who caught it with the practiced ease of someone who'd learned to read the dragon-god's body language. "Wear that, it will tell me if you need me."

Imay's face burst into a huge smile as she put the necklace over her head. At its end was a large, faintly glowing red jewel.

"If it turns white, I'm on the way," Ophidian assured her. And then he was gone, his last look for Krea Wymarc — a glance full of warning and meaning. On the chair nearest the door there suddenly appeared a bundle of clothes.

"Oh, very clever," Wymarc murmured, moving into the room and shutting the door. She went to the chair and started dressing herself. "Imay, it might be best if you rode my back." The zwerg princess gave her a startled look. "As a wyvern." Imay relaxed and nodded. Wymarc turned to Bethany Margiss. "I think it is too early for you to stretch your wings this night — would you object to riding on Ellen Annabelle?"

Bethany Margiss paused in pulling up her leggings long enough to give Ellen a wary look. The smallest in the room smiled at her, saying, "Annabelle is a full-grown wyvern, so it won't be a problem."

"Okay," Margiss allowed. Bethany had given her assurances and memories of when Skara Bethany had ridden before. She smiled at Ellen Annabelle. "This should be fun!"

"Less talk, more speed," Wymarc snapped.

Reedis found the bedroom by following his nose. Nelly always wore a certain scent that Reedis found heavenly. He smiled as he opened the door carefully and confirmed that he'd found the right room. And then… he froze.

He stood there looking at the dim shape lying under the covers. Could he? Should he?

"If you don't get in here right this second — and close the door — I'm going to freeze!" Nelly murmured from under the covers. As Jarin Reedis moved inside and closed the door, she added, "I've laid out bedclothes for you, they should fit."

Reedis found them, and started dressing, glad that the night kept his flushed expression from Nelly's probing eyes.

"Jarin," Nelly called from the bed, "be a pet and warm the room up. Not too quickly, it's all I can do to keep my eyes open."

Jarin, with a triumphant mental grumble to Reedis, did as requested.

Reedis, now dressed for bed, moved to the far side of the bed and tentatively lifted the covers.

"Please get in," Nelly said. "I'm afraid that it's all I can do to keep my eyes open." Reedis slipped under the covers and arranged his head on the bed, facing Nelly's eyes. "And cuddle," she said, reaching an arm around him. "I could do with a good cuddle."

"Too much blood," Molle said in a low voice as she examined the wounded girl in front of her.

"Will she live?" Chandra asked fearfully, the ground beneath them rumbling as a reflection of her worry.

"No one will live if you bring this place down around us," Queen Diam chided her. Drake had left the room at the first sight of the zwerg, nodding thankfully to the queen and Chandra. Hamo and Granno had arranged guards outside the tavern. Captain Welless had taken the whole scene in one quick glance, nodded toward Hamo, and ordered his soldiers back to their quarters.

"We should talk, later," Diam had told him just before he decamped.

"Drake!" Chandra called out. The dark youngster had popped his head back in, his eyes only for Margaret's bloody form. "Don't go too far, we may need you to fetch things."

Drake nodded and made to withdraw once more but Molle — the zwerg healer — stopped him. "We need fresh sheets, a soft comforter, hot water — that much for starters."

"Arnica?" Drake asked, surprising the others with his knowledge of the herbal.

"Not yet," Molle said in an approving tone, "but soon, perhaps."

Drake withdrew.

"She's so big," Lissy said, moving to the far side of the bed and kneeling beside it, "I'd forgot how big she really is."

A sound from the street caught Lissy's attention. And then the sound of running feet. Before they arrived, a bright light shot into the room and straight to Lissy's outstretched hand.

"They're here!" Lissy shouted to her mother. She turned her head and shouted through the door. "We're here!"

"Hurry!" Molle said, casting a worried look to her queen.

Imay was the first through the door. She was followed by a teenage albino girl. Then a girl of no more than ten who looked exhilarated, frozen, and fearful all at once. The last one in was a mere child, just out of infancy.

"Perhaps it's best if you —" Queen Diam began but the girl cut her off with an upraised hand and an expression that seemed far beyond her years. "Oh, Ellen!"

"We came as quick as we could," Ellen said, moving beyond the others and kneeling down, opposite Lissy. She gave the zwerg princess a quick smile and a nod. When she looked at Margaret's bloodied body, she hissed. She turned up flaming eyes at the others. "Who did this?"

"My father," Chandra said in a cold voice. "And who are you to ask?"

"Ellen Annabelle," the girl replied, dismissing the older teen with a glance. She moved to grab Margaret's bloodied hand where it lay down over the edge of the bed.

"Don't!" Chandra growled and the building shook. "Only the healer —"

"She's the healer, Chandra," Diam told her in a quiet voice. "This is Ellen Annabelle."

"She's just a girl!"

"And you're just an earth mage," Ellen replied, glancing back up toward her. She stood up and moved around the bed to crouch beside Lissy, putting a hand on the small zwerg princess' shoulder comfortingly.

"You know, I like her," Krea Wymarc said to Ellen Annabelle. "She's got spirit."

"She needs sense," Annabelle said with Ellen's mouth. To Ellen she said, "What can we do?"

"We have an oath," Ellen reminded her. She glanced around the room and raised a hand, pointing. "I don't know you —" she pointed at Molle, swiveled her hand to point at Chandra "— or you." She dropped her hand. "You have to leave."

"Ellen!" Annabelle hissed. Ellen's expression changed to one of startlement as her older twin soul explained, "That's not how it's done!"

"Well, it's either that or father comes and kills them," Ellen said.

"Molle is my healer," Diam said. "And what oath?"

"The same oath I swore, mother," Imay said. She purposefully kept her eyes from Ellen. "There are some things that cannot be known."

"My sister is dying," Chandra groaned. She glanced at Molle. "Won't you please help her?"

"Her wounds are beyond my powers," Molle told her in a sad voice. She glanced to Ellen Annabelle. "She is your best hope."

"Come, child," Diam said, reaching a hand toward Chandra. "Let's leave it to the healers. Your sister, who is dear to us, won't come to any harm."

But Chandra would have none of it, twisted out of Diam's grip and running toward Ellen. She reached for the girl but stopped when Ellen raised a hand with a hot flame burning at her fingertip.

"I don't want to kill you," Ellen told her coldly, "but I will if you don't leave this room."

Chandra started to reply just as hotly but Wymarc sighed and waved a hand. The earth mage's eyes grew wide and she collapsed on the floor. Ellen glanced around her to Krea Wymarc, brows raised in question.

"I don't like to advertise," Wymarc said, sounding both diffident and pleased at the same time. "We all have our powers, you know." Ellen's glance darted to the fallen teen. "She's asleep, that's all." She gave Ellen a challenging look. "Will you let her sleep here, beside her sister?"

Ellen pursed her lips tightly then nodded. She glanced to Lissy. Diam saw the look and motioned toward her daughter. "It's okay, it'll be boring. You can come and tell Imay all about everything."

The young zwerg princess brightened at the notion and slid away from Ellen, running to grab her mother's and sister's hands. Diam stood with them on either side of her for a moment, then backed out of the door. "Molle, perhaps you should come, too."

Molle nodded and stood up, backing away from Ellen while keeping a respectful distance from Krea Wymarc.

Krea Wymarc nodded to Bethany Margiss to close the door and stepped forward to kneel beside the stricken Chandra, repositioning her more comfortably. Satisfied, she turned to Ellen Annabelle. "That was uncalled for, you know. If you'd left it to me —"

"Or me," Annabelle agreed with Ellen's voice.

Krea Wymarc inclined her head in a nod, continuing, "We could have done that without so much drama."

Bethany Margiss followed the exchange with an expression of growing dread. She moved to Ellen Annabelle and knelt down beside her, laying a hand on her shoulder. She turned to Krea Wymarc and said, "She doesn't know what to do."

Ellen crumpled against her, her hand against her face doing nothing to stifle the sound of her sobs. "She's going to die and I can't help her!"

"Can't or won't?" Wymarc demanded.

"Shush!" Krea said with the same voice. "That's just wrong, Wymarc and you should know better."

"And should we?" Annabelle asked, turning Ellen's gaze on the older twin soul. Wymarc's expression altered. "That zwerg out there, Molle, she knows what's needed. She'll know — whether she's in this room or not — just what we must have done." She nodded toward the sleeping form of Chandra. "So will she."

Wymarc sighed. She met Annabelle's expression frankly. "So it will be, every time, you know," she told the twin soul pair. "Every time you use your magic, more people will know."

"But not everything," Bethany spoke up with Margiss' voice. The other two twin souls — Krea Wymarc and Ellen Annabelle — turned to her. "They'll know that healing was done but they won't know how."

"We could mask it," Annabelle said with sudden enlightenment.

"Make it smell different, seem more like witchcraft," Krea added in agreement. She patted her pockets and pulled out a small packet, tossing it Ellen Annabelle. She turned to Bethany Margiss. "Got anything else?"

"This is lavender," Ellen said, identifying the packet by its scent. Wymarc nodded.

"Rosemary," Margiss said, tossing a small packet toward Ellen. She turned to Krea Wymarc and explained, "I like to use it in cooking."

"Those will do," Wymarc declared.

"That's a disguise," Ellen agreed but her tone dropped as she added, "But I still don't know what to do."

"You touch her, you feel her pain, you draw it out and make it go away," Margiss told her in a slow, halting voice.

"Use your tears, child," Wymarc added. Ellen pulled her hands from her face and saw that they were wet, covered with tears.

"If you try, and nothing works, she can't be worse," Krea added.

Ellen nodded and pushed herself up to her feet. She leaned over Margaret but did not touch her. She placed her hands on either side of the teen's shoulders. She closed her eyes. She was grateful when she felt Bethany Margiss lay her hands on her shoulders, comfortingly. She smiled when she smelled the mixture of lavender and rosemary filling the room.

"Take my power," Margiss told her. "Add it to yours."

Ellen felt a surge through from the older girl's larger hands on her shoulders and — suddenly — she felt a surge of blue light magic seep through her. She thought it purple and pushed the magic through her wet hands onto the torn skin of the girl beneath her.

*Heal. Mend. Be whole.* Ellen moved her hands, her eyes still closed, slowly and steady over Margaret's body. She felt the pain but Annabelle soothed her, absorbed it. *We know pain, it is nothing to us.*

Ellen's hands moved lower, further down the back, down the legs — one hand for each leg — and slowly she made her way down to Margaret's ankles. The magic flowed through her, doing what she begged, healing, closing, mending, fixing, *helping* — and Margaret was whole.

Bethany Margiss caught her as, with a cry of anguish, Ellen Annabelle collapsed. She caught her and moved her away from Margaret's torn body, lowering her to the ground and going down with her, turning under her so that Ellen's head rested against her chest. She was crying — they both were crying but Ellen knew that the tears were not of sorrow.

From beyond her, on the bed, Ellen Annabelle heard a faint motion, a muffled groan, and a startled breath.

"You're safe," Krea Wymarc spoke out loud. "You're safe and with friends." She knelt down by Chandra's still form and touched the girl's temples. Chandra's eyes blinked and she looked up at Krea, startled. Wymarc told her, "Your sister is safe and whole."

"Margaret?" Chandra cried, rising to her feet and gazing at the body on the bed.

"Stay still!" Wymarc ordered as Margaret started to move. "We need to get you clothed, and fed immediately."

"I'm very thirsty," Margaret muttered to the pillow beneath her. Her whole body tensed as she asked her most feared question. "Father?"

"He's gone," Wymarc assured her in a cold tone. She turned to the door and called through it. "We need clothes! And soup!"

Grateful cries and thundering feet answered her.

# Epilog

A light spluttered in the darkness. General Michael Armand's eyes flew open and he reached for the knife under his pillow.

"You won't need that," an old — and familiar — voice assured him.

"Oliver?"

"Come, we haven't much time," mage Ingam Oliver said, throwing a bundle down onto Armand's chest. "Get dressed and hurry."

"What?" Armand said, sitting up and pulling the bundle toward him. Travel clothes. "Ingam, what is it?"

"Do you want to live?" Ingam Oliver, formerly commander of the Soria Army, asked his former apprentice.

"Who would think of killing me?" Armand demanded in reply.

"Oh, you're still woolly headed from sleep," Ingam replied with a touch of frost in his voice. "*Think!*"

"Why would the king want me dead?" Armand said, rising from his bed and pulling on the clothes with practiced fingers.

"And who is his greatest threat?" Ingam asked. "And how do you serve him, alive?"

"A dead traitor is worth more, you think," Armand said, fumbling into his trousers and pulling the warm tunic over his head. He glanced around for shoes, saw them beside the bed — sturdy riding boots — and pulled them on. "This is my uniform, surely it will stand out?"

"You're inspecting the guard," Ingam told him. "When you get to the gates, you'll have them opened and we'll ride out." His lips twitched. "When you don't come back is when someone will start to wonder."

"And by then we'll have found a change of clothes," Armand guessed. He frowned. "But where? And what then?"

"Where? Pinch or the shore, you chose," Ingam told him. "There are always those who need a good leader —"

"Only a winning leader," Armand muttered, moving to his coat rack and pulling on his overcoat.

"A losing leader who learns, costs less but knows more," Ingam told him.

Armand accepted that with a quick nod and gestured for Ingam to lead the way.

"The Pinch? Go over to the Emperor?" Armand guessed. Ingam nodded. "The shore? Seek employment in the navy?" He frowned and shook his head before Ingam Oliver could shoot him an outrage look. "No, head westwards or south for finer pickings."

"Think fast, you'll need an answer in half an hour," Ingam warned.

"That soon?"

"That late," Ingam replied grimly. "I think, if it weren't for the king's dalliance with the queen, he'd have had you in irons sooner." Ingam waved a hand and Armand felt magic settle over him.

"What did you do?"

"A simple blurring," Ingam said. "People who know you will forget, people who don't won't think twice of our passing."

General Armand grunted thanks. Ingam raised a finger to his lips, pushed one of the double doors open and peeked around it. A moment later, he stepped through, beckoning the general to follow.

## END

# Wyvern Rider

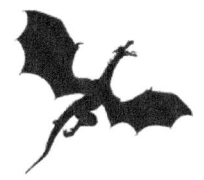

# Book 19

Twin Soul series

# Dedication

**For Buffy:**

**The best animal companion**

**anyone could ask for!**

# Chapter One

Peter Hewlitt, the spymaster, climbed the steps to the landing of the Reedis Memorial Academy two at a time early that morning. He dodged students who eyed him warily, grabbing one long enough to ask, "Mage Margen?"

"Follow me," a young girl said, waving a hand high enough for him to spot it. She couldn't have been more than twelve, not much older than the students Hewlitt had spied at Margen's classroom back the palace. Before Vistos. The girl turned to eye him suspiciously. "You seem a bit old."

"Your powers of observation are well-developed, I see," Hewlitt said.

"Miss Marcks!" Mage Margen's voice boomed from down the corridor. "I trust you are as ready with your skills as you are with your wit this morning!"

"Yes, sir, of course, sir!" the young girl, Miss Marcks, replied with a bob of her head and a glare toward Hewlitt. "It's just —"

"I can see, Miss Marcks," Mage Margen said sternly. "And I should *like* to see you in your place and ready to learn."

"Of course, sir!" Miss Marcks replied crisply, speeding up her pace but not before dropping a lingering glare on Hewlitt. She rounded the corner into the classroom just as mage Margen appeared in the doorway. She jerked a thumb to point back toward Hewlitt, saying in an undertone, "There's a stranger here, sir, I thought you should know."

"He *is* strange, Miss Marcks," Margen replied, his lips twitching, "but I can assure you he is not a stranger to me." Margen nodded toward Hewlitt, adding, "You're awfully eager this morning."

"I am worried," Hewlitt confessed, crossing the distance between the two. "There was enough trouble yesterday with Vistos but —" he stopped, glancing around the corridors to be sure that they were alone "— news early this morning has added an urgency to our mission."

Margen's brows creased. "To check up on the children?"

The sound of footsteps moving purposefully from down the hall distracted them. Hewlitt turned around in time to see Jarin Reedis and Principal Kendral moving quickly toward them.

"That," Hewlitt said as the others entered earshot, "and perhaps more."

"I have a school to run, and the mage here has classes to teach —" Nelly began.

"I know," Hewlitt agreed. He turned to Jarin Reedis. "But I don't know if the arrival of a dragon and a spy would be welcome by the mage's former students."

"And I would like to make some acquaintances down there," Nelly agreed, "perhaps see about setting up another establishment in Sorellay."

"Sorellay?" Margen repeated thoughtfully. "I suppose it's a decent enough size town to be able to take advantage of a school of magic."

"It's a port town, with plenty of traffic," Hewlitt agreed. "And it's a central point for the movement of grain and cattle in the south coast."

"But I can't just leave the children alone," Nelly declared. "They're paying to learn."

"Rather, their parents," Margen observed.

"Do you have any promising apprentices?" Nelly asked Margen.

"The King took my most promising pupils," Margen replied with a sour look at Hewlitt. He frowned. "After that, Miss Emer is perhaps my most —"

"I can do it!" a girl's voice cried gladly from inside the room.

"I can, too!" Miss Marcks added just as loudly.

"Hmm…" Margen considered the possibilities with an expression just bordering on terror. Finally, he shrugged and glanced toward Nelly. "They *could* manage for a class, perhaps two."

"Enough for the morning?" Hewlitt asked. "I doubt we'll be gone longer than that."

"Mother," Nelly declared suddenly. The three men turned to her in confusion. She gave them a small smile. "I can ask mother to help."

"My dear," Reedis said carefully, "I do not recall your mother being well versed in the ways of magic, so I —"

"Not magic," Nelly cut him off, "managing."

"Actually," Peter Hewlitt declared, "from all that I've heard about your mother, I would have to agree. It would take more than a school full of magicians to overwhelm her."

"Miss Marcks, Miss Emer!" Margen called. The two girls came rushing out, beaming from ear to ear.

"Well, they certainly seem eager," Nelly observed. She gazed at them menacingly. The two girls took a step back and toward each other. "Would you be willing to do this? My mother has run grown men out of her tavern, so she won't put up with any mischief in my school."

"I can't talk for Sarah but I know that *I* can manage a whole morning," Bree Emer declared resolutely.

"I can manage," Sarah Marcks declared staunchly.

"Well then, if we can get your mother to agree to this imposition —"

"I think we can," Hewlitt said, "seeing as she'll be a partner soon enough."

"Partner?" Reedis said with a barely concealed squeak. His last memory of Mrs. Kendral was of her waving a large poker in his direction and screaming about the destruction of their larder. The memory caused Jarin to snort in glee.

"Well, I'm sure that where Nid Kendral ventures, his wife can't be far behind," Hewlitt observed.

"I've met Mrs. Kendral once, I think," Margen said, his tone cautious.

"Good, then why don't you and Mr. Hewlitt go persuade her while Reedis and I see to things here," Nelly said.

Margen's expression grew more doubtful but, before he could respond, Peter Hewlitt grabbed him by the arm and pulled him down the corridor. Somewhat bewildered, Margen called over his shoulder, "Miss Emer, Miss Marcks, consult with Miss Kendral on your tasks for the morning!"

"Don't worry, if there's any trouble before you get back, Margen," Reedis said, "I'll let Jarin — *the dragon* — deal with any miscreants."

Silence fell abruptly throughout the school and Reedis smiled at the two substitute teachers and their principal. Nelly gave him a reproving look but he could tell her heart wasn't really in it.

"He's gone," Ophidian declared when he returned from a quick survey of the village. He'd arrived only a few moments after Margaret had been healed, his arrival heralded by the brilliant glow of Imay's necklace. The zwerg princess had been consulting with her mother when the glow had interrupted their conversation.

"You were worried, scared," Ophidian had said when Imay had first arrived, "I felt it."

Imay and Queen Diam had quickly filled him in on the nature of the emergency and Ophidian had needed no prodding to take off immediately to search for Torvan Brookes. He'd paused when he'd felt Ellen Annabelle use her magic — and a fainter magic of another — to heal the girl, Margaret. Imay had grabbed his arm in worry and had shaken her head at him, glancing toward her mother the princess. Ophidian had let out his worries with a sigh and a nod that promised that he and the zwerg princess would talk, later.

The exchange had not gone unnoticed by the zwerg queen but Diam was too smart to reveal that to the dragon god.

"What would you have done if you'd found him?" Imay asked him in a small voice.

"I do not tolerate such behavior," Ophidian replied shortly.

Queen Diam shot him an incredulous look. Before he could respond, the door from the bedroom opened and Krea Wymarc stepped through. She glanced to Imay who gestured to her mother and Granno. "Krea Wymarc, may I make you known to my mother, Queen Diam, and our trusted general, Granno?"

"Diam, it's been a long time!" Wymarc cried, moving forward to grab the small queen in a tight hug. Over her shoulder she informed the surprised Imay, "I knew you mother when she was little and —"

"Ahem!" Queen Diam coughed, moving away from Krea Wymarc and nodding pointedly toward her daughter.

Wymarc laughed, turning back to Imay. "Well, let's just say that we had some interesting times." Wymarc used Krea's hands to gesture to their human body. "Of course, I had a different twin at the time—" she broke off as a young man, a teenager, opened one of the other bedroom doors and peered out.

"My sister?" he asked the group hopefully.

"She is well," Krea said, pointing toward the open door. "I'm not sure if she's dressed, however."

"She is," Chandra said, emerging from the room and looking at the young man. "Come on in, I'm sure she'll want to see you."

"She's lucky to be alive," Wymarc muttered, casting a quick glance toward Ophidian. "Very lucky."

"Molle said there was nothing she could do," Diam noted.

"Some things we could teach you," Wymarc said. "But this was a major healing." She sighed theatrically, like she was drained. "It took the combined efforts of many." Imay, glanced between her mother and Ophidian before nodding in firm agreement.

"May I offer my congratulations?" Diam said, gesturing toward the open door. Wymarc glanced to Ophidian but the dragon god shrugged and waved the zwerg queen on her way. Diam reached for Wymarc's hand in passing and the two entered the room together.

Behind them, Ophidian chuckled. Imay shot him a quizzical look but the dragon god merely shook his head, saying, "I'll let her tell you." Then, cryptically, he added, "Or one of them."

Margaret was sitting up, dressed in soft pajamas with pillows propped behind her back. She looked exhausted, her eyes were red from crying, but she was smiling at her brother and sister, consoling them in soothing tones. Every now and then she'd glance toward little Ellen and Margiss, looking confused. She brightened when Krea Wymarc entered with Queen Diam.

"The god Ophidian says that your father has left," Queen Diam told the three children as soon as she could, her eyes tight on Margaret's eyes. She saw how the young woman reacted to the news.

"He was mad at me —" Margaret began apologetically. "I shouldn't have —"

"Anger does not require dismemberment," Diam replied forcefully. "And you are not obligated to apologize for the actions of another."

"But —" Margaret began.

"She's right," Ellen told her with feeling. Margaret frowned at her. Ellen was not to be deterred. "I saw your back. That was uncalled for."

"I agree," Diam said.

"He said that I shouldn't have negotiated with you —"

"Enough, child," Wymarc said, moving fully into the room and coming to stand behind Ellen and Margiss.

Margaret's look betrayed her surprise at being called a child by someone who looked only a few years older than herself.

"Margaret Waters, air mage," Diam said, drawing attention to herself, "may I make you known to the twin soul wyvern, Krea Wymarc, her companion wyverns Ellen Annabelle, and Bethany Margiss?" She waved from the others to Margaret. "Ladies, may I make you known to a powerful magic user and kind heart?"

"You're — you're wyverns?" Drake Fisher said, standing back, his eyes going wide.

"Don't wyverns eat people?" Chandra asked, stepping to stand beside him, both taking positions in defense of their bed-ridden sister.

"Only when we're *really* hungry," Wymarc said with a flash of her eyes.

"Wymarc, please!" Krea said with the same voice. "They're scared and they don't know any better!"

"Wymarc," Diam said, "to my certain knowledge hasn't eaten anyone in the last hundred years or more."

"How do you know?" Margaret asked, glancing fearfully from Krea Wymarc to Queen Diam.

"Because," Diam said with a chuckle, "for nearly a hundred years I was her rider."

"What?" Imay cried from the doorway, with a look of pure amazement.

"What's a rider?" Ellen said to Krea Wymarc.

"You haven't told them?" Diam demanded of Wymarc.

"There hasn't been time," Wymarc said defensively. "And I didn't want to frighten them."

"Time?" Diam repeated, her brows creasing thoughtfully. "Frighten them?" She glanced toward Ellen Annabelle and Bethany Margiss and then back to Wymarc. A suspicious look warped her features. "Wymarc, just how *old* are these two?"

"Father," Wymarc called through the door, "I think you might want to join us." When she got no response, she called again, "Father?"

Imay glanced about her and, in surprise, reported, "He's not here."

# Chapter Two

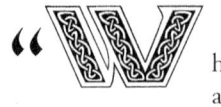"hy, Ophidian, how nice to see you!" Avice called as the dragon-god appeared with a stern-looking man in tow. "What brings you — uninvited, as always — to our humble abode?"

"Where's Terric?" Ophidian demanded, glancing around the large dining hall. "Is he in the garden?"

"And what need do you have of Terric?" Sybil asked from the kitchen.

"I wish to make him an offer," Ophidian said.

"An offer, really?" Terric said, arriving suddenly in front of Ophidian. His brows furrowed as he spotted the other man. With a bite to his tone, he added, "You bring a mortal in here and have me speak?"

"Terric, god of Death, permit me to introduce to you Sentonius Dakken," Ophidian said, waving a hand to indicate the blonde, blue-eyed man standing beside him. His lips quirked as he added, "You perhaps would recall Merus Dakken."

"Oh, another of your get!" Terric said, sounding relieved. He nodded toward the twin soul dragon who nodded back. "And my apologies on your friend Merus," Terric said, "if I recall correctly, his loss was unexpected."

"Sentonius had been our rider for a long time," Dakken replied with a growl. "He has done well, since."

"Well, good," Terric said. He returned his attention to Ophidian. "What do you want?"

"I wish to offer a temporary trade," Ophidian said.

"A trade?" Terric's brows rose. "I'm not in the habit of —"

"Quenkorian has made a four-power mage," Ophidian said.

"A four-power mage?" Avice said. "Are you certain?"

"Torvan Brookes, formerly known as the Steam Master, found his true calling," Ophidian said grimly. "He was always attracted to power and pain; he lost control and gave way to it completely." Quickly he detailed what he'd learned of Margaret Waters and her punishment.

"How do you know he did this?" Sybil challenged.

"Magic has a smell, at least for me," Ophidian said. "And some magics, the stench they leave is unmistakable."

"If he has created a four-powered mage, he has a purpose for him," Terric said grimly. He looked to Avice. "You remember the last time?"

His mate, the god of Life, nodded. Terric returned his attention to Sentonius Dakken. "And so why bring him? What trade?"

"Since that interloper —" Ophidian began.

"Lyric?" Avice interjected.

Ophidian nodded. "Since she came to your house, the defenses have been weakened."

"Anyone who wants to deal with me will get only what they deserve!" Terric declared with a chuckle.

"You are not the only thing of value here," Ophidian replied. He nodded toward the library behind them. "And, last time, books were destroyed that may not have copies elsewhere in the world."

Terric's eyes narrowed at Sentonius Dakken. "Pardon me for saying this but you don't look the scholarly type."

Sentonius barked a laugh which Dakken cut off. "My current form confuses many," the dragon replied. "But consider Merus, if you please."

"Hmm," Terric grunted, accepting the dragon's words. He turned his attention to Ophidian. "A trade?"

"No living man may destroy a four-power mage," Ophidian said. "And," he added grimly, "I believe that this one has *five*."

"What, you want me to raise the dead?" Terric barked in surprise.

"Not raise, just loan," Ophidian replied.

Avice started laughing, raising a hand and pointing a finger at Terric. "You should see your face!"

"Sentonius was a guard before Dakken recruited him," Ophidian explained. "Since, he's learned magic but he applies it in a special way."

"To guard," Avice guessed.

"You may think that you are safe from intrusion but Lyric proved otherwise," Ophidian reminded them. "I would prefer you not be molested."

"So you would trade the services of your dragon-get, for what?" Terric asked. His brows were raised in curiosity. They lowered slowly as a possibility presented itself. "Oh, no! You can't mean —!"

"I only ask because I can guess what will come," Ophidian said. "I need guards for Ellen Annabelle and Margiss Bethany."

"Annabelle is —?" Avice began in surprise.

"A wyvern, saved by the tears of Ellen, shed on my fingers," Ophidian said.

"So you've got your power back?" Sybil asked, her tone dubious.

"Through Ellen only," Ophidian said.

"We've met Annabelle," Terric said. "She was a good person. This Ellen —"

"She was a street urchin and doomed to die young except that Captain Ford —"

"I remember her!" Terric declared. Everyone stopped to look at him. He flushed and quickly explained, "I wanted to learn more about Captain Ford, after his death. So I had a chat with his memories."

"His memories?" Sentonius Dakken asked.

"This is not something that is repeated," Ophidian warned harshly. The twin soul dragon nodded once in understanding. Ophidian accepted the commitment with a jerk of his chin and turned back to Terric. "His memories?"

"Well, he wasn't going to need them where he was going," Terric said defensively. "Ellen reminded him of himself. He gave her something —"

"Elementals from the zwerg caves of the shattered hills," Ophidian said. "Annabelle enticed them and gave them to Ford as —"

"Partial payment for her passage," Terric finished. "So the girl survived? How did that happen?"

"Captain Ford, mostly," Ophidian said. "She was set by him to spy on Rabel —"

"Hrrmph!" Terric grumbled. "Your latest violation of the rules of life."

"Rabel, of course, took her under his wing and started to teach her magic," Ophidian continued amiably. "When a poisoned quarrel was shot at Ellen, Annabelle leaped in front of it, saving the girl's life —"

"At the cost of her own," Terric recalled sourly. "And then your Ellen used *your* magic to bring her back to life."

"As a wyvern," Ophidian corrected. "And became the wyvern's twin soul."

"They must make quite a pair," Sybil said approvingly. She cocked an eye toward Ophidian. "And their power is —?"

"To heal," Avice said with a catch in her voice.

"Annabelle was poisoned," Ophidian said. "The poison lives in her veins and causes her permanent pain."

"And your Ellen keeps her alive with her love," Avice said, smiling. "And together, they can make poison or —"

"They can heal wounds," Ophidian finished. "So, can you spare me your dead for their protection?" He nodded toward Sentonius Dakken. "I guarantee that you shall be equally rewarded."

"There is more," Avice said, sending Ophidian a sharp glance.

Ophidian sighed. "Mage Vistos worked with Quenkorian. He developed a sweet that poisons the soul —"

"Yes, we're aware of it," Avice remarked dryly. "He used it on Skara Ningan."

"He tried to poison Margen's granddaughter, Margiss —"

"And so now she is a wyvern, too?" Avice guessed.

Ophidian nodded. "Bethany Margiss."

"And what is *their* power?" Avice prompted.

"I'm not quite sure," Ophidian admitted. "Healing, certainly but it seems like they are able to heal the soul."

"You are saying that you've begotten a Soul-Healer?" Sybil cried.

Ophidian nodded. "So, perhaps you see why I want them protected." He glanced around. "Where's Bryan?"

"Here, as always," the Ferryman said, dropping two gold pieces into his father's hand. Terric accepted them with a grateful smile. Bryan said to Terric, "Is he asking to take your two souls off your hands?" Before Terric could reply, he added, "If so, I heartily approve. Your Walpish is always beating me at chess."

"I said you needed more practice," Avice told her son in the tone used by mothers through all generations — gods or no.

"Thomas, Skara!" Terric called. The two dead humans came sauntering through the door from the garden.

"My lord?" Thomas asked. He caught sight of the others. "Great god Ophidian, to what do we owe the honor?"

Ophidian glanced to Terric who gave him the barest of nods in agreement. Ophidian smiled. "Colonel Walpish, Assassin Ningan, how would you like the job of a lifetime?"

"A lifetime?" Thomas Walpish replied with a sly grin. "I'd say that you are too late for that, great god."

"You know what I mean," Ophidian grumbled.

Skara nudged Walpish with her elbow. "Why did you think to call upon our services, great god?"

"The god who killed you has created a five-powered mage," Ophidian explained.

"And how may we aid you?" Thomas asked.

"Torvan Brookes, who was the Steam Master, accepted Quenkorian's staff not a day past. There are two twin soul pairs who —" he broke off, continuing in a software voice, "— all my children are dear to me. But Ellen Annabelle is the only wyvern who can create new wyverns."

"And dragons?" Dakken asked.

Ophidian shrugged. "That remains to be seen. I know also that she has created a centaur from a wounded horse and a dead girl —"

Terric hissed and Ophidian shot him a look.

"The two just lately have repaired the damage done to another mage — Margaret Waters — by her adoptive father, Torvan Brookes."

"You think he will want revenge?" Skara asked.

"Him, or Quenkorian," Ophidian said.

"We're dead, my lord, how can we help?" Thomas asked.

"For now, you are as alive as the distance between one heartbeat and the next," Ophidian said.

"Technically, between the last heartbeat and eternity," Terric muttered, eyeing his gardeners darkly.

"But you are alive," Ophidian said. Terric nodded in agreement. "You are also dead."

"Yes, my lord?" Thomas said questioningly.

"He wants to tell you but he cannot," Avice said with a small smirk. She jerked her head toward Terric. "Only he can tell you."

"If you wish to keep a secret, we shall not press you," Skara said respectfully to Terric.

"What the dragon god cannot tell you is that no living soul may kill a four-powered or five-powered mage," Terric admitted with a sigh. He turned his gaze on Ophidian. "Mind you, until this moment, I thought that meant that only Gaban the Mighty had the power to defeat a four-powered mage but now…"

"You're reconsidering the prophecy," a sorrowful voice declared. Thomas and Skara started at the sound of the voice coming from beside them. Hansa, god of fate, stepped forward, turning his head to the two undead and then back to Ophidian. "Always mucking things up, aren't you?"

"And it's good to see you, too, brother!" Ophidian declared cheerfully. "Especially seeing as you just confirmed my suspicion!"

"You think I didn't *know* that!" Hansa harrumphed. He grimaced at Ophidian, nodded toward the others, gave Thomas and Skara a baleful look and warned them, "Even the dead must take care when dealing with the gods!"

And then he disappeared.

"Cheerful, as always," Ophidian said with a grin toward the empty space. He turned his attention back to the two undead. "And now that we've cleared that up, what say you?"

"They should train, too," Sentonius spoke up, glancing appraisingly at Walpish and Ningan. "Learn magic," Dakken added approvingly. He glanced to Ophidian and winked at Terric, "*More* magic!"

"Magic?" Ophidian murmured to his brother god. Terric looked flustered and Avice laughed.

"How do you think he beats me at chess?" Bryan asked.

"I *read*, Bryan," Thomas Walpish declared, waving a hand toward the library.

"Books on magic, no doubt," Bryan replied, adding under his breath, "And to think, *I* invented the game. *Shah mat*, it was in the old days. Kings would play me for weeks trying to win their lives back —" he broke off, casting a wary look at his father.

Terric chuckled. "But you never told them that you did not have that power."

"Weelll," Bryan said with an unrepentant shrug, "it helped pass the time."

"And it was amusing," Avice guessed.

"That, too," Bryan conceded.

"They are all — with the possible exception of Annabelle Ford — young girls," Ophidian said entreatingly to Thomas and Skara. "Margaret Waters was whipped — her whole backside — until she was in tatters —"

"We'll go," Thomas said, reaching a hand toward Skara who took it firmly and added a nod of her own.

"Good," Ophidian said. He nodded once toward Terric, and Avice, and disappeared.

"If you please, my gods," Sentonius Dakken said with a nod to each, "I should like to see to your stables and place wards."

"Wards?" Avice asked.

"One can never have too many wards," Sentonius told her gravely.

Avice raised an eyebrow and waved a hand invitingly, gesturing toward the stables.

"When you're done, would you care for a game of chess?" Bryan asked hopefully.

"We'd be delighted, great god," Dakken chuckled.

# Chapter Three

"What are you doing here, child?" a voice called out in the darkness. "It's cold tonight and this is no place for you." The man gestured to the camp beyond him. "The prisoners are tough soldiers —"

"I'm looking for my father," Babette Collet replied firmly. "This is the last camp. I've searched all the others."

"Your father?" the guard repeated.

"Captain Louis Collet," Babette replied, lifting her head in pride. "He served with the second company, first battalion under General Adkins. His battalion commander was Colonel Molet."

"Come back in the morning!" the guard called.

"It's been days and I haven't seen him," the girl cried, her face twisting in sorrow. "My mother died and he's the only one —" She broke off with a sob and raised her arms entreatingly. "Do you have a daughter, sir?"

The guard's expression shifted and he twisted his head to look quickly behind him. Then he shouldered his weapon, and waved her through. "If anyone asks," he warned her, "you didn't come this way."

Babette smiled at him and rushed through, scampering out of sight behind him as she ducked behind the nearest of the tents.

The guard shook his head. This was the fourth urchin he'd let slip pass in the past few days; none of them had come back with good news.

"Beastly cold, isn't it?" Colonel Lewis said as he stepped up by the giant wheel — the helm, the airmen called it, slapping his hand against his shoulders in an attempt to warm up. The helmsman spared him a look, relaxed when he realized it was only the cavalryman and turned his attention back to his steering. A moment later, he allowed, "It's warmer by the fire, sir."

"Fancy a break?" Lewis asked affably. The helmsman gave him a startled look. Lewis continued relentlessly, "We're how many thousands of feet up? Nothing to hit. All I have to do is keep the front pointed in the right direction while you warm up. Nothing to it." He moved forward, arms outstretched, ready to take the wheel.

"It is beastly cold," the helmsman allowed.

"You'll only be gone a few moments," Lewis agreed. "Here," he reached for the wheel, "let me try."

The helmsman reluctantly stood back. He spent a few moments correcting Lewis' style and then he sprinted off, toward the warm glow of the coal fire that powered the steam engine.

Lewis smiled to himself. *I always wondered how hard it could be to steer one of these!*

It took just a little more skill than keeping a horse moving in the right direction — less, if you considered that you didn't have to kick the airship to get it moving. Lewis peered ahead into the dark, whitened by the occasional flurry of snow. He couldn't see a thing.

"The eagleman Ikar, Your Highness!" a page's piping voice squeaked as the doors to Prince Paulus' throne room opened.

"Enter and report!" Jenid Paulus ordered from his throne. The harsh-faced Ikar rushed in, trailed by another hawk-faced eagleman, and both knelt. "Rise and report," Paulus ordered with a flick of his fingers.

"We are back from our scouting mission to the Jasram Plains, Your Highness," Ikar said.

"And?"

"We found nothing —"

"But the reports were of a wyvern! What of that?"

"Long gone, Your Highness," Ikar replied.

"So what *did* you see?" Paulus demanded.

"We kept to the heights to get range and speed," Ikar replied. "Our eyes see far. All across the plain we saw nothing moving."

"And you think to waste my time with *that?*" Paulus screeched.

Ikar spread his hands, palms down. "It is what we saw."

The other eagleman bobbed his head up, and nerved himself to say, "We scared the wyvern away, Your Highness."

Paulus glared at the man but said to Ikar, "You let your minions talk?"

Ikar punched out, catching the other eagleman in the jaw and sent him sprawling. He returned his attention to the Prince, "Not more than once."

Paulus chuckled. "So what do we do now?"

"Your Highness, what the loud-mouthed chick did not report, because he is too dim-witted to see, is how much we didn't see," Ikar replied.

Paulus cocked an eyebrow up.

"There was no signing of trading, of tilling, of *anything*," Ikar said.

"Perhaps they're all dead," Paulus replied. "That was the plan, after all."

"So I understand," Ikar replied. Meanwhile, the other eagleman — Ostan — shuffled back upright, spitting out a tooth and a pool of blood which he caught in his outstretched hand.

"But?" Paulus leaned forward in his throne encouragingly.

"I wonder if that was what we were supposed to see, Your Highness," Ikar replied.

"What do you suggest?"

"I think we need to get down to the ground —"

"That was why I sent you, if you recall," Prince Paulus interjected, his expression clouding.

"If I had a troop of cavalry with me, we could have landed and had them launch us," Ikar replied. "But… landing on a flat plain — we cannot get airborne again." He shrugged. "And my report to you would take weeks, rather than days to return."

Paulus' expression hardened into a frown. "Thinking above your station, are you, eagleman?"

Ikar shook his head quickly. "No, Your Highness. I merely offer a suggestion."

"It is not your place to offer suggestions," Paulus said, waving them away. "If I want you, I'll call for you."

Ikar touched his head to the ground, waved a hand at the other eagleman, who repeated his gesture and then the two of them slowly backed away.

"If there are no hexine, I'm ruined," Paulus said after long thought.

"Your Highness, if I may," a dark-robed man stepped forward from the shadows. "There may be another explanation."

Paulus turned toward the mage and gestured for him to explain.

"Perhaps the wyvern has been taking the hexine," the mage suggested.

"Taking them?" Paulus snapped. "Where?"

The mage raised his arm and pointed through the ceiling.

Paulus' eyes bulged as he followed the hand upwards.

"Where were you?" Wymarc asked when she spotted Ophidian entering the room. Ophidian gave her a smug look and shook his head, glancing around to the others in the room. Margaret Waters was dressed and sitting up at the side of her bed, sipping a wholesome smelling soup. The dark girl with the fierce temperament was kneeling beside her, urging her on with soft, kind words.

The dark boy — who looked nothing like his 'sister' was standing against a wall, arms crossed, eyeing everyone suspiciously. Ophidian's lips twitched and he gave the lad a silent salute.

"The girl is Chandra, earth mage," Wymarc informed him, following his gaze. "The boy is Drake —" she put an emphasis on his name with a wry look at the dragon god "— Fisher, fire mage."

Ophidian nodded to each in turn.

"You're looking awfully pleased with yourself," Diam, who had been outside, talking with her family, said when she noticed his return. Her voice sharpened as she added, "What's up?"

"Before we get lost in another of father's —" Wymarc began haughtily.

"You're here!" Bethany shouted, jumping up from the others and racing toward an empty space behind Ophidian. "How did you —?"

"Bethany Margiss, what are you —?" Ellen Annabelle asked as she tried to comprehend her friend's sudden movement. Her jaw dropped. "How did *they* get here?"

"You're dead, I saw it," Bethany said sorrowfully. "I —" she gestured to her body, Margiss' body, "— I wouldn't have left you —"

"Would someone tell me *what* is going on?" Wymarc demanded loudly in Krea's voice, turning the young albino girl's eyes accusingly toward Ophidian.

"I made a deal," Ophidian told her.

"A deal?"

Ophidian nodded and pointed to Ellen Annabelle and Bethany Margiss. "The girls are going to need protection. They're going to need to learn to defend themselves —"

"Yes, yes!" Wymarc interrupted, raising Krea's hand dismissively. "We all know that! What has that got to do with —" She broke off, suddenly pointing toward the shadows on the floor "— who is here?"

"It's Skara!" Bethany cried, wrapping her arms around thin air and squeezing. "Skara and the colonel!"

"Who?" Diam demanded, glancing toward Bethany and suddenly taking a step back, arms outstretched to force her daughters protectively behind her. She glared at Ophidian. "A new trick?"

"They're the best," Ophidian agreed with a dip of his head. He turned to the others. "Who all sees our friends?"

"I see two people," Margaret said in a dead voice, "a man and a woman."

"As do I," Imay agreed. A hiss of surprise from beside her indicated that Lissy also saw them.

"I don't know what you're talking about," Granno grumbled, his eyes heavy with accusation for the dragon god.

"I see them," Molle said with a sad shake of her head. She gave Ophidian a hard look. "Why do you rob the dead of their rest?"

"I don't," Ophidian replied. He waved a hand toward the shadows and said a soft word. The two figures appeared to all. "Skara Ningan and Thomas Walpish have agreed to aid us, temporarily."

"Are you alive again?" Bethany squeaked, hugging Skara tighter.

Skara reached down and stroked Margiss' hair. "No, child, our time has run."

"Except for the very last bit," Thomas Walpish added. He glanced toward Ellen Annabelle. "The time after our last heartbeat."

"Who must know?" Ophidian said, his eyes on Ellen Annabelle.

"Imay is oathsworn already," Annabelle replied with Ellen's child voice. "It is unfair to force her to keep an oath from her mother." Her eyes darted to Lissy. "Or to Lissy." She turned to Margaret Waters. "She —"

"Wait!" Wymarc said, stepping between Ophidian and the rest of the group. "It is time to explain more, father."

"Really?" Ophidian teased her. "I think oaths should come first."

Wymarc pursed Krea's lips until the albino girl won back control of her body. "Ophidian, what is she going on about?"

Ophidian laughed. "Very well, those who are willing to swear their lives to me, step into this room or remain inside."

Imay glowered at him and shot a beseeching look to Wymarc, who nodded in encouragement, adding, "Granno should know, too."

"He's past due telling," Imay agreed, reaching to snag her bodyguard's arm and drag him in. "Lissy —"

"She deserves to know," Ellen said. "And —"

"I'm a princess," Lissy said, raising her head regally.

"You two," Ophidian pointed toward Chandra and Drake, "I think you would like to be here."

"At what price?" Chandra demanded. She glanced toward Margaret. "And what of our sister?"

"That is why you should come here."

"Captain Welless —" Imay began.

"I've made an oath already," Captain Welless said, moving away from the door.

"You may want to rethink that oath," Thomas Walpish warned him. Welless stopped and gave Walpish a hard look. Then he nodded and joined the others. "I remember you."

Thomas Walpish smiled.

"Hamo, come along," Diam ordered as the taller man started to move away. "It'll be crowded but I'm pretty sure you'll find it worth your loyalty."

"I don't —" Ophidian began, frowning at the half-zwerg.

"Father," Wymarc interrupted, "I think we should take all the help we can get."

Ophidian eyed her for a moment then turned back to Hamo Beck. "If you wish."

The room wasn't as crowded as it should have been. Wymarc glanced knowingly toward her father, the dragon god and waited for the others to notice. She saw that Ellen Annabelle — probably Annabelle — was the second to catch on. Margaret Waters, surprisingly, was the third.

"The size of the room doesn't matter," Ophidian said as the others started muttering among themselves. "I don't like being crowded."

"I recall," Diam said drolly.

"This is no time for levity," Wymarc told Diam reprovingly.

"Quenkorian has given Torvan Brookes a five-power staff," Ophidian told them. Wymarc gasped, Diam cut off a cry, and the others looked alarmed.

"Nothing can stand against a five-powered staff," Wymarc said. "Not earth —" she nodded toward Chandra "— not fire —" a nod to Drake "— nor air —" a nod to Margaret "— nor water."

"What about me?" Ellen Annabelle asked.

"The fifth power is for you," Wymarc told her with sympathy in her expression.

"What is the fifth power then?" Margaret asked.

"Pain," Bethany Margiss replied immediately. "Torvan Brookes was all about pain."

"He's not the only one," Ellen Annabelle said, reaching to clasp hands with Bethany Margiss.

"He will attack when you are alone," Wymarc said, her eyes going first to Ellen Annabelle and then to Bethany Margiss.

"His god doesn't know about you, and that is your first defense," Ophidian said. "It won't last."

"What about them?" Drake asked. "They're just girls —"

"They are wyverns," Wymarc said. She glanced toward Ophidian. "And, I think now would be a good time to get oaths, don't you agree?"

"Those who stepped into the room took the oath," Ophidian told her with a grin. He nodded toward the group. "If they hadn't meant it, they would have burst into flames."

"Really?" Chandra asked, her eyes alight with wonder.

"He's a god," Margaret reminded her. She glanced toward Ophidian. "And one of the first."

Wymarc snorted but Ophidian ignored her.

"Ellen Ford did it," Ophidian said softly. All eyes turned to the little girl. "When an assassin —" he nodded toward Skara "— tried to kill her with magic, Annabelle Ford intercepted the dart and took the poison."

"That was Jenthen Barros," Skara Ningan said. She glanced apologetically to Ellen Annabelle. "We trained together under Vistos."

"Who is, happily," Thomas Walpish piped up, "quite dead."

"Ellen did it," Ophidian repeated, his eyes flashing at the interruptions. "When Annabelle died, she challenged me —"

"Father could heal, once," Wymarc interjected.

Ophidian glared at her for a moment before continuing, "— to heal Annabelle." He shrugged. "I could not —"

"Then how?" Lissy asked, eyes wide. Her mother grabbed her shoulder warningly. Lissy glanced up toward her in curiosity, then realized her mistake and curtsied to Ophidian. "I'm sorry, great god," she said, "but your story is awe-inspiring."

Ophidian accepted the apology with a nod and a grin. "As I was saying, I could not," Ophidian repeated himself. He nodded to the smallest child in the room, Ellen. "But Ellen taught me how to use her tears —"

"And we brought Annabelle back as a wyvern," Ellen said. "But she was insane with the pain of the poison —"

"Vistos' poison," Skara muttered darkly, her hand going to her jaw in memory.

"So Ellen," Annabelle now took control of the child's voice, "called me back and we became a twin soul."

Ellen smiled at the memory.

"And then they discovered that they could make wyverns on their own," Bethany said, pointing toward herself in Margiss' body. She nodded toward Skara. "First with Skara and then —" she shook her head regretfully "— with Margiss when Quenkorian killed Skara." Her eyes went to the assassin, still not believing her presence.

"They discovered more," Ophidian said.

"They can heal," Margaret Waters guessed.

"And kill," Annabelle said, using Ellen's voice, an expression on her face so grim that no child could ever make it.

"You healed Margaret?" Chandra asked, moving toward Ellen Annabelle and going to her knees in front of her. When Ellen Annabelle nodded, Chandra said, "How may I repay you?"

"I had help," Ellen said defensively, nodding toward Bethany Margiss. "Bethany's power is different —"

"Yes, I was wondering about that," Ophidian murmured. Diam and Molle gave him thoughtful glances.

"All the wyverns have their own unique powers," Wymarc said. Quickly she added, "We try to keep them secret, lest they be used against us."

"Or cause you to become targets," Thomas Walpish guessed.

"Riders, father," Wymarc interrupted in consternation, "we need to tell them about riders." Ophidian glanced toward her. "*Now.*"

Ophidian nodded and smiled at her, turning to Diam. "Queen Diam, why don't you tell them?"

# Chapter Four

"Come in then," a gruff voice called from the outside of a crowded tent. Rough hands pulled Babette Collet into the tent. It smelled of too many men and too few baths. Babette, who herself had not seen water for many days, found the odor easy enough to ignore. What she could not ignore, however, were the grim faces on the men in the tent, particularly the one standing at the front.

"I am General Dartan," he said, catching Babette's eyes, "who might you be?"

"If it pleases you, sir, I am Babette, the daughter of Captain Collet," Babette said meekly.

"Captain Collet!" "I heard of him, good man!" Many other voices rumbled in agreement.

"I was looking for my father," Babette said. A motion caught her attention and she noticed that there were four other girls in varying ages standing beside the general.

"So are they," General Dartan affirmed, pointing to the other girls. He turned toward a small, ratty man. "So, Amuir, do you need more?"

The man frowned at Babette and then at the other girls. He turned to the general and shook his head. "There are more than enough questions for me," he said. "But, general, do you really want an answer to this question?"

"What question?" Babette asked with a frown.

"Do you want to know where your father is, child?" General Dartan asked. When Babette nodded, he gestured toward the ratty man again. "Mage Amuir can cast a spell, using you as a guide, to help us find him."

"Why not the others?" Babette said, pointing to the group of girls.

"I'll use them, too," Amuir told her. He pointed to the group. "Come here, join them." He spoke to the girls even as Babette moved to join them. "You all hold hands, now. Start of your missing ones. Don't speak but imagine them the last time you saw them in uniform."

Babette grabbed a hand from either side of her and closed her eyes. She imagined her father in his uniform, smiling at her and assuring her that the silly Kingslanders were not going to harm anyone. "You have nothing to fear, *ma chere*."

She smiled at the memory. She felt the others, caught a faint aura of their thinking.

The mage nodded toward her, saying, "This one has a touch of the gift."

"She does?"

"Magic is all around," Amuir said. "Some stumble into it. She's one."

*Me?* Babette thought to herself in surprise.

"Settle down, get back to your thinking," Amuir warned her. "Your power aids mine when you think."

Babette thought once more. And she felt…

"Hearts pull," Amuir said, almost like he was chanting. "Let the love of these girls for their parents pull their hearts toward them. Let their love find them."

Babette added, in her own mind, *Please!* She wondered which god she was praying to, the god of love, perhaps?

"Ouch!" one of the girls cried. "It bites!" Another yelped in pain.

Babette felt as though her heart was pulling out of her chest. She moved, pulled by the feeling, trying to ease the pain by following its tug.

"Let her go," Amuir's voice called to the crowd. "She knows where she is going."

"Someone follow her," General Dartan ordered. "Mullich, you are the best at keeping hidden, you do it."

"Yes sir," a man's voice replied. Babette didn't hear him following her. She felt the fabric of the tent on her face and brushed it aside, daring to open her eyes. In front of her, overlaid on her sight, was a thin pulsing light blue line. It pointed back toward the village. She followed it.

She followed it through the streets, past the barracks, out through the new gate by the metal rail lines, across the bridge and out to the fields where the enemy had camped. The line grew stronger, thicker, wider as she crossed the bridge and it veered away, toward the sea. But it stopped abruptly at a mound.

"This is the mound the queen was buried on," Babette said, wondering what could have led her here. She didn't know the queen, had never ever seen her. Why would —

A dim light blue shape formed from the magic that had led her to this place. It took a form, a shape. It was a person. He was in uniform. There was a hole in his chest.

"Father!"

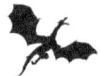

Queen Diam gave the dragon god 'a look.' She'd been a queen for a while — as well as a mother — and she knew full well how to give 'a look.' The god stared back at her and decided to be amused. Diam held his gaze for a long moment then snorted, her eyes twinkling.

"Very well, great god," Diam said, "seeing as I am *not* a rider, nor one of your get —"

"Oh, be that way!" Ophidian said with a wave of his hand. Diam grinned at him. He turned to the others. "What I tell you now, no one else should hear from your lips." He looked from one to another in the room until they all nodded in agreement, stopping with Skara and Thomas.

"What about us?" Thomas demanded, "shouldn't we be sworn as well?"

"If you wish," Ophidian said.

"You're dead, he can't force your oath," Wymarc said, waving Krea's hand airily.

"I shall keep your secrets," Skara told Ophidian stoutly.

"As shall I," Thomas added.

"Thank you," Ophidian said to them. He nodded to Krea Wymarc. "As my daughter said, I cannot force the dead to take oaths."

"Which is all for the better, as he'd be intolerable otherwise," a small boy spoke up.

"Why are you here?" Ophidian grumbled.

"He's keeping an eye on us," Thomas said, nodding to the boy who smiled as he nodded back. Glumly, Thomas added, "Or perhaps just me."

"I always said that you'd get interesting," Aron, god of judgment said in agreement.

"You just never said that I'd die beforehand," Thomas grumbled, beckoning with an arm for the boy to join him.

Aron moved to his side and looked up at him, telling him solemnly, "I judged that you would not take the news well."

Thomas snorted softly in amusement. Then he turned his gaze back to Ophidian.

"Many thousands of years ago," Ophidian began, "when I was a young god and the world was not the way it is now —"

"Are you going to take forever, brother?" Aron interrupted. "Should I come back in an hour?"

Ophidian gave him a quelling look. "I thought that men — zwerg, humans, mer folk, and all the others that walked the world — were being treated poorly."

"You were bored," Aron corrected. "You wanted to make things 'interesting', as I recall."

"I thought that keeping humans as toys and pets to do with as we please was not what was intended for us," Ophidian replied loftily.

"There was a great battle," Wymarc broke in.

"The gods fought," Queen Diam added, cocking a grin at Krea Wymarc. "They fought for thousands of years."

"And I became sorely wounded," Ophidian said. "My blood fell like rain and I feared that I would be defeated."

"You nearly were," Aron added softly. "You nearly bled to death."

"And you shed tears of rage and sorrow," Diam said. She raised a finger and pointed it at Wymarc. "And she was the first tear."

"And when I hit the ground, I became a wyvern," Wymarc said with Krea's voice.

"But it wasn't enough," Aron added. "As a wyvern you were too close to the gods, too powerful and too weak at the same time."

"There was a girl nearby, she saw me," Wymarc said. "She came to me, even in her fear."

"And you bonded and became the first twin soul," Diam finished for her.

Wymarc nodded, with Krea's eyes hooded in memories — and pain — from thousands of years before.

"And the dragons?" Drake Fisher asked in a small voice.

"They are my blood," Ophidian said. He nodded toward Wymarc. "Wymarc was the first to return to me, the first twin soul. When I realized what had happened, I found souls for my dragon children."

"And then he fought back," Aron said. He smiled. "It was such a battle and the other gods were totally amazed."

"Some were appalled," Ophidian admitted.

"But the power — and the courage — of the dragons and wyverns, of their special powers, of their dedication to their father — it made the difference," Aron countered.

"With the aid of his blood and sweat," Wymarc said, pointing a finger at the body she was in, "Ophidian was able to convince more gods to agree with him."

"And so the God's War ended," Aron agreed. "And humans — zwerg, mer, normal, and all others — were granted the ability to work magic."

"And thrive and grow in knowledge," Ophidian said, nodding in agreement.

"It was a good thing," Aron said. He frowned as he added, "I was wrong to oppose you."

Thomas Walpish gasped and looked down at the young god who shrugged guiltily.

"Everyone can make a mistake," Skara said, resting a hand consolingly on the boy's shoulder.

"But twin souls can die," Wymarc said, her voice going dark.

Ophidian nodded. "Can and do," he agreed.

"And so, because their human partners could not stand the thought of their immortal partners grieving their loss," Diam said, "they convinced their wyvern and dragon halves that they needed to have someone with them at all times, in case the worst occurred."

"A rider!" Imay said, her eyes going wide. She glanced at Krea Wymarc. "But then —"

"It was complicated, quick, and unforeseen," Wymarc said with Krea's voice. She glanced at Ophidian but the dragon god was content to let her explain. "Diam had been my rider for a long time but when she met —"

"I met your father," Diam said to Imay in a soft, sad voice.

"I released her," Wymarc said. "Both Annora and I hated to do it but we were so happy for you and we knew you were destined for the throne."

"Around the same time, I discovered the boy dragon in the frozen wastes," Ophidian said.

"In the bitter north," Wymarc continued, "a baby boy named Jarin was near death. He was joined with the foundling dragon."

"You came to me, asked me and Annora to take him under our wing." She frowned. "You suggested we bring him to Rabel Zebala —"

"Father!" Krea cried, taking over her voice. "But why?"

"Because Rabel Zebala and I had talked over the years," Ophidian said. "Annora and Wymarc knew it and thought perhaps they could find the dragon a twin soul either in him or —" he nodded toward Krea "— in his daughter."

"Only there was an airship," Wymarc said. "It shot us out of the sky —"

"And I found you," Krea said with her own voice. "If you'd had a rider, what would have happened?"

"The rider would have taken the mortal soul's place," Diam said softly.

"And when there is no rider?" Thomas asked with a frown.

"I remember Pallas, and how Arolan trapped her in the bitter north," Annabelle said with Ellen's piping voice.

"Pallas was another dragon?" Margaret asked.

"She was another wyvern," Wymarc replied. She narrowed Krea's eyes as she added, "And something happened to *her* rider and twin soul."

"Yes," Ophidian agreed, stroking his goatee thoughtfully.

"The plan is not young," Aron said. "Balance can take a long time."

"This is connected to Quenkorian?" Ophidian said, peering down at the boy god.

"They are connected," Aron said. "Or so it seems to me."

"You're worried about me," Annabelle said, catching Ophidian's gaze. "You're worried about what would happen if anyone were to hurt Ellen."

"Nobody's going to hurt me!" Ellen swore with her own voice. And then her voice caught. "But, if they did — you'd be alone and in pain!"

Bethany Margiss moved swiftly to grab the smaller person from behind in her arms. "We'll take care of you."

"It is best to be prepared," Wymarc said firmly. The others looked at her. "It is a horrible pain to deal with the loss of your twin soul."

"There is more to it," Diam spoke up. The others looked at her. She smiled and her eyes lit. "The rider gets a chance of a lifetime, to fly in the air on the back of a wyvern —"

"Or dragon," Ellen spoke up. Diam cocked an eyebrow in her direction, so she explained, "I did it, with Rabel and Jarin."

"Be that as it may," Diam said, nodding to Ellen Annabelle, "the gift goes both ways. While the twin souls are paired, the rider is also a partner and the three become more than family."

"The riders protect their wyverns," Skara said, glancing to Thomas.

"And the wyverns protect their riders," Wymarc said in counterpoint.

"And there is much danger," Aron said. "To both rider and dragon."

"You tell us this because you want riders?" Bethany Margiss said to Ophidian. A slight nod of his head answered her. Her face screwed up and she pointed to herself, "But we're too small!"

"You'll get bigger," Wymarc assured them. "You are young now —" she sent a nod in Ellen's direction as well "— but you'll get bigger, older —"

"Wiser," Diam added.

"— and you'll be able to carry more than one person," Wymarc continued.

"Jarin had no problem carrying me and Rabel," Ellen said in agreement. She nodded to Bethany Margiss, adding, "And Annabelle is grown up, so as a wyvern we're big enough to carry others easily."

"You want us to become riders?" Drake said to Ophidian. He glanced at the twin souls in the room. "How do we choose?"

"You don't," Wymarc said, pointing to Ellen Annabelle and Bethany Margiss, "*they* do."

"Actually," Diam said, "I thought it was mutual."

"If the rider says no," Wymarc said. "But it is the wyvern who asks."

"Except with these two," Diam said. She glanced to Ophidian and asked, "This is their first time, isn't it?"

"They're new," Margaret Waters said with a sudden leap of insight.

"There hasn't been a new wyvern in over a thousand years," Aron said. He gave his brother, the dragon god, a sorrowful look, as he added, "Because Ophidian can't cry."

"Ellen did it for me," Ophidian admitted.

Aron's eyes widened and he gave Ellen a sad look. "They will kill you as soon as they know."

"They can try," Ellen growled. Annabelle added, "We're hard to kill."

"And they can heal," Diam said. "That is a rare gift."

"Bethany Margiss can heal as well," Ellen Annabelle said, nodding toward the taller girl.

"But you heal differently," Diam said, glancing at the girl. She turned her head to Molle, the healer, who nodded in agreement.

"I help the mind," Bethany Margiss said.

"There's more," Ophidian said, nodding to Ellen Annabelle. "Tell them about the south."

The small girl sighed. Annabelle took her voice as she explained, "We went south to visit my old home."

"That's where you got the elementals?" Diam asked.

Annabelle nodded. "I was raised with Queen Alva of the Shattered Hills," she said. "When we got there, we startled some humans and... one died."

"Balance," Aron murmured so softly that only Thomas and Skara heard him.

"There's more," Ophidian cautioned.

"The girl was dead," Annabelle said sadly. "But a horse had gone lame — broken forelegs —"

"You didn't!" Wymarc swore. Annabelle glanced her way but Wymarc turned her gaze to Ophidian. "Don't tell me she made a centaur!"

"She had no choice," Ophidian said. "And it's not all bad."

"Only if you're a god," Wymarc muttered darkly.

"You can bring the dead back to life?" Diam asked Ellen Annabelle in hushed tones.

"No," Ophidian said firmly, "she can't. She can meld two souls, in broken bodies, into one whole."

"And make centaurs," Wymarc added.

"Centaurs do it all the time," Aron said with a smirk.

"Actually, not so much," Ophidian corrected him. "There's been trouble in the south."

"Oh, I bet that Kahlas —" Aron began then clapped a hand hastily over his mouth.

Ophidian turned to Bethany Margiss, Ellen Annabelle, and Krea Wymarc. "I'd feel better if you had riders," he told them. He nodded toward Skara and Thomas. "You can't pick them but they can train your riders and help guard you."

"Because Quenkorian is going to find out and he's going to try to kill them," Diam said darkly.

"Him and others," Aron agreed.

"What about Jarin Reedis?" Ellen Annabelle asked. "Shouldn't he —?"

"He should get a rider, certainly," Ophidian agreed. "In fact, I intend to approach him immediately after we're done here."

"About time," Wymarc murmured. "Reedis is not much better than Jarin, you know."

Ophidian shot her an amused look.

"Choosing a rider is not forever," Diam said. "You can try it out, see if it works for you." She nodded toward Krea Wymarc. "And when times change, you can always go your separate ways."

"I know you're supposed to ask," Margaret Waters said in a small voice to Ellen Annabelle, "but I would be honored if you chose me."

"Would you?" Ellen cried in surprise. "Even though I'm only a little girl?"

Margaret nodded firmly. Ellen rushed to her and grabbed her in a hug, looking up at the older girl and swearing, "And if it doesn't work out, that'll be okay. I mean —"

"Hush," Margaret said, hugging her back, "that's enough of that." Ellen hushed. Margaret pushed her back so she could meet her eyes. "Annabelle, is this all right for you?"

"I've always wanted a little sister," Annabelle admitted, moving Ellen's body back to hug the older girl tightly.

"You are a fire mage, are you not?" Wymarc said to Drake. Startled, he nodded. Wymarc smiled with Krea's white face. "How do you feel about flying with us?" Catching the boy's look, Wymarc added, "I know a thing or two about fire."

"I should like that," Drake said formally. He nodded to Krea, "If that is acceptable to you, Krea."

"It might get interesting," Krea said thoughtfully, "there's a boy, you see."

"I am sure you have many suitors, Miss Krea," Drake said with a bow. "I did not mean to interfere —"

"You're not thinking of *that* boy!" Wymarc swore to Krea.

"And what if I am?" Krea snapped back out of the same mouth. She gave Drake an apologetic look. "Sometimes Wymarc and I don't always agree."

"Age brings wisdom," Wymarc said to Drake. She sighed. "But we'll both have to accept Krea's decisions on matters of her heart."

"I agree," Drake said with a bow. "I would be honored to be your partner in the sky."

"'Rider' will do," Wymarc said with a sniff. She pointed to Krea's body. "Just remember that I'm older than I look."

"*Much* older," Krea added with a wink.

"Bethany Margiss," Diam said, catching the young twin soul's attention and nodding toward Chandra, "may I make you known to Chandra the earth mage?"

Bethany Margiss nodded, looking glum.

"Did I tell you how she got our attention when she needed help for her sister?" Diam plowed on resolutely. Margiss shook her head. Diam smiled. "She's an earth mage, she broke the ground under our entrance, shattered our gates and forced her way inside, shouting for help for her sister."

Bethany turned with big eyes toward Chandra. "I'm too small," Bethany said softly, "I can't carry anyone yet." She pointed to her body. "My body's about the same size when I'm a wyvern."

"You'll get bigger," Diam reminded her.

"You helped save my sister?" Chandra said. Bethany Margiss nodded.

"And she pulled the cursed teeth from those infected by Vistos' cursed sweets," Skara spoke up. She smiled at Bethany Margiss. "I was Bethany's twin soul until Vistos murdered me."

"But then, you should be her rider," Chandra said backing up a step.

"I'm dead," Skara said, shaking her head, "so that's not an option."

"Did you really shatter the ground to save her?" Margiss asked. "What sort of spell did you use?"

"You know magic?" Chandra asked warily. Margiss nodded. "My grandfather is mage Margen —"

"Wait, I *know* him!" Chandra cried excitedly. "He worked with father —" Her voice caught. "I mean, he worked with my step-father."

"You know him?" Margiss asked.

"He taught me the boom spell that I used to shake the ground," Chandra explained. She smiled at the memory. "He was kind and gentle."

Margiss smiled. "He is."

Ellen Annabelle moved to join them, saying, "Annabelle's big enough, we could carry two."

Chandra glanced to Bethany Margiss. "If you don't mind?"

"We'll get bigger," Bethany Margiss promised. Chandra smiled at the twin soul girl.

"I would like to see that," she agreed shyly, extending her hand to the smaller girl. Bethany Margiss smiled as they shook their new rider's hand.

Queen Diam sidled over to Ophidian and murmured softly, "That all seemed a bit too simple."

Ophidian frowned and started to answer her but just then, a small piece of torn parchment appeared in the air above his hand and fluttered down. With a grumble, Ophidian took the piece of paper and read what was written on it. Silently he passed it over to Queen Diam who read it quickly. Her eyes widened. Wordlessly, she passed it back to the dragon god.

"My brother and his little games," Ophidian said, tossing the paper out of his hand and turning it to ash with a burst of flame.

"Well, at least we know," Queen Diam said.

"Don't say it!" Ophidian begged but it was too late, his words were in unison with Diam's: "It was fate."

# Chapter Five

"I saw the ghost, too," the man who'd shadowed her, Ives Murat, affirmed when Babette reported back, her face tear-stained, to the tent much later. Murat's words were enough to set the whole tent roaring with the men's anger.

"They murdered them!" "In cold blood!" "Unarmed men!" "We'll be next!"

"Quiet," General Dartan said in a firm voice that carried. He nodded to Babette. "We must get confirmation, child," he told her gravely. "Where there are bodies, particularly bodies with holes from bullets, they must also have been musketeers."

Babette looked confused. The general took pity and explained, "Someone did this, some of their men. We must find one who was there, get their confession."

"I'll go," Murat offered, moving to stand beside Babette. "She'll need muscle."

General Dartan shook his head. "First, let us get our proof," he said to his men.

"And when we get proof, what then?" Murat demanded.

General Dartan smiled dangerously. "There are rules for war," he said. "If they are broken, the rules change."

"They've only got one division here," one of his lieutenants agreed with a knowing look.

General Dartan nodded and turned his gaze back to Babette. "Find one of the men, get the confession. Can you do that, child? For you father?"

"Yes."

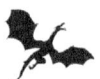

"Rabel stood as my friend when they took my body to Fixer," Ibb told Tracker as they examined the crushed caravan from a safe distance. With the grinding of gears that was his version of laughter, he added, "He is older than he looks."

"And you'll let him learn our secrets?" Tracker asked suspiciously.

"Some of which I taught him," Rabel said pointing from himself to the Ibb.

Again the metal man gave a gear-grinding laughter and rotated his head up and down in agreement.

"But this magic of... twisting the world... this I have trouble comprehending," Rabel admitted.

"I believe it was one of the gods who first suggested it," Ibb said.

"Was it one of the Three Impossibilities?" Tracker asked.

"It was," Ibb agreed. The metal immortal explained to Rabel, "When we first set out to create ourselves, the gods told us that three things were impossible. Twisting the world was one of them." Ibb gave a short gear-grind chuckle. "But we proved them wrong."

"Which is how your caravan can be a backpack," Rabel guessed. "But what was done with this caravan... it wasn't something you've seen before."

"True," Ibb agreed. "And the one who did it —"

"She fooled you," Tracker said. "She took our tests and somehow fooled you."

"And now she's twinned herself to the first *kitsune* who took a twin soul," Ibb said.

"She did?" Tracker cried angrily. "We must find her and bring her to justice."

"And free my Meiko," Hana Renn called in a firm voice. She stood beside Angus and Nestor Pallas. She waved a hand toward Ibb, Tracker, and Rabel. "We came to help."

"What can a girl —?" Tracker began airily.

"Don't say it," Ibb warned.

Hana waved her hands and rose on a cone of air, flying over the ruined caravan and lowering herself until she was almost touching it. She frowned and pointed, telling the others, "Did you see this book?"

"No," Rabel admitted, "what book?"

"I can't tell," Hana admitted, still hovering. "I can only make out a part of the cover and the pages. It's all crushed in one of the cracks here."

"A crack?" Ibb said, his metal eyebrows lowering harshly. He turned to Rabel. "Do you recall a crack?"

"No," Rabel replied with an equally worried look.

"It's getting bigger," Hana added, pointing. Ibb, Tracker, and Rabel rushed to the far side of the caravan where Hana hovered.

"I can see it," Tracker said. She leaned forward and her blue eyes twirled in her face, extending and spiralling out of her head. "It is hard to recognize…"

"The crack is getting bigger," Rabel said, raising a hand in a warding gesture. He turned to Ibb. "Is this a problem?"

"Very much so."

"There, there, dear, no worries," Moira Kendral assured her daughter. She waved at the party standing in front of her. "You just do what you need to do and come back when you're ready." Her jaw tightened as she added, "And we'll look at the books when you get back."

"Of course, mother," Nelly Kendral said, trying to keep her voice steady. *The books!*

"Although," Mrs. Kendral said thoughtfully, glancing around, "I don't see why we all had to go to the roof for this conversation."

"Not so much for the conversation as for the departure," Peter Hewlitt assured her with a grin. He gestured toward Jarin Reedis who had been trying to keep as still, silent — and invisible — as possible. Peter nodded to Jarin Reedis who, with an indrawn hiss of trepidation, jumped over the side of the building.

"By the gods!" Mrs. Kendral exclaimed. "Why did he —?" She broke off as a large black dragon appeared hovering with deep slow wingbeats just at the side of the roof. Mrs. Kendral turned to her daughter. "He's a dragon?" Nelly nodded. "And you're going to ride him?" Nelly nodded again. She gulped, took a running leap and landed on the dragon's neck. She turned to her mother with a huge grin. "And I'm going to marry him, too!"

Mrs. Kendral's eyes bulged and she gasped for a response but Margen and Hewlitt both followed Nelly's example and jumped on Jarin Reedis' back. With a triumphant roar, the black and red dragon beat his way up high in the sky and disappeared toward the south.

"Well," Mrs. Kendral said to herself as the group disappeared, "life with those two certainly won't be boring, will it?"

After one final glance at the dark smudge high up in the sky, Moira Kendral turned back to the stairs and the — to her — quite simple task of managing a bunch of unruly, over-educated soon-to-be mages. *Really, rather restful,* she thought as she made her way down to the ever-increasing level of noise that indicated boisterous spirits and an improperly developed sense of freedom.

They flew for nearly two hours. Nelly would exclaim at each new vista that came into their view. Peter Hewlitt would peer with wide eyes at the landscape below, particularly the snow-covered fields and the small, quaint villages. The rail line was not always visible — snow covered some of the tracks and tree cover obscured other parts — but they had no real trouble following it.

And they had absolutely no question about when it ended.

Jarin let out a loud cry of alarm when they spotted it: the rail lines were abruptly all tumbled in an untidy mess, the train following on sat idly, smoke circling up from its chimney. The construction had ended just about three miles from the next large town.

"That's Sorellay," Hewlitt said, pointing toward the distant line of houses and the open port.

Jarin let out another worried cry and began spiralling downwards, looking for a good place to land.

He found it not far from the end of the rail line.

"They've seen us," Margen said, pointing to a knot of people who were all gesticulating wildly at the sight of the black dragon.

"You'd better land out of sight," Hewlitt suggested.

"We don't want any trouble," Nelly added in agreement.

Jarin snorted but complied, landing behind a downslope and disgorging his passengers before turning, once more into his human shape.

Nelly took one look at him and with a sympathetic cry, passed him the extra jacket that she'd brought just for this purpose. Reedis smiled at her and donned it hastily, still looking rather blue around the mouth and shivering. Nelly hugged him tight and kissed him all over his face, saying, "You were magnificent!"

"Thank you," Jarin replied, looking pleased.

"We should get going, before they send someone looking," Margen said, heading off toward the train on the other side of the hill.

"Captain Elwes, you have your orders!" Prince Paulus bellowed as he waved the troop on their way. It wasn't a full troop of cavalry, only a platoon which meant that it was too small a command for a captain. But Jaweer Elwes knew better than to argue — at least, if he wanted to keep his head.

Captain Elwes gave his liege a jaunty salute, turned his stallion and kicked the horse into a quick gallop, racing up along the column of horses to take the lead. He passed the wagon midway to the head of the column and gave it a dark look — the birdmen were bedded inside, getting their "beauty rest," as he liked to call it.

Forty cavalry, two birdmen. It was a small force, even for a reconnaissance patrol. The covered wagon held not just the birdmen but supplies meant to last them for more than three weeks.

Elwes wasn't really worried about supplies, Prince Paulus ruled the realm, he could invoke His Highness' name and get whatever he wanted… or there would be consequences — like cold steel and dead bodies.

"You won't learn everything in a day," Wymarc consoled Drake as they walked to the outskirts of Korin's Pass. "In fact, I'd be surprised if it doesn't take you a year to really feel comfortable being a rider."

Drake frowned. "I'll be faster."

"Maybe," Wymarc allowed. "But I would prefer it if you just did your best rather than pushing yourself too hard."

Drake looked down at the young girl walking beside him and forced himself to remember that he was talking to the thousand year old wyvern that lived inside the same body as the albino girl.

"Right now, today, all we want to do is practice getting aboard the wyvern, staying on, and learning how to fly," Wymarc told him. She glanced all around her and stopped. "This is a good place."

"Margaret, Chandra, we'll take turns first and then we'll see if I can handle the both of you," Ellen Annabelle said. She gave Bethany Margiss an encouraging look. "Bethany, you can follow us and keep an eye on what we're doing. You might have some suggestions to make it easier."

"I think I'll fly lower," Bethany Margiss declared.

"Lower?" Ellen Annabelle repeated.

"That way, if someone falls, I might be able to catch them."

"Nobody is going to fall!" Wymarc declared stoutly. She turned to the others. "Now you're all going to get a chance to fly, so pay attention." Captain Welless gave her a wary look. "You too, captain," she told him. "There's no reason you shouldn't at least know what your limits are."

"And me?" Lissy asked wistfully.

"That depends upon your mother," Wymarc replied, glancing toward Queen Diam. Diam gave her a rueful look and then nodded toward her youngest daughter.

"I trust Wymarc with my life," Diam said, her eyes going to Granno, her longtime friend and bodyguard, who was doing all he could to contain himself.

"I'm going to jump in the air," Wymarc said, "and change into a wyvern." She glanced around to be certain everyone heard her and understood. Casting her eyes at Drake, she continued, "After that, I'll land and beckon for you to mount. The easiest way is to throw your upper half over my back and then twist until your legs are on either side of me." Drake frowned. "You'll be riding just above my wings, so have a care." Cautiously, Drake nodded. Wymarc turned to the rest of the group. "I'll take Drake up and return him to the ground after our flight." She wagged a finger at Ellen Annabelle. "You wait, young lady, until I return before you think about doing anything."

"Can I watch?" Bethany Margiss asked.

"As a wyvern?" Wymarc asked. When the young twin soul girl nodded, Wymarc pursed her lips thoughtfully.

"I don't see why not," Ophidian said. "I plan on doing the same."

"You, I'd expected," Wymarc told the dragon god. She nodded toward Bethany Margiss. "Very well, but wait until we're in the air before you change. I don't want one of us bumping into the other."

"Of course!" Bethany promised.

Wymarc took one final look around at the group, nodded firmly, and stalked off further away from the village. She increased her speed, jumped up — and was a wyvern. With a screech of pleasure, she thrust her wings down hard and leapt higher into the sky. She circled over them and cried in pure pleasure as she turned and dove toward the earth once more.

"Show off," Diam murmured, her eyes glistening with pride and old memories. She nodded to Ellen Annabelle. "She always prided herself on her skill and speed."

"She's beautiful," Annabelle agreed with Ellen's voice.

"Annabelle's beautiful, too, mother," Imay assured her.

Diam smiled and nodded, saying nothing.

Wymarc landed and turned her gaze toward Drake Fisher. The teenager nodded to himself and strode forward. He reached for the wyvern's back and leaped up in one graceful movement.

"Oh, nicely done!" Diam said.

Wymarc twisted her neck around to eye the fire mage for a moment then straightened her head, took an awkward step and jumped up into the air. With three strong downbeats of her wings, the two were racing into the sky.

"She's fast," Ellen said.

"I've seen you fly, Annabelle," Ophidian said, "and you do nearly as well." He turned his gaze to the wyvern high in the sky and added softly, with pride in his voice, "But Wymarc's always been the fastest aloft."

"Watch me!" Bethany Margiss cried, leaping forward and jumping into the air. For a moment the girl seemed destined to fall back to the ground but then she changed and, with two strong flaps of her wings, surged upwards, crying in joy.

Ophidian sighed theatrically. "I'd better go after her." He didn't falter as he changed shape and roared mightily as his wings bore him skywards.

Above him, Bethany Margiss squeaked in surprise and side-slipped to get more distance between herself and the huge dark dragon that was Ophidian.

"If they don't come down in the next few minutes, you might consider going after them," Queen Diam said warningly to Ellen Annabelle.

"We'll wait," Annabelle replied even as she felt Ellen's impatience bubbling up inside their body. More to Ellen than the rest, she added, "We have patience."

"Okay," Ellen said aloud, "but Margaret is being left out."

"I can wait," Margaret said, her eyes heavenward, following the thring winged shapes as they grew smaller in the afternoon sky. She spread her hands out at her side, wondering if she could use her magic to lift her off the ground. It certainly would be something. She lowered her gaze and said to Annabelle, "Have you ever heard of a mage flying?"

Ellen's lips twitched into a smile. "Ellen hasn't seen her do it but I've seen Hana Renn fly," Annabelle replied. She twisted Ellen's face into a sad frown as she added, "Hissia and Hanor gave her the ability themselves to make up for her loss."

"Her loss?" Chandra asked, having been close enough to hear the whole conversation.

"Later," Annabelle said. "It is a sad story as yet without an ending."

"Hana is nice," Ellen said, taking control of her mouth back from Annabelle. She glanced up to the sky. "Oh! They're taking too long!"

As if she'd heard it, Wymarc screeched high in the sky and began a steep descent. Bethany Margiss cried in surprise and turned to follow the larger wyvern back to the ground. Ophidian, with a boastful cry of his own, merely circled above, lord of all he surveyed.

When Wymarc touched back on the ground, she wriggled her shoulders — wings. Drake took the hint and cautiously leaped off her. When he reached the ground, he raced to her head, to say, "That was amazing! If I were to die today, I could not be happier."

"Savor it, Wymarc," Chandra advised, glancing affectionately toward her stepbrother. "Drake doesn't do happy." She cocked her head consideringly and tilted an eyebrow toward Margaret. "You know, I think this is the first time I've seen him happy."

Margaret nodded in agreement.

Ophidian swooped down from the sky, touched ground and was his cinnamon-skinned self in a moment.

Wymarc transformed to Krea and glanced over to him. "Well?"

"It went well enough," Ophidian allowed. "It's not as if you haven't done it before, so pardon me if I don't wax as lyrical as your erstwhile rider."

Wymarc made Krea's face frown. Krea took over her body once more and said to Ophidian, "Well, I thought she did just great!"

"I'm sorry, Your Majesty, but that's the best we can do at this time," Mannevy reported to King Markel the next day. "The *Wasp* can't possibly reach the capital until tomorrow and it will take the same amount of time on the return journey."

"But — what about a train?" King Markel asked, grasping for any possibilities. "Aren't they faster?"

"Actually, sire, I believe that in most circumstances airships are faster," Mannevy said. "And, in any event, we have got tracks laid from our new capital here in Sarskar to your old capital in Kingsland yet."

"I thought we'd *paid* for that already!" King Markel fumed.

"Paid, yes, sire, but built —" Mannevy shrugged "— not yet."

"So you are telling me, your liege lord, that you cannot have me crowned for another…" the king paused and counted on his fingers "… three days at least?"

"Probably four, sire, if we're being honest," Mannevy replied.

Queen Rassa gave her new king an exasperated look.

King Markel threw up his hands. "I know, I know," he cried. "But he's been with me quite a long time now."

"Clearly, you keep him on because of his great talent," Rassa said, acid dripping in her voice.

King Markel leaned toward her and lowered his voice to say, "We should talk of this later."

"Your Majesties," Mannevy said, pretending he hadn't heard, "if that will be all?"

"Yes, go, go! Leave us!" King Markel said, waving his first minister out of the chambers with an irritated gesture.

First Minister Mannevy bowed low, turned and quickly left the chambers.

"Really, my love, if that is the best your old kingdom can offer, it's a wonder how you managed to win the war," Rassa said after the chamber doors were firmly shut.

"I had to do it all myself," King Markel said with a sniff.

Rassa stroked his cheek in sympathy, saying, "Well, now you have *me* to help you." Markel sighed and leaned into her caress.

# Chapter Six

"Margen!" Peter Hewlitt called as the mage crested the top of the rise. Margen turned back to him. "You may have trouble being recognized."

"Yes," Margen called back, "I'd thought of that." He paused and waved for the others to catch up.

At the top of the rise, Peter Hewlitt surveyed the scene stretched before them. Margen saw the way the spymaster squinted and pulled forth a telescope from inside his robes, saying, "Try this."

Hewlitt accepted the spyglass with alacrity and re-scanned the vista in front of them. When he finished, he swore and passed the glass to Margen. Reedis and Nelly gave him inquiring looks.

"The tracks are scattered, the rail ties — some are laid badly and others are scattered," Hewlitt explained.

"Where are Margen's mages?" Reedis asked.

"No sign of them," Hewlitt said. "But there's a shack with smoke rising from a chimney, I expect they're there." He frowned. "Or maybe the railmen."

"We won't learn more standing here," Nelly said, trudging forward determinedly. Hewlitt shot Reedis a look but the twin soul mage merely shrugged and stepped off after his betrothed.

"There's some men coming," Matt Evans said, peering out of the dirty waxed paper window that he had insisted the railmen install when they'd taken shelter here. Outside it was still cold and the ground was covered in fresh snow from the night before but the wind was light — nothing like the howling gale of the night before.

Freddie Fennimore nudged him aside to get a look of his own. "Three men and a woman." He turned to the silent third of their group. "Did you hear that, Babs, there're people coming."

Barbara Garrett didn't even twitch at his words, lying as she'd been put on the cot in the corner, her fists clenched tightly. Freddie sighed and glanced toward the rail foreman, Mr. Gossett.

Norman Gossett rose from his rough hewn chair and peered out the window. "They don't look rough," he said to his lads who had remained at the table. He glanced toward the still form of Barbara Garrett and added, "Maybe they can help."

"I said it before and I'll say it again: you shouldn't have tried to attack him," Albert Sorstrom growled. "Him a mage and all."

"He shouldn't a-done that to the girl," Norman growled in reply. Three others at the table looked nervously between the rail boss and Sorgstrom. "It don't matter that he's a mage, he shouldn't have done it."

"Bloody well broke her, he did," Dennis Travers tittered in amusement. Sorstrom and Gossett exchanged looks — they both found Travers' behavior to be more than a little 'off.' "Ain't never seen nothing like it, just whipped her raw through her coat and all."

"Leave off," Kenster Jarvin growled, glancing sympathetically to the still form lying motionless in the bed. "She can her you."

"She can't hear nothin'," Travers said, giggling again. "'Can't hear nothin' 'cuz he took her mind."

Jarvin sprang from his chair, ready to punch Travers. Travers backed away, hands up defensively. But he wasn't smart enough to keep his mouth shut. "What?" he cried in mock innocence. "I'm jus' saying what we all know." He glanced toward the bed. "Poor tike."

Matt Evans jerked away from the dirty window and tapped Freddie Fennimore on the shoulder. "Come on, they're almost here."

Freddie gave the other mage a worried look but followed. They were trailed by Norman Gossett who warned, "You just let me do the talking, young sirs."

"Someone's coming out," Hewlitt said as they approached the shack. He gestured for the others to halt but mage Margen brushed past him, a determined look on his face. Jarin Reedis followed, saying to Hewlitt, "I don't really think they'll challenge a dragon, do you?"

Hewlitt grunted and followed along. Nelly took a few quick steps to catch up to Reedis, grabbing his arm with both of hers in a possessive manner. Reedis looked over to her and smiled, placing his other hand over hers.

"That's close enough!" a gruff man called, stepping in front of the two mages that Margen just barely recognized as his former students.

"Freddie, Matt, it's me!" Margen said.

"Who?" Matt asked. Freddie said nothing, his expression pensive.

"Mage Margen," Margen replied. He raised his hand and moved it in a curious twisted loop. A purple smoke appeared in the center, twisting itself. "Surely you recognize my mark?"

"I never saw that before," Freddie said. "And you're not mage Margen, you're too young."

Margen's expression fell. "Where's Barbara?"

"Who wants to know?" the gruff man demanded. He nodded toward the mages. "These two have been through enough, I won't have them hurt."

"Hurt?" Margen repeated. He took a step back and peered more intently at Freddie and Matt. "Did Brookes *hurt* you?"

"Beat them," the gruff man said. "Beat them and threatened their lives if they weren't faster laying the track." He gestured toward the shambles of rail and timber in the distance. "Me and my men, we laid in on him, scared him away."

"Torvan Brookes?" Peter Hewlitt asked, his expression wary.

"You know him?" the gruff man said. He took a step forward, threateningly. "You want trouble, my boys will sort you out soon enough." He pointed back to the two teen mages. "What these two can't do, my men'll handle."

"We're not here for trouble," Nelly said, moving forward, her hands raised, palms out. "We came here to check on mage Margen's students." She nodded to them. "We were worried about them."

"Too late to be worried," the gruff man said, spitting on the ground in emphasis. "The damage has been done."

"Barbara?" Margen asked in a small voice.

"He beat her," Freddie said with tears in his voice. "He beat her until we all attacked him and pulled him away." He shook his head, his eyes watery. "She hasn't so much as moved since."

"I must see to her," Nelly said, storming forward. Jarin Reedis matched her move. He jerked a thumb toward Margen. "I am Jarin Reedis, the airship mage. This *is* mage Margen. He made a deal with my father, the god Ophidian, after mage Vistos cursed his granddaughter and tried to kill us all."

"Well, actually," Nelly said conversationally, "that was the god Quenkorian who tried to kill us. Vistos was merely his lackey."

Reedis smiled at his wife and shook his head fondly.

"Who are you, then?" the gruff man demanded of Hewlitt.

"I am Peter Hewlitt, the king's spymaster," Peter replied. The gruff man's eyebrows rose and he took an involuntary step back. "And you are?"

"I'm Norman Gossett, the rail boss on this line," the gruff man told him. He ducked his head. "I didn't mean no harm, sir." He gestured toward the scratch-built shack. "It's just that with all that's happened, can't be too careful."

"So I see," Hewlitt agreed. He extended his hand. Gossett took it slowly in his own, like a man expecting to be bitten by a snake. "You fought a mage and won?" Hewlitt said as he released the other's hand. "I appreciate the difficulty that must have presented."

"No difficulty," Gossett said firmly. "Me and my men were fighting mad for what he did to the two lads, when he lit into the girl, we didn't stop to think."

"Anger can be its own power," Hewlitt said in agreement. They reached the door to the shack. The others had already entered. Hewlitt gestured for Gossett to precede him. Gossett nodded and stepped through.

Inside, Hewlitt pulled a scented handkerchief to his nose — a trick he'd learned from first minister Mannevy — to keep his senses from being dulled by the acrid smells of smoke and unwashed bodies. His eyes darted around the large single room, picking out the railmen at the table, frowning at the wax paper window, scowling at the cot.

"She needs help," mage Margen said as he knelt beside Barbara Garrett's stiff form. He turned to Hewlitt and their eyes met. "She needs a healer."

"Perhaps more," Nelly added, standing besides the girl's head. Nelly glanced up to Reedis. "Her mind's gone wandering."

"What?"

"I've seen it among soldiers or sailors when the terrors of fighting get to be too much for them," Peter Hewlitt said. His jaw clenched as he added, "But I've never seen the likes of this." He turned to Jarin Reedis. "We must warn your father."

"This is the darkest of magic, the foulest of deeds," mage Margen said in agreement. He raised his eyes toward Hewlitt. "The court healer, is she up to this?"

Hewlitt shook his head slowly. A moment later he spoke. "Torvan Brookes was a man who got results," he said, shaking his head, "I never guessed at the methods he used."

"He must be stopped," Margen swore. "He must be stopped now." He turned to Jarin Reedis who was standing behind Nelly.

Reedis touched Nelly's shoulder softly where she knelt beside the broken girl. Nelly reached back and touched it with her own hand before pushing it off her shoulder. "Go!"

"Are you sure?"

"She needs more help than I can give," Nelly said. "Go find it!"

"I'll stay with her," Margen said.

"Would you mind if I came along?" Peter Hewlitt asked diffidently. Reedis gave him a look. "I don't often make it a habit of talking to gods but I believe I should tell some things to your father myself."

"We'll be safe enough here," Margen said. He smiled at Matt and Freddie. "These two lads are strong and there's some things I could teach them quickly that will help."

"I'll be back as soon as I can," Reedis promised, gesturing for Hewlitt to follow him and rushing out the door.

"It'll be days before they can get anywhere," Gossett grumbled as they exited the shack.

"You should go and tell them, then," Nelly said, her jaw clenched.

"I'll just do that," Gossett said, giving the young woman a foul look. Some of his men followed him.

"Why did you say that?" Freddie asked worriedly. "He's protected us and you make him look like a —"

"By the gods!" the men outside shouted. "Stand back, stand back!" "He's huge!"

Nelly smiled sweetly. "My husband is a dragon," she said. "Now, why don't you be a dear and get us a pale of clean water? Or, failing that, get a bucket of clean snow and put it near the fire."

Freddie Fennimore moved as if stung.

A long moment later, amidst the sound of low voices, the railmen returned to the shack. Norman Gossett cleared his throat loudly and said in Nelly's direction, "I see what you mean, miss."

Nelly turned and smiled at him. "Yes, I rather thought seeing it would settle any questions you might have."

"How may we help you?" Albert Sorstrom asked fervently.

"She needs to be kept warm," Nelly said. "There's not much we can do beyond that, I'm afraid."

"I'll cut some wood," Sorstrom declared. He turned back toward the door and was eagerly followed by several more railmen, all eagerly proclaiming their willingness to help.

"How did you do that, miss?" Matt Evans asked in an awed tone. "Are you a mage?"

"I *teach* mages."

Jarin Reedis gave an irritated roar as he appeared over Korin's Pass. He had gone to Ophidian's castle first only to be told that he needed to come here instead and he was worried, tired, and *hungry*.

He was also confused. As he spiralled down toward the ground, he saw figures moving back and forth, brandishing — or pretending to brandish? — swords and fighting… shadows?

He was glad to reach the ground and turn back into Reedis.

"Ophidian!" he called, turning in a slow circle, trying to locate the dragon god. "We need help!"

Two girls paused in their shadow fights and turned toward him. Another, older girl, gave him a frown.

"Lissy!" he called with a huge smile plastered on his face as soon as he spotted the young zwerg princess. "Queen Diam!"

Diam rushed over and smiled at him in return, catching her youngest daughter by the hand and dragging her along.

"How's my air—" Reedis broke off abruptly as Queen Diam frantically shook her head. He recovered quickly, asking, "How is your kingdom, good queen?"

"Busy, as always," Queen Diam said. She waved an arm, indicating the present scene, adding, "And things *here* are much vexing."

"Have you seen Ophidian?" Reedis asked. "One of Margen's students was *beaten* by Torvan Brookes —"

"Father beat someone else?" a young, dusky skinned girl asked suddenly, her brows lowered sharply.

"He beat Margaret near to death," Ellen Annabelle said, moving to join them, lowering the — yes, it was a blade she bore — thin rapier to her side.

"Can you come?" Jarin Reedis implored her. "This girl, she doesn't speak, she doesn't move, she — she looks broken."

"I don't know if I can help," Ellen Annabelle said, waving another, older girl over to join them. "Bethany Margiss might be better."

"Can you *both* come?" Jarin Reedis asked. "The sooner this girl gets help, the better, I think."

"Father?" Ellen Annabelle called, glancing around.

"Here," Ophidian said, suddenly appearing right beside Jarin Reedis. Reedis gave him a sour look, saying, "Have you been here this whole time?"

"Along with some friends," Ophidian said with a grin. He waved his hand and a man and a woman appeared beside him. "You *have* met Skara Ningan and Thomas Walpish, haven't you?"

"You're alive?" Reedis cried, rushing to grab the two. He turned to Ophidian, "But how?"

He was answered as he passed right through the two he'd tried to hug. His brows rose and he turned back, standing between their shades and looking to Ophidian. "Not alive?"

"Not dead, yet, either," Ophidian said. He gave Reedis a considering look. "And you're the first one to pass through them like that."

"It was not a pleasant experience," Thomas Walpish admitted.

"Sorry," Jarin Reedis muttered ruefully. He turned to Ophidian. "This girl worked for Torvan Brookes and he beat her senseless."

"I know her," Bethany Margiss said. "We should help her."

"You can take Chandra," Ophidian declared, "Bethany Margiss is still too small for a rider."

"We tried," Bethany Margiss declared ruefully.

"You'll get bigger," Chandra assured her. She eyed Jarin Reedis. "I am Bethany Margiss' rider."

"Rider?" Jarin Reedis said in confusion. He cast a glance toward Ophidian.

"All wyverns and dragons have riders," Krea Wymarc said, moving to join them in the aggressive walk that was undeniably Wymarc and not the more diffident Krea. "That way, if anything happens to their twin soul —"

"The rider can take their place," Reedis guessed, feeling suddenly very tired. To Jarin, he thought, *Why didn't you have one with you?*

"We were trying to get a rider for me when *your* airship shot us down," Jarin replied aloud.

"Sorry," Reedis said. He thought about a rider, about someone who would — "Nelly."

"Yes," Jarin said. His thoughts were a jumble, matching Reedis' but the two agreed that if something were to kill Reedis, it would be nice to know that both Jarin and Nelly were together.

"That can be dangerous," Wymarc warned with Krea's voice. Jarin Reedis looked at her. "I've seen it work very well, but sometimes…"

"Then we'll have to make sure this isn't one of those times," Jarin said with Reedis' voice.

"Where is this girl?" Ophidian asked.

"I'll take you," Reedis told him, moving away from the others and turning back into a dragon, still on the ground. Jarin and Reedis were both rather pleased that they could pull it off.

It took longer than the twin soul pair would have preferred to arrange the distribution of riders and wyverns — Jarin was surprised to see a young man climb aboard Wymarc. He was slightly less surprised to see a girl — a teenager — climb aboard Ellen Annabelle. The girl, Chandra, and the two ghosts climbed on his back.

Ophidian leapt and changed into his dragon form, beckoning Jarin Reedis to show the way. Jarin climbed slowly, carefully, worried about the people riding his back, particularly the ghosts. Wouldn't the breeze blow them away?

It didn't, and soon they were skyborn, racing south.

# Chapter Seven

Alain Casman was worried. He was a stranger with the centaurs and the hexine, an outsider in their camp. Janzie treated him roughly, with no attempt to hide his disgust. His sister, Mayze was a bit more tolerant. All the others in the camp kept their distance from him. And, if the strange voice at night wasn't real, Alain was going insane.

"Those horses won't feed themselves!" Janzie called gruffly. "Get that hay spread out and then get ready for breakfast."

And that was another thing — Alain had never worked before eating in the morning. His stomach grumbled and he felt miserable. Thinking back on it, Alain Casman wasn't sure he could remember a single happy moment from the day he'd decided to honor his sister's plea to flee with her northwards. His time with Queen Airivik as "Britches" and "No Britches" was a stomach-churning haze of half-remembered shameful feelings and drug-muddled memories. He was glad that he'd repaid Madame Parkes' "kindness" with cold steel, that he had freed himself from his thrall and rescued his sister from a slow trap into slavery… and worse. But none of that brought him happiness.

Janzie shoved his shoulder roughly and Alain spun around with an angry look.

"I *said,* feed the horses!"

"I'm sorry," Alain said, eyes downcast, "I didn't sleep well last night."

"Didn't sleep well, eh?" Janzie said. His expression changed and his eyes narrowed. "Why?"

"I dreamed someone was talking to me," Alain said.

Janzie's eyes bulged and he turned on his heel to shout, "Mayze! They're talking to the *boy!*"

Before Alain could react, Mayze rushed over and stood in front of him. "They talked to you?" She demanded, continuing in a rush, "What did they say? Who said it? What do you know?" And then, before he could answer, she went on, speaking for herself. "Why did they talk to him? Does he know something? Is it the blood?"

Janzie seemed to understand that last question because he said, "Wait! Do you mean centaur or human?"

"Both, maybe," Mayze said, nodding to herself. "I wonder why they didn't talk to the girl."

"She's confused enough, being part horse and still new," Janzie said with a frown. "Or maybe…"

"Maybe it's because he's male," Mayze said. She turned her attention back to Alain. "Was it a male voice or female?"

"It was a woman's voice," Alain declared. "She said, 'Mother moon looks down on you.'"

"'Mother moon'?" Mayze repeated. She looked at Janzie. "See, I told you something was up!"

"I never argued the point," Janzie said, raising his hands defensively. He turned his eyes on Alain but kept speaking to Mayze. "Do you think she's answering us?"

"Something has to give," Mayze said cryptically. "Either that or…"

"Yeah," Janzie agreed, with feeling.

"Or what?" Alain demanded. "Are you saying that I didn't dream? That someone —" he broke off and turned toward the covered enclosure that housed the hexine. One of the six-legged beasts was looking right at him, meeting his eyes and nodding her head slowly. Alain trotted over to her. "You spoke to me? Really?"

The hexine nodded again. *You needed help. Still need it.*

"What's your name?" Alain asked.

*I am Seena,* the hexine mare replied. *Are you the one?*

"The one what?"

*The one who will free us?*

"I've only just freed myself," Alain said ruefully.

*Then you've had practice,* Seena replied, sounding serenely confident.

Alain rocked back on his heels. "I suppose I have, at that."

*And freed your sister, too, if your memories were true,* Seena replied. *Twice. And now she's been reformed in a centaur's shape.* The large hexine turned to nudge the other hexine standing beside her. *Do you doubt now, Leetar?*

*My question still is: how is he going to get us up?* A deep, bass male voice replied. *It's one thing for prophecy, another for action.*

*Have faith,* Seena said.

*Too many have died for me to still have faith,* Leetar replied with a sorrow so great that Alain whimpered at the feeling. The male hexine turned to face the rear of their enclosure. *I can only think now of our daughter, and her future.*

*You'll see,* Seena said. *Have faith in Kahlas, my love. She brought these two here, she has a reason.*

"Kahlas?" Alain asked out loud.

"What do you know of Kahlas?" Janzie demanded harshly.

Bethany loved flying. She was in her element. She could feel Margiss' worry and tried to console her just as Margiss had tried to console *her* about their new human body. They soared to join the others, Bethany's winging beating faster than the others to keep up with them.

*I'll get bigger,* Bethany promised Margiss. *We'll have our own rider ourselves.*

*Of course we will!* Margiss agreed firmly.

Ophidian, the great dark dragon shape, swerved toward them and, with a startled cry, they jerked away and down, fearing a collision.

*Stay put!* Ophidian chided them. *I need to show you something.*

*Show?* Margiss repeated, surprised that they could hear the god's voice in their minds. Bethany reminded her that Ophidian was, after all, a god, and could do many things. Admittedly, this was new.

*Last time you rode on Annabelle, so you didn't have to know how to go places,* Ophidian told them. *This time, you need to* see *where you're going to get there.*

See? Bethany wondered. How could they *see* someplace they'd never been. As if in answer, a scene — an image clearer than a dream but not quite as clear as eyesight — formed in their minds. Bethany cried with joy.

*Make the scene real,* Ophidian instructed.

While Margiss spent a moment pondering on that strange instruction, Bethany did as the god told her —

— and they were suddenly high in the air over an entirely different part of the world. Bethany cried in delight even as Margiss worriedly suggested that they should look around, fearful that they'd come to the wrong place.

A cry above them revealed that Ophidian had followed. Shortly, they were joined by the others — Jarin Reedis, Ellen Annabelle, and Krea Wymarc.

*Well done*, Ophidian told them, indicating that they should lead the way to the ground.

Bethany was reluctant to leave the glories of the air and her fabulous wings but Margiss reminded her that they were going to see Barbara Garrett, Freddie Fenimore, and Matt Evans — old classmates. Bethany accepted this and pulled in her wings, diving toward the ground. Margiss shrieked inside her head the whole way down until Bethany gently unfolded their wings, cupped air and brought them to a jarring halt.

*Ow!* Bethany cried as the force of their speed tried to tear her wings out of her body. Margiss, feeling triumphant, said nothing. Beyond the wrenching pain, they suffered no further damage and shortly were just inches above the snow-covered ground. Bethany touched the ground with one talon-foot and a moment later Margiss walked forward toward the shack.

"My arms!" Margiss cried, rubbing her shoulders painfully.

*Sorry*, Bethany said, not realizing that the exertions of the one form would be carried to the other. *Maybe we'll have time —* she broke off abruptly. *Do you feel that?*

Margiss did and picked up the pace until, regardless of their sore arms, they were running toward the shack.

They ran toward the sound of silent agony.

Tiko Amushi was a very careful person. She'd had to be to live as long in her trade. She'd left the boat with its dead behind her several days before, climbing the sheer cliffs from the shore to the heights with the knowledge that any mistake would be her last.

She hadn't expected to find Ophidian's castle at the top. She'd hidden as soon as she realized her location — to be caught by the dragon-god was to die, she was certain.

But he had servants... perhaps she could suborn them. If she could find his treasure room or — better — his library, her fortune and fame would be assured. Who would not be thrilled to hear the tale of one who had stolen from a god?

Her stomach demanded sustenance and she had to agree that it had first call on her actions: a corpse was not capable of much. So she'd searched for a quick entrance nearest the kitchens. She'd found it, found some small breads that could be safely 'liberated' to her stomach and then she'd rested. She would be careful, she would take her time, and she would be rewarded beyond her wildest dreams.

That was her plan.

It didn't work that way.

It didn't work that way because the library was also a workshop. Tiko crept along in the shadows of the castle's corridors until she heard voices. Instead of ducking away from them, she crept toward them, certain that she could handle any mere mortals.

But when she stepped into the largest room she'd ever seen, her senses overloaded and she could only stand there, just inside the entrance, jaw dropped as she tried to make sense of what her eyes and ears were showing her.

The voices were coming from the ground level, just a few hundred yards from her location. Her eyes bulged as she spied the metal shapes moving around a strange object. A young man moved up beside them, giving her a scale on which to measure the metal people. *Immortals*. Here.

And the object? It looked like one of their caravans only it was destroyed, crushed by forces she could only imagine. If it had been whole, it alone would have been worth more than she could hope to gain. And Tiko Amushi knew how to control a caravan. Her master would be ecstatic. This one, however, was destroyed. Perhaps if she could learn how it was wrecked…?

"What are you doing here?" a voice cried from above her. Tiko looked up and saw a young girl, who looked like kin, hovering in the air. The girl turned her head and shouted, "Pallas! We have an intruder from the Western Kingdom!"

"What do you want me to do with her?" a man's voice replied.

"We should put her on ice, don't you think?" the girl said.

*On ice?* Tiko thought to herself. And then a huge flying serpent, blue-white in color, swooped down toward her, opened its jaws and… Tiko thought no more.

"Father can thaw her when he wants," the man's voice rumbled dully through the layer of ice in which Tiko's frozen form was encased.

"Where did she come from?" another man's voice asked. "And why did she come here?"

"Who sent her?" a female metal voice asked.

"Hana, can you move her?" the first male's voice asked. "She's in the way where she is."

"Of course," the girl said. She wafted the frozen Tiko over to a corner at the far side of the room.

"She looks rather decorative," the male serpent said thoughtfully.

"I can see you making a garden of ice sculptures."

Tiko's ears stopped working, her heart stopped beating, and her frozen body heard no more.

Peter Hewlitt was glad when he heard footsteps approaching. In the hour since the others had left, the girl seemed to have gotten worse, fainter, weaker. He'd discovered, to his dismay, that she was particularly susceptible to the sound of his voice. Apologetically, Matt Evans had explained that Peter's voice was similar to that of the Steam Master's, blocking and moving into Hewlitt's space to force the spymaster to move away.

"Who's that?" Travers demanded when he heard the approaching sounds.

"They're back," Hewlitt said, moving toward the door.

Travers jumped in front of him, blocking his way. "Don't do that! It can't be them, it's too soon!"

Hewlitt was the king's spymaster. With two quick jabs, he had the railman on the ground, holding his sides and writhing in agony.

Nelly was unsympathetic, looking up from her kneeling position beside the stricken girl, she tsked, saying to the groaning Travers, "Really, you should know better!"

The door burst open and a young girl strode in, moving with determination.

"Margiss, what are you doing here?" Freddie Fennimore said.

"It's Bethany Margiss now," Bethany replied with Margiss' voice. She moved past him and knelt beside Nelly, nodding to the older woman before turning her attention to Barbara. She stroked the girl's hair softly and said, "We're here, we came as soon as we could."

Nelly found herself suddenly crying and didn't understand why until she saw tears rolling down the young girl's face and realized that her knee was touching Margiss'. The moment she pulled away from her, the intense pain and emotion left her. "How do you do that?"

"Do what?" Bethany Margiss replied, still intent on Barbara. "Barbara, dear, we're here. We're here to help."

Others entered the room and Nelly was relieved to have Jarin Reedis touch her shoulder lightly in an unspoken inquiry. Nelly knelt back and stood, turning to embrace the twin souled man who hugged tightly in return.

"She's broken," Travers said with a soft giggle, rising from the floor while keeping his distance from Hewlitt.

"So are you," Annabelle said with Ellen's voice. She turned back to Bethany Margiss and gestured toward Barbara. "I need to tend to her wounds."

Margiss nodded and moved over. Margaret hissed as she took in the other girl's state. She took an involuntary step back and turned away. Ellen Annabelle shot a look in her direction but, with a firm nod, put the older girl's discomfort out of her mind and returned her gaze to the injured Barbara.

Annabelle knelt down and turned back to the rest of the room. "She's going to want her privacy."

The men glanced at each other uncomfortably.

"I can make a fire," Ophidian promised. The railmen, who up until that moment had not noticed the dragon god, found themselves moving hastily to the door without quite knowing why. Soon, only Ellen, Margiss, and Nelly remained behind.

"Can you stand guard?" Ellen said to Skara who had just that moment walked through the door.

"Who are you talking to?" Nelly said, giving the young twin soul a surprised look.

"She can't see me," Skara said to Ellen. She made a face. "I think only those who have seen death can see me."

"Well, she saw you die," Bethany Margiss told her. She touched Nelly's hand. "Nelly Kendral, meet Skara Ningan."

Nelly's eyes widened as she could suddenly see the other woman. "You were the one they killed!"

"Yes," Skara admitted dourly. "Thomas is outside with the men."

"But the door didn't open!" Nelly said, glancing from Skara to the door behind her.

Skara grinned impishly. "Yes," she said, "pretty amazing, isn't it?"

Nelly nodded mutely.

"One of the perks of being dead," Skara said.

"Shh!" Annabelle hushed. "We need to roll her over, lift her shirt —"

"Or cut it —" Margiss said.

"Lift it unless you've got a replacement," Annabelle continued. She glanced to Bethany Margiss. "I may need your help with the healing."

"Healing?" Nelly said.

"It's a secret far too many people are beginning to know," Skara said with a sour glance toward Ellen Annabelle. "Little Ellen brought Annabelle back to life as a wyvern and twinned with her."

Nelly looked at the little girl with respect. "You did?"

Ellen nodded, her cheeks flushed.

"She can heal others," Bethany Margiss agreed.

"You took those poisoned teeth," Nelly pointed out.

Margiss nodded and jerked a hand toward Ellen. "She does physical healing better than me."

"And you?"

"She heals the mind," a new voice spoke up. The five women turned to the sound and saw a woman dressed in pale colors standing before them. Skara moved to protect the others but Bethany Margiss stopped her with a curt gesture.

"Goddess," Bethany Margiss said, bowing her head quickly and glancing for the others to do the same.

"Goddess?" Skara said questioningly, not moving from her defensive position.

"Kahlas," the goddess replied. She smiled at Margiss. "Well sensed, newborn."

"Please," Ellen Annabelle begged, "let me heal this one."

"That's why I'm here," Kahlas agreed, though she kept her eyes on Margiss. She waved for Ellen to proceed. Ellen made an imploring gesture to Nelly who quickly caught on that the seven year-old body was not suited to turning the older teenaged body over. Gently she helped Ellen and Margiss roll the injured girl over.

"Allow me," Kahlas said, moving forward. With a wave of her hand, the back part of Barbara's shirt disappeared, revealing ugly welts. Margaret turned around and made a horrified sound.

"You were worse," Bethany Margiss told her. Margaret's eyes went dark. "We can help her, don't worry."

Margaret nodded and moved to stand behind Ellen Annabelle. Ellen reached back a hand. Margaret took it and the younger girl squeezed it once in comfort and let it go.

"You can add your magic to hers," Kahlas said to Margaret in a kindly tone. "Just touch her and think to add your strength."

"My magic is mostly air," Margaret said.

Kahlas nodded. "I know."

Margaret gulped as she recalled that she was talking to a god. She touched Ellen's shoulder. The little girl patted her hand once in assurance then moved her hands to hover over the injuries on Barbara's back. Bethany Margiss moved closer to Ellen Annabelle and laid a hand on the smaller girl's arm, closing her eyes.

Ellen turned to Kahlas, "Is there anything else I should do?"

Kahlas smiled at her. "I don't know," Kahlas told her. She glanced toward Margaret. "Your friend might know better."

"I was in too much pain to even think," Margaret admitted ruefully. She gently squeezed Ellen's shoulder. "Whatever you did last time worked."

Ellen nodded in understanding, eyes still closer.

Fortunately, Barbara's physical injuries were less than Margaret's had been. In a few scant minutes, the wounds closed, the skin healed, and bruises disappeared. Ellen let out a deep breath and leaned back against Margaret, exhausted.

"It is the mind that will be more difficult," Kahlas said, magically returning the back half of Barbara's shirt to her body.

"What do I need to do?" Bethany Margiss asked, moving closer to the still form on the cot.

"You need to come with me," Kahlas said. "Ophidian?"

"I hear you," the dragon god said, standing inside the room as though he'd never left. "What do you propose?"

"I am one of the guardians of the mind," Kahlas said. She nodded toward Bethany Margiss. "If she wishes it, I could teach her much."

"In exchange for what, exactly?" Nelly said, moving to stand by Bethany Margiss.

"Oh! Aren't you a proper guardian!" Kahlas said, her lips turning up in delight. She turned to Ophidian. "Do you claim her?"

"My heart belongs with Reedis," Nelly snapped back. In a softer voice, she added, "And Jarin, his twin soul."

"So you are half-dragon but not wholly so," Kahlas said to herself. She met Nelly's eyes. The woman stared back unflinchingly.

"Miss Kendral, you should know that Kahlas is the goddess of the moon and the inner eye," Ophidian said in a tone that was mild but conveyed a warning.

"I am not afraid of gods," Nelly replied staunchly.

"Yes," Ophidian agreed with a sigh, "I'd noticed."

Kahlas laughed. She waved a hand toward Nelly. "I mean no harm to you and yours, mage."

"I'm not — I mean, I don't —" Nelly stammered. She broke half and gave the goddess a quick curtsy. "Thank you."

"Back to this deal," Skara Ningan said, moving to stand by Nelly protectively. The school principal gave her a grateful look.

"The dead walk?" Kahlas said, turning to Ophidian.

"I made a deal," Ophidian said, nodding toward Ellen and Margiss. "They need protecting."

"That is why I am here," Kahlas said. She nodded toward Bethany Margiss. "She has potential, as you know, but she is untrained."

"You offer to train her?" Skara demanded. "How?"

"Why is it a concern of yours, dead human?"

"She was once my twin soul," Bethany spoke up quickly, her eyes flashing. "I love her as a sister, if not more."

Skara's face burst into a huge grin. She nodded, eyes misting, in fervent agreement with the young twin soul.

"Spymaster Hewlitt," Kahlas' voice rose to carry through the door and into the winds outside the hut.

"Am I wanted?" Hewlitt replied, knocking on the door. "Miss Kendral?"

"Come," Nelly replied.

Hewlitt opened the door and strode through, followed on his heels by Margen and, oddly, Travers.

"Yes, yes, I see you," Kahlas said as soon as Travers caught sight of her. She turned to Ophidian and gave him the sort of exasperated expression that only one god can give to another. Ophidian buried his grin in a thin-lipped grimace.

"Do you recall a young lad lately in the service of the queen?" Kahlas demanded of the spymaster, her eyes still on Bethany Margiss.

"The one she alternately called 'Britches' and 'No Britches'?"

"What?" Nelly demanded. She turned to Hewlitt. "How old was this lad?"

"He had a sister," Kahlas continued, ignoring Nelly's outburst. She turned to catch Hewlitt's eyes. "They had fled from Jasram to prevent her from marrying against her will."

"I was not aware of that," Hewlitt said, pursing his lips in thought. He glanced to the goddess. "Casman?"

Kahlas nodded.

"Casman!" Ophidian said. He turned to Kahlas. "Now things become clearer."

"It helps that I can see the whole world, not just the parts that interest me at one particular moment," Kahlas said high-mindedly.

"Which reminds me," Ophidian began, "I have —"

"Yes, I know," Kahlas said. "And it would be best not to forestall her journey much longer."

"Ibb said —"

"You speak with the metal ones?" Kahlas interjected. When Ophidian nodded, she continued in a lower tone, "I cannot scry what they think."

"Understandably," Ophidian agreed. "But Ibb and Tracker are helping me on a project which might help your pet on her way."

"She's no pet!" Kahlas replied hotly. When she noticed the satisfaction in Ophidian's eyes, she shook her head. In a soft tone, she continued, "If you'd just asked me, I would have told the same."

"But now I know," Ophidian replied.

"Are you two going to keep entertaining yourselves for the rest of the day?" Jarin Reedis demanded as he walked in. "Or is something of import going to be said, or some action taken?"

"Oh, *he's* your son!" Kahlas said to Ophidian with glee.

"She's getting around to making us an offer," Bethany Margiss said, glancing toward Margen. "I think she wants us to join her on the moon."

"Yes, exactly," Kahlas agreed. She turned to Ophidian, noting the other's growing ire. "At least, at first. After…"

"Can you help her?" Margaret Waters spoke up, moving to stand beside Bethany Margiss but pointing toward Barbara Garrett. The young teen was sleeping peacefully, her muscles unclenched.

"And him?" Nelly said, nodding toward Travers.

"And you want help for your Casman children," Hewlitt guessed.

"Oh, look, it's Kahlas!" Wymarc said acidly as Krea Wymarc stepped through the door. She turned back to the remaining railmen and said, "You'd best stay outside, unless you want to go mad."

"Oh, hello, Wymarc," Kahlas said. "Didn't recognize you in the new body?" She scanned Krea's albino form quickly and scowled. "Bit of a step down for you, isn't it?"

"You dare!" Wymarc hissed, her words echoed by Jarin Reedis.

"Kahlas, really," Ophidian said in a mild voice. "Were you not once all white yourself?"

"And I remember the scorn applied to me by a young daughter of yours," Kahlas said, nodding coldly toward Wymarc.

"I apologize," Krea said. "Wymarc was younger then and hadn't the chance —"

"*I* apologize," Wymarc said, taking control of Krea's voice. "I was wrong." She lifted her eyes up to meet Kahlas'. "Will you forgive me?"

Kahlas' eyes widened in shock. A moment later she said, "Of course I'll forgive you." She turned back to Ophidian. "They *do* grow up, don't they?"

Ophidian acknowledged this with a dip of his chin. "As to your offer…?"

Kahlas turned back to Bethany Margiss and knelt down. "Young wyvern, yours is a gift given only rarely and it could help so many. Would you please let me teach you all that I can?"

"The last one was… Aldara," Ophidian recalled.

"Aldara the Addled?" Wymarc snapped, her eyes going wide. She looked beseechingly to Ophidian. "Father, you can't —"

"Aldara lived a long time a very long time ago," Kahlas said, "when the gods themselves were very different." Kahlas looked over to Bethany Margiss. "She had my training but she was overwhelmed in the end." Kahlas made a gesture toward Ophidian. "During the God's War."

"Could this happen to Bethany Margiss, too?" Skara asked in a small voice.

"It could," Kahlas agreed. "Nothing is guaranteed." She nodded to Bethany Margiss, adding, "And there are gods arrayed against you. There are gods who like to break men's minds, to hurt, to maim —"

"Please, goddess!" Travers begged. "Please."

"And sometimes," Kahlas said with a wave toward Travers who broke off and curled up in a ball, whimpering, "sometimes they bring it on themselves."

"What else?" Nelly demanded. "You threaten this child's sanity, tell her that gods might want to torture her, why are you here?"

"It's the children," Hewlitt said, nodding to Kahlas. Kahlas turned her head toward him and tilted an eyebrow upwards. "The children of the moon."

"Too many are dead," Kahlas said in agreement, her voice sad. She glanced over to Ophidian. "Your children live, grow and prosper…"

"That is because of her," Ophidian said, nodding to Ellen Annabelle. She turned bright red. Ophidian added softly, "And because *humans* took pity on her and helped her live."

"That is what I'm asking for," Kahlas said. "Pity."

"You know Hana, don't you?" Krea spoke up. "You are the goddess of the —"

Kahlas stopped her with an upraised hand. "Not many people know, it is a secret, perhaps forever."

"Not if we can help it," Krea spoke up fiercely. "I gave a vow —"

"And *that* too, should be kept a secret," Kahlas warned. She turned her eyes back to Bethany Margiss. "What I am offering is a chance to learn to help injuries of the brain and the mind, a chance to heal the inner eye, a rare gift only suited to those with rare talents."

"And if she refuses?" Skara demanded.

"And what of Chandra?" Bethany Margiss demanded.

"Who?"

"Her rider," Wymarc explained. She jerked her head toward the door. "She is, apparently, sensible to —"

The door opened and Chandra stomped in, glaring at Ophidian, then Kahlas.

"Chandra Earthshaker, may I make you known to Kahlas, goddess of the moon," Ophidian said with a chortle.

"Earthshaker?"

"She broke the gates of the zwerg kingdom in the north, looking for someone to help me," Margaret Waters explained, beaming with pride toward her adopted sister. She waved a hand toward Bethany Margiss. "You don't get one without the other."

Kahlas turned wide eyes toward Ophidian. "You would have me take an *earth* mage to the moon?"

Ophidian shrugged. "Not my choice."

Skara shot Chandra an inquiring look. The dark girl explained, "I was keeping the others from entering." She nodded toward Kahlas. "Besides, there was far too much drama already."

"It's the children who worry you," Hewlitt spoke up. Chandra shot him a look which he ignored. "What is going on in Jasram?"

"A very good question," Kahlas allowed. "Are you not the king's spymaster?"

"I have enough to do, keeping up with what is going on in the kingdom," Hewlitt admitted, spreading his hands in a gesture of helplessness.

"Kingdoms, now," Kahlas reminded him. Hewlitt accepted the correction with a grimace and asked, "But the children?"

"They, too, are broken and need help only *we* —" she gestured between herself and Bethany Margiss "— can give."

"She'd be safer," Ophidian said diplomatically.

"On the moon?" Chandra asked. She turned to Kahlas. "Would my magic not work there?"

"'Earth' includes anything you can touch," Kahlas told her. "You magic would work perfectly well up there — perhaps too well."

"How do we get there?" Bethany Margiss asked. She glanced toward Margen. "And could others visit?"

"I'm afraid that we'll be rather busy down here," Margen told his granddaughter apologetically. "But it is a chance of a lifetime, to journey to the goddess' home in the sky."

"Mr. Travers," Bethany Margiss said, moving toward the man. Travers craned his head back over his shoulder and looked up to her. "Let me see if I can help you."

Travers whimpered and turned his head back to the ground but he did not resist when Bethany Margiss touched him lightly on the neck. She gave a hiss of pain before clenching her jaw but she did not flinch away from the man. She made a quick gesture behind her back with her hand and said softly, "Chandra, can you make the ground shake, softly?"

Chandra's eyes widened. She moved toward Bethany Margiss, knelt and closed her eyes. Softly, gently the shack began to shake.

Travers let out a whimper, then a sigh. Bethany Margiss muttered soft, soothing nonsense words to the man and then, sat back, taking her hand from his neck and turning to Chandra. "You can stop now."

"You are good," Kahlas said. "I can feel his ease from here."

"He'll never be completely better," Margiss said, her eyes moist, "but I did what I could."

"His injuries are hard to heal," Kahlas said in agreement. One corner of her lips twitched upwards. "He calls to me often and I do what I can, give him dreams and comfort."

Bethany Margiss nodded and stood, grabbing Chandra's hand in her own. "I would like to learn more."

Kahlas raised an eyebrow toward Ophidian.

"I do not release any oaths or vows," Ophidian warned his sister god. "And you *will* keep in touch."

"As you say," Kahlas agreed. She raised her hands, palms up to the two girls.

"Grandfather?" Margiss called out.

"Go!" Margen told her, smiling fondly. "You know how to contact me."

Margiss' eyes widened and she smiled fiercely. She reached forward and placed her hand, palm down, in Kahlas'. Chandra's hand joined the goddess' other hand.

And the three vanished.

## END

# King's Crown

# Book 20

Twin Soul series

# Dedication

**For Miguel Sandoval.**

**An incredible son, husband, and father.**

**A true fighter.**

# Prolog

**P**eter Hewlitt, Kingsland's spymaster, was glad when he heard footsteps approaching the scratch-built shack where he'd been on guard. In the hour since the others had left, the girl seemed to have gotten worse, fainter, weaker. He'd discovered, to his dismay, that she was particularly susceptible to the sound of his voice. Apologetically, Matt Evans had explained that Peter's voice was similar to that of the Steam Master's, blocking and moving into Hewlitt's space to force the spymaster to move away.

"Who's that?" Travers demanded when he heard the approaching sounds.

"They're back," Hewlitt said, moving toward the door.

Travers jumped in front of him, blocking his way. "Don't do that! It can't be them, it's too soon!"

Hewlitt was the king's spymaster. With two quick jabs, he had the railman on the ground, holding his sides and writhing in agony.

Nelly was unsympathetic, looking up from her kneeling position beside the stricken girl, she tsked, saying to the groaning Travers, "Really, you should know better!"

The door burst open, and a young girl strode in, moving with determination.

"Margiss, what are you doing here?" Freddie Fennimore said.

"It's Bethany Margiss now," Bethany replied with Margiss' voice. She moved past him and knelt beside Nelly, nodding to the older woman before turning her attention to Barbara. She stroked the girl's hair softly and said, "We're here, we came as soon as we could."

Nelly found herself suddenly crying and didn't understand why until she saw tears rolling down the young girl's face and realized that her knee was touching Margiss'. The moment she pulled away from her, the intense pain and emotion left her. "How do you do that?"

"Do what?" Bethany Margiss replied, still intent on Barbara. "Barbara, dear, we're here. We're here to help."

Others entered the room and Nelly was relieved to have Jarin Reedis touch her shoulder lightly in an unspoken inquiry. Nelly knelt back and stood, turning to embrace the twin-souled man who hugged tightly in return.

"She's broken," Travers said with a soft giggle, rising from the floor while keeping his distance from Hewlitt.

"So are you," Annabelle said with Ellen's voice. She turned back to Bethany Margiss and gestured toward Barbara. "I need to tend to her wounds."

Margiss nodded and moved over. Margaret hissed as she took in the other girl's state. She took an involuntary step back and turned away. Ellen Annabelle shot a look in her direction but, with a firm nod, put the older girl's discomfort out of her mind and returned her gaze to the injured Barbara.

Annabelle knelt down and turned back to the rest of the room. "She's going to want her privacy."

The men glanced at each other uncomfortably.

"I can make a fire," Ophidian promised. The railmen, who until that moment had not noticed the dragon god, found themselves moving hastily to the door without quite knowing why. Soon, only Ellen, Margiss, and Nelly remained behind.

"Can you stand guard?" Ellen said to Skara, who had just that moment walked through the door.

"Who are you talking to?" Nelly said, giving the young twin soul a surprised look.

"She can't see me," Skara said to Ellen. She made a face. "I think only those who have seen death can see me."

"Well, she saw you die," Bethany Margiss told her. She touched Nelly's hand. "Nelly Kendral, meet Skara Ningan."

Nelly's eyes widened as she could suddenly see the other woman. "You were the one they killed!"

"Yes," Skara admitted dourly. "Thomas is outside with the men."

"But the door didn't open!" Nelly said, glancing from Skara to the door behind her.

Skara grinned impishly. "Yes," she said, "pretty amazing, isn't it?"

Nelly nodded mutely.

"One of the perks of being dead," Skara said.

"Shh!" Annabelle hushed. "We need to roll her over, lift her shirt —"

"Or cut it — " Margiss said.

"Lift it unless you've got a replacement," Annabelle continued. She glanced to Bethany Margiss. "I may need your help with the healing."

"Healing?" Nelly said.

"It's a secret far too many people are learning," Skara said with a sour glance toward Ellen Annabelle. "Little Ellen brought Annabelle back to life as a wyvern and twinned with her."

Nelly looked at the little girl with respect. "You did?"

Ellen nodded, her cheeks flushed.

"She can heal others," Bethany Margiss agreed.

"You took those poisoned teeth," Nelly pointed out.

Margiss nodded and jerked a hand toward Ellen. "She does physical healing better than me."

"And you?"

"She heals the mind," a new voice spoke up. The five women turned to the sound and saw a woman dressed in pale colors standing before them. Skara moved to protect the others, but Bethany Margiss stopped her with a curt gesture.

"Goddess," Bethany Margiss said, bowing her head quickly and glancing for the others to do the same.

"Goddess?" Skara said questioningly, not moving from her defensive position.

"Kahlas," the goddess replied. She smiled at Margiss. "Well sensed, newborn."

"Please," Ellen Annabelle begged, "let me heal this one."

"That's why I'm here," Kahlas agreed, though she kept her eyes on Margiss. She waved for Ellen to proceed. Ellen made an imploring gesture to Nelly who quickly caught on that the seven-year-old body was not suited to turning the older teenaged body over. Gently, she helped Ellen and Margiss roll the injured girl over.

"Allow me," Kahlas said, moving forward. With a wave of her hand, the back part of Barbara's shirt disappeared, revealing ugly welts. Margaret turned around and made a horrified sound.

"You were worse," Bethany Margiss told her. Margaret's eyes went dark. "We can help her, don't worry."

Margaret nodded and moved to stand behind Ellen Annabelle. Ellen reached back a hand. Margaret took it and the younger girl squeezed it once in comfort and let it go.

"You can add your magic to hers," Kahlas said to Margaret in a kindly tone. "Just touch her and think to add your strength."

"My magic is mostly air," Margaret said.

Kahlas nodded. "I know."

Margaret gulped as she recalled that she was talking to a god. She touched Ellen's shoulder. The little girl patted her hand once in assurance, then moved her hands to hover over the injuries on Barbara's back. Bethany Margiss moved closer to Ellen Annabelle and laid a hand on the smaller girl's arm, closing her eyes.

Ellen turned to Kahlas, "Is there anything else I should do?"

Kahlas smiled at her. "I don't know," Kahlas told her. She glanced toward Margaret. "Your friend might know better."

"I was in too much pain to even think," Margaret admitted ruefully. She gently squeezed Ellen's shoulder. "Whatever you did last time worked."

Ellen nodded in understanding, eyes still closer.

Fortunately, Barbara's physical injuries were less than Margaret's had been. In a few scant minutes, the wounds closed, the skin healed, and bruises disappeared. Ellen let out a deep breath and leaned back against Margaret, exhausted.

"It is the mind that will be more difficult," Kahlas said, magically returning the back half of Barbara's shirt to her body.

"What do I need to do?" Bethany Margiss asked, moving closer to the still form on the cot.

"You need to come with me," Kahlas said. "Ophidian?"

"I hear you," the dragon god said, standing inside the room as though he'd never left. "What do you propose?"

"I am one of the guardians of the mind," Kahlas said. She nodded toward Bethany Margiss. "If she wishes it, I could teach her much."

"In exchange for what, exactly?" Nelly said, moving to stand by Bethany Margiss.

"Oh! Aren't you a proper guardian!" Kahlas said, her lips turning up in delight. She turned to Ophidian. "Do you claim her?"

"My heart belongs with Reedis," Nelly snapped back. In a softer voice, she added, "And Jarin, his twin soul."

"So you are half-dragon, but not wholly so," Kahlas said to herself. She met Nelly's eyes. The woman stared back unflinchingly.

"Miss Kendral, you should know that Kahlas is the goddess of the moon and the inner eye," Ophidian said in a tone that was mild but conveyed a warning.

"I am not afraid of gods," Nelly replied staunchly.

"Yes," Ophidian agreed with a sigh, "I'd noticed."

Kahlas laughed. She waved a hand toward Nelly. "I mean no harm to you and yours, mage."

"I'm not — I mean, I don't — " Nelly stammered. She broke half and gave the goddess a quick curtsy. "Thank you."

"Back to this deal," Skara Ningan said, moving to stand by Nelly protectively. The school principal gave her a grateful look.

"The dead walk?" Kahlas said, turning to Ophidian.

"I made a deal," Ophidian said, nodding toward Ellen and Margiss. "They need protecting."

"That is why I am here," Kahlas said. She nodded toward Bethany Margiss. "She has potential, as you know, but she is untrained."

"You offer to train her?" Skara demanded. "How?"

"Why is it a concern of yours, dead human?"

"She was once my twin soul," Bethany spoke up quickly, her eyes flashing. "I love her as a sister, if not more."

Skara's face burst into a huge grin. She nodded, eyes misting in fervent agreement with the young twin soul.

"Spymaster Hewlitt," Kahlas' voice rose to carry through the door and into the winds outside the hut.

"Am I wanted?" Hewlitt replied, knocking on the door. "Miss Kendral?"

"Come," Nelly replied.

Hewlitt opened the door and strode through, followed on his heels by Margen and, oddly, Travers.

"Yes, yes, I see you," Kahlas said as soon as Travers caught sight of her. She turned to Ophidian and gave him the sort of exasperated expression that only one god can give to another. Ophidian buried his grin in a thin-lipped grimace.

"Do you recall a young lad lately in the service of the queen?" Kahlas demanded of the spymaster, her eyes still on Bethany Margiss.

"The one she alternately called 'Britches' and 'No Britches'?"

"What?" Nelly demanded. She turned to Hewlitt. "How old was this lad?"

"He had a sister," Kahlas continued, ignoring Nelly's outburst. She turned to catch Hewlitt's eyes. "They had fled from Jasram to prevent her from marrying against her will."

"I was not aware of that," Hewlitt said, pursing his lips in thought. He glanced to the goddess. "Casman?"

Kahlas nodded.

"Casman!" Ophidian said. He turned to Kahlas. "Now things become clearer."

"It helps that I can see the whole world, not just the parts that interest me at one particular moment," Kahlas said high-mindedly.

"Which reminds me," Ophidian began, "I have —"

"Yes, I know," Kahlas said. "And it would be best not to forestall her journey much longer."

"Ibb said —"

"You speak with the metal ones?" Kahlas interjected. When Ophidian nodded, she continued in a lower tone, "I cannot scry what they think."

"Understandably," Ophidian agreed. "But Ibb and Tracker are helping me on a project which might help your pet on her way."

"She's no pet!" Kahlas replied hotly. When she noticed the satisfaction in Ophidian's eyes, she shook her head. In a soft tone, she continued, "If you'd just asked me, I would have told you the same."

"But now I know," Ophidian replied.

"Are you two going to keep entertaining yourselves for the rest of the day?" Jarin Reedis demanded as he walked in. "Or is something of import going to be said, or some action taken?"

"Oh, *he's* your son!" Kahlas said to Ophidian with glee.

"She's getting around to making us an offer," Bethany Margiss said, glancing toward Margen. "I think she wants us to join her on the moon."

"Yes, exactly," Kahlas agreed. She turned to Ophidian, noting the other's growing ire. "At least, at first. After…"

"Can you help her?" Margaret Waters spoke up, moving to stand beside Bethany Margiss but pointing toward Barbara Garrett. The young teen was sleeping peacefully, her muscles unclenched.

"And him?" Nelly said, nodding toward Travers.

"And you want help for your Casman children," Hewlitt guessed.

"Oh, look, it's Kahlas!" Wymarc said acidly as Krea Wymarc stepped through the door. She turned back to the remaining railmen and said, "You'd best stay outside, unless you want to go mad."

"Oh, hello, Wymarc," Kahlas said. "Didn't recognize you in the new body?" She scanned Krea's albino form quickly and scowled. "Bit of a step down for you, isn't it?"

"You dare!" Wymarc hissed, her words echoed by Jarin Reedis.

"Kahlas, really," Ophidian said in a mild voice. "Were you not once all white yourself?"

"And I remember the scorn applied to me by a young daughter of yours," Kahlas said, nodding coldly toward Wymarc.

"I apologize," Krea said. "Wymarc was younger then, and hadn't the chance —"

"I apologize," Wymarc said, taking control of Krea's voice. "I was wrong." She lifted her eyes up to meet Kahlas'. "Will you forgive me?"

Kahlas' eyes widened in shock. A moment later she said, "Of course I'll forgive you." She turned back to Ophidian. "They do grow up, don't they?"

Ophidian acknowledged this with a dip of his chin. "As to your offer…?"

Kahlas turned back to Bethany Margiss and knelt down. "Young wyvern, yours is a gift given only rarely and it could help so many. Would you please let me teach you all that I can?"

"The last one was… Aldara," Ophidian recalled.

"Aldara the Addled?" Wymarc snapped, her eyes going wide. She looked beseechingly to Ophidian. "Father, you can't —"

"Aldara lived a long time, a very long time ago," Kahlas said, "when the gods themselves were very different." Kahlas looked over to Bethany Margiss. "She had my training, but she was overwhelmed in the end." Kahlas made a gesture toward Ophidian. "During the God's War."

"Could this happen to Bethany Margiss, too?" Skara asked in a small voice.

"It could," Kahlas agreed. "Nothing is guaranteed." She nodded to Bethany Margiss, adding, "And there are gods arrayed against you. There are gods who like to break men's minds, to hurt, to maim —"

"Please, goddess!" Travers begged. "Please."

"And sometimes," Kahlas said with a wave toward Travers who broke off and curled up in a ball, whimpering, "sometimes they bring it on themselves."

"What else?" Nelly demanded. "You threaten this child's sanity, tell her that gods might want to torture her, why are you here?"

"It's the children," Hewlitt said, nodding to Kahlas. Kahlas turned her head toward him and tilted an eyebrow upwards. "The children of the moon."

"Too many are dead," Kahlas said in agreement, her voice sad. She glanced over to Ophidian. "Your children live, grow, and prosper…"

"That is because of her," Ophidian said, nodding to Ellen Annabelle. She turned bright red. Ophidian added softly, "And because *humans* took pity on her and helped her live."

"That is what I'm asking for," Kahlas said. "Pity."

"You know Hana, don't you?" Krea spoke up. "You are the goddess of the —"

Kahlas stopped her with an upraised hand. "Few people know, it is a secret, perhaps forever."

"Not if we can help it," Krea spoke up fiercely. "I gave a vow —"

"And *that*, too, should be kept a secret," Kahlas warned. She turned her eyes back to Bethany Margiss. "What I am offering is a chance to learn to help injuries of the brain and the mind, a chance to heal the inner eye, a rare gift only suited to those with rare talents."

"And if she refuses?" Skara demanded.

"And what of Chandra?" Bethany Margiss demanded.

"Who?"

"Her rider," Wymarc explained. She jerked her head toward the door. "She is, apparently, sensible to —"

The door opened, and Chandra stomped in, glaring at Ophidian, then Kahlas.

"Chandra Earthshaker, may I make you known to Kahlas, goddess of the moon," Ophidian said with a chortle.

"Earthshaker?"

"She broke the gates of the zwerg kingdom in the north, looking for someone to help me," Margaret Waters explained, beaming with pride toward her adopted sister. She waved a hand toward Bethany Margiss. "You don't get one without the other."

Kahlas turned wide eyes toward Ophidian. "You would have me take an *earth* mage to the moon?"

Ophidian shrugged. "Not my choice."

Skara shot Chandra an inquiring look. The dark girl explained, "I was keeping the others from entering." She nodded toward Kahlas. "Besides, there was far too much drama already."

"It's the children who worry you," Hewlitt spoke up. Chandra shot him a look, which he ignored. "What is going on in Jasram?"

"An excellent question," Kahlas allowed. "Are you not the king's spymaster?"

"I have enough to do, keeping up with what is going on in the kingdom," Hewlitt admitted, spreading his hands in a gesture of helplessness.

"Kingdoms, now," Kahlas reminded him. Hewlitt accepted the correction with a grimace and asked, "But the children?"

"They, too, are broken and need help only *we* —" she gestured between herself and Bethany Margiss "— can give."

"She'd be safer," Ophidian said diplomatically.

"On the moon?" Chandra asked. She turned to Kahlas. "Would my magic not work there?"

"'Earth' includes anything you can touch," Kahlas told her. "You magic would work perfectly well up there — perhaps too well."

"How do we get there?" Bethany Margiss asked. She glanced toward Margen. "And could others visit?"

"I'm afraid that we'll be rather busy down here," Margen told his granddaughter apologetically. "But it is a chance of a lifetime, to journey to the goddess' home in the sky."

"Mr. Travers," Bethany Margiss said, moving toward the man. Travers craned his head back over his shoulder and looked up at her. "Let me see if I can help you."

Travers whimpered and turned his head back to the ground, but he did not resist when Bethany Margiss touched him lightly on the neck. She gave a hiss of pain before clenching her jaw, but she did not flinch away from the man. She made a quick gesture behind her back with her hand and said softly, "Chandra, can you make the ground shake, softly?"

Chandra's eyes widened. She moved toward Bethany Margiss, knelt and closed her eyes. Softly, gently, the shack began to shake.

Travers let out a whimper, then a sigh. Bethany Margiss muttered soft, soothing nonsense words to the man and then sat back, taking her hand from his neck and turning to Chandra. "You can stop now."

"You are good," Kahlas said. "I can feel his ease from here."

"He'll never be completely better," Margiss said, her eyes moist, "but I did what I could."

"His injuries are hard to heal," Kahlas said in agreement. One corner of her lips twitched upwards. "He calls to me often and I do what I can, give him dreams and comfort."

Bethany Margiss nodded and stood, grabbing Chandra's hand in her own. "I would like to learn more."

Kahlas raised an eyebrow at Ophidian.

"I do not release any oaths or vows," Ophidian warned his sister god. "And you *will* keep in touch."

"As you say," Kahlas agreed. She raised her hands, palms up, to the two girls.

"Grandfather?" Margiss called out.

"Go!" Margen told her, smiling fondly. "You know how to contact me."

Margiss' eyes widened, and she smiled fiercely. She reached forward and placed her hand, palm down, in Kahlas'. Chandra's hand joined the goddess' other hand.

And the three vanished.

# Chapter One

"Well, *that* was exciting," Ophidian said as Kahlas, goddess of the moon, Bethany Margiss, twin-souled healer, and Chandra 'Earthshaker' vanished from the hastily-built shack in which they'd all been conversing. "Let it not be said that my sister doesn't know how to make an exit."

His expression changed when he glanced toward the cot where Barbara Garrett lay, sleeping peacefully, and frowned. "Hmm, apparently she forgot —"

He broke off as the girl's form grew transparent and then invisible, and the blanket thrown over her collapsed.

"I was wondering about that, too," Nelly said, before suddenly pressing her hands to her face and exclaiming, "Oh, heavens! Look at the time! We must get back to mother!"

"Drake!" Wymarc cried as she turned and banged the hut's door open. "Get ready, we're leaving!"

"But what about the railway?" Norman Gossett pleaded.

"Yes," Hewlitt added, glancing toward Ophidian, "what about the railway?"

"You know," Ophidian said in a dangerously soft voice, "I don't owe you anything."

"No," Hewlitt agreed hastily. "In fact, you have been too kind. But I cannot help but think that you, the god of change, are not uninterested in seeing what happens when the rail lines connect all the cities and towns of Kingsland."

Ophidian gave him a look.

"I suspect he's right, you know," Margen chimed in. "Think of all it could do."

"And the airships!" Reedis added. "What wonders will they bring!"

"With airships, why would you need rails?" Ophidian asked slyly.

"Rails for heavy goods moving slowly, airships for lighter goods moving fast," Hewlitt replied immediately. Ophidian looked surprised. The spymaster shrugged. "I have been thinking about this a lot, recently."

"Apparently," Ophidian agreed drolly.

"How long would it take to finish the line to Sorellay?" Hewlitt asked Gossett, the rail boss.

Gossett shrugged. "Without magic —"

"With magic," Margen interrupted. He glanced toward Margaret. "I'd heard it said that you are something to behold, young lady."

Margaret blushed.

"And it wouldn't hurt to learn from the best," Drake piped up faithfully. He glanced at Matt Evans, the other air mage.

"It would be a learning experience," Margen agreed. He glanced toward Nelly. "But, my dear —"

"If you wish to stay here, mage, I think I could take a hand at teaching," Wymarc allowed.

"She's very good," Ellen Annabelle quickly added. "And I'll be safer here than I would at the school."

"Weelll," Nelly said slowly. She glanced at Jarin Reedis. "Do you suppose you could teach a class?"

"Your school *is* named after him," Jarin said.

"I'd be delighted," Reedis allowed. "I can teach balloon magic."

"He can," Ellen Annabelle agreed, "he taught us."

"He did?" Ophidian repeated. He glanced toward Reedis. "And why is this the first I've heard of it?"

"Well, I wouldn't say that you're too busy talking to hear anything," Wymarc replied. "I'll say instead that perhaps you were too *involved* in other matters."

Ophidian fumed at her. Wymarc, with a thousand years' experience, met his gaze staunchly.

"So it's settled," Nelly declared, grabbing Reedis' arm and pulling him out the door. "We'll go back to school — mother will be *much* relieved — and leave you to it."

"And you?" Ophidian demanded of Hewlitt.

"Can you carry... four?" Hewlitt asked Ellen Annabelle. The young girl nodded firmly. Hewlitt smiled at her. He turned to Ophidian. "If it pleases you, I shall remain here. I have never seen railway track laid and I would relish the experience."

"Be careful, spy, you've all the makings of a decent mage," Ophidian warned. Before Hewlitt could react, the dragon god disappeared.

"Sire, I have good news," first minister Mannevy said as he entered the royal chambers that afternoon.

"Finally," Queen Rassa muttered.

"The airship has returned?" King Markel guessed, frowning as he tried to remember their previous conversation. "You found more money?"

"Not... exactly," the first minister temporized. "However, I *have* discovered a way in which we can get you coronated immediately."

"And how is that?" King Markel said. "You told me that we didn't have enough money."

"And we do not," Mannevy agreed. "But, as we know we will shortly have enough money to pay for the coronation, I discovered a number of your new subjects who were willing to loan us the funds on the promise of the gold when it arrives."

"Why not just take it from them?" Markel wondered.

Mannevy gave him a pained look. "The thought had crossed my mind, sire," the first minister admitted, "but I thought perhaps you might want to be able to have future dealings with these good people."

"We can always declare them traitors later," Queen Rassa allowed, "and take *all* their money."

"Indeed," Mannevy allowed, looking even more pained, "that is possible. However, I advise against it as it would bring suspicion on the integrity of the crown."

"As long as I *get* my crown, I don't care," King Markel said. He smiled at his minister and rubbed his hands. "When can we do it?"

"Arrangements still take time, sire," Mannevy warned. "But, with this news — perhaps tomorrow evening?"

"Excellent!"

"You can teach?" Mrs. Kendral said when Reedis and the rest returned. When mage Reedis nodded affirmatively, Mrs. Kendral waved him down a corridor. "Room Three."

Reedis shot a look at Nelly who pursed her lips to speak but she was cut off by her mother, who told her, "You have several parents waiting in your lobby."

"My lobby?" Nelly squeaked. She didn't know she had a lobby.

"Angry?" Wymarc asked.

"Hopeful," Mrs. Kendral replied enigmatically. She frowned at Wymarc in Krea's body. "Were you hoping to teach as well?"

"Krea is young, but Wymarc is thousands of years old," Reedis told his future mother-in-law.

"Ah!" Mrs. Kendral responded. She gestured down the hall. "If you can take on the class in room Five, then."

"Of course," Krea Wymarc replied, hastening away.

"Well, that's settled," Mrs. Kendral said primly. She turned to her daughter. "If you can manage here, dear, I shall take myself off to the Steam Master's office."

"Office?"

"Yes," Mrs. Kendral said. "I am *very* interested in his bookkeeping."

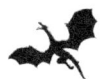

"The Steam Master said you were the best," Freddie said as he walked with Margaret Waters to the ruins of their construction site. "He used to give Barbara *such* a hard time. He'd always say, 'Margaret can do it better! Why can't you be like her, rich girl?'"

Ellen, who was walking beside them, touched Margaret on the arm. The taller girl looked down at her and Ellen smiled.

"I don't think I am that great," Margaret said, reaching down to take Ellen's hand. "I just do my best, is all."

"That's what Barbara did," Matt Evans said softly. He was trailing just behind them. Further back were the rail crew, mage Margen, and the spymaster, Peter Hewlitt.

Margaret stopped and dropped Ellen's hand, smiling apologetically. To Freddie, she said, "I always call on the gods before I start."

She glanced at the jumble of railroad ties, at the scattered lengths of steel rails. She turned back to the rail boss, Mr. Gossett. "How is the track to be laid?"

"Straight for the next league," Mr. Gossett replied. "But you don't have to worry about all that —"

"A league I can manage," Margaret told him. She eyed the sky. "It will be getting dark soon enough. We'll lay the league and see what comes next."

Gossett gave her a wide-eyed look. "Whatever you say, miss," he said, his tone doubtful.

Margaret turned to Ellen and smiled. She took three steps forward and knelt on one knee. She closed her eyes and brought her arms up imploringly. "I call upon the gods of the air. Hissia, Hanor, hear my plea!"

She stood, her arms still outstretched. "Please help me show my friends your power. Please let me bear your servant."

"Really?" a voice spoke up from behind her. "But did you not swear service to that child there?"

Margaret spun around and bowed to the goddess of air, Hissia. "She saved my life."

"And now you are hers," Hissia sniffed.

"She was in pain, I helped," Ellen said, moving forward and bowing her head to the goddess.

"You have chosen her as your rider," another voice, male, spoke up from behind Ellen.

"If something happens to me, I want Annabelle to have the best," Ellen said, turning to face Hanor, the god of air. She waved a hand toward Margaret. "And I think she *is* the best."

"She's got you there, dear," Hissia said, amused. She gave Ellen a probing look. "You smell of Rabel."

"He helped me, I am learning from him," Ellen agreed politely. She raised her eyes toward Margaret. "As I hope to learn from Margaret."

"You are a healer, is that not enough?" Hanor asked.

"We are becoming a sorcerer," Annabelle said with Ellen's voice. "There are those who would cause hurt and find our power a source of dread."

"There are more who would see you dead than you guess," Hanor said.

"We stand as their guardian," Thomas Walpish said, moving forward to stand stalwart in front of Ellen. Skara Ningan took her place beside him.

"Oh!" Hissia's eyes widened. She looked to Hanor. "It seems Death has taken an interest in this affair."

"Please, great gods," Margaret said, clasping her hands together and bowing, "we wish only to help." She waved at the timbers and the rails. "With these tracks we can join this country together, make it easier for people to meet, to learn, to honor you."

"Honor us?" Hanor repeated, his tone doubtful.

"When the trains move, the air rushes past," Peter Hewlitt said as he strode forward to join the group. "Then everyone can feel your power."

"Hmm," Hanor allowed, glancing toward Hissia to gauge her reaction.

"I would only honor you," Margaret said beseechingly.

"And your vow to this girl?"

"These women," Annabelle corrected gently with Ellen's voice. "We asked Margaret to be the rider, the one who would bond with the wyvern should anything happen —"

"Enough," Hanor said, waving the girl to silence. "Do you not think, little Ellen, that we didn't hear you call the new-made wyvern to you? That we did not know that you pulled her from the skies with nothing more than your will?"

"And love," Ellen said. "She gave her life to save me."

"And love," Hissia said in agreement.

Hanor, god of air, leaned forward and spoke down into Ellen's ear, "We saw it all, little one, never fear."

"Could we learn your magic, too?" Ellen asked in reply. She pointed to herself and moved her hand in such a way that it included both her and Annabelle.

Hissia knelt down so that her words focused on Ellen's other ear. "Of course."

"Ophidian is our brother in many ways," Hanor allowed. The two gods straightened back up. "Watch and learn, little one."

"Margaret," Hissia said to the older girl, a smile playing on her lips.

"Oh, thank you!" Margaret replied, jumping up with joy. "I'll do my best, I promise!"

"It's all we ask, wyvern rider," Hanor replied. He smiled at her and then slowly blew away. Hissia followed a moment later.

Margaret leaned down to whisper in Ellen's ear, "They're still here."

"I guessed," Annabelle replied.

Margaret straightened up and turned to the others. "All honor to Hissia and Hanor. They shall allow my magic today."

The others knelt and bowed their heads, shouting, "All honor!"

Margaret turned back away from them and surveyed the job at hand. She crouched once more, raised her arms above her head and then dropped them straight in front of her. Winds twirled in circles from the ends of her hands. The winds tore through the snow in front of her, raising it in giant whorls that filled the sky. The snow swirled higher and higher and fell away, revealing the bare frozen ground in a long straight line. A line that ran a full league — straight — in front of her.

She heard Norman Gossett's gasp of astonishment and allowed a small smile to cross her lips.

With a shout of joy, Margaret lifted the timber rail ties high in the air, laying them out in the sky with a precision that warmed her heart. She turned toward bare ground and lowered her arms, flicking down them at the last moment.

The timbers, laid out like a giant fence in the sky, fell with precision on the ground below.

Shouting with joy, Margaret used her aching arms to raise long lines of rails from the second car and then laid them out on top of the rail ties.

She knelt and bent her head low toward the ground. "Hissia, Hanor, great is your power."

She heard shouts from behind her, shouts of amazement and awe. She rose with a weary sigh then turned toward the approaching men.

But her eyes were on little Ellen as she asked, "How was that?"

"That was beautiful," Ellen Annabelle told her, moving forward to wrap the larger girl in a tight hug. "You are amazing."

"Well, me and the gods," Margaret said, chuckling.

"Always the gods," Ellen agreed.

"Not always," the wispy voice of Hanor corrected her. Ellen's eyes widened and the air god wavered back into sight. He smiled down at her. "Sometimes even gods need to be reminded of their power."

"Like you with your father," Hissia said in agreement.

"We do what we can because the gods love us," Ellen told them solemnly. She waved a hand toward the straight line of track. "We should call this the air line."

"The 'air line'?" Hanor repeated, glancing toward the air goddess.

"That would please us," Hissia agreed. And, with a final nod, the two gods vanished.

# Chapter Two

"There are some places where being a wyvern is a disadvantage," Wymarc said with a long sigh later that day.

"Like in the classroom?" Reedis guessed, nodding in agreement. "I only managed to teach six of the twelve in my class how to lift a cloth bundle."

"Yes, it's hard," Wymarc agreed. Under her breath she added, "Eight."

Reedis' hearing was better than the twin soul wyvern had imagined, for his eyebrows rose in surprise and admiration. "Really? However did you manage —?"

"Centuries of training," Wymarc told him. Reedis' brow fell again in dejection. "Did you tell them the story?"

"What story?" Reedis asked.

"The story of how you built the first airship," Wymarc said.

"I did," Reedis admitted. He smiled in memory. "They were quite amazed, I could tell." His brows creased as he thought to ask, "And you? Did you tell them a story?"

"I did," Wymarc admitted.

"Really?" Reedis prompted.

"I told them the story of how you shot me out of the sky," Wymarc said coldly.

"Oh."

"But I think what helped most was that I identified the natural leaders of the class and challenged them to be the first to learn," Wymarc said, deciding — partly in response to Krea's groans — not to upset the man too much.

"Oh!" Reedis said. "I wish I'd thought of that."

"It took me a century to figure it out," Wymarc admitted.

"Did you have fun?" Nelly asked as she trotted out of her office in response to their voices in the hall.

"I did," Wymarc admitted. "There's something especially *satisfying* about knowing that you've taught."

"There is," Reedis agreed. He beamed at his fiance. "And it's all because of you!"

Nelly blushed and bobbed her head shyly. "Well after dinner, if the two of you would consider teaching *me* what you taught the others —"

"It would be my pleasure," Wymarc told her fondly.

"Mine, too," Reedis added with a grin.

"Mother should be back by then," Nelly said, turning toward the front doors. She frowned. "And Margen, too."

"I suspect that he and Ellen Annabelle are engaged in a little creative air magic right now," Wymarc said.

"Really?" Reedis asked in surprise.

"I saw the track Margaret laid through Korin's Pass," Wymarc said. "I don't doubt that both of them are... *intrigued* with the notion."

"Or jealous," Jarin said with Reedis' voice.

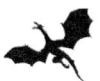

Moira Kendral had never used magic. She didn't need to because she found other people who could do it for her.

"My magic lies elsewhere," she would say when asked. And it did.

"Hello?" Moira called out at the door. "Is anybody there?" No reply. She tried again, just to be certain, "Hello?"

Nodding to herself, Moira Kendral waved the cabbie away. The cabbie gave her a worried look but flicked the reins and his horse broke into a brisk walk, heading back from the docks toward the center of the town and, hopefully, a new fare.

Moira pushed the door open and peered inside the large building beside the rail station. It was dark. It was dirty.

"Have to do something about that," Moira muttered to herself as she strolled through the doors. She reached into her handbag, felt about and pulled a small bundle from it. "Light!"

The little fire demon responded immediately, rising from her hand and illuminating her way.

"Thank you," Moira said as the little demon led the way further into the darkened chamber. It always pays to be polite to staff, Moira reflected. She'd had the demon for more years than she cared to admit, feeding it at the tavern's fire or bringing it up to the bedroom to sleep in the fireplace. It was a simple creature, wanting little, and Moira treasured it. "Take a look, if you'd like. But no fires, please!"

The fire demon bobbed up and down in front of her in acknowledgement, then sped off. Moira waited a moment, following its path to see what its light disclosed. "Do you see a fireplace?"

The fire demon sped forward, darting into nooks and crannies, its light fading as it was hidden from her and then reappearing a moment later, continuing its journey. When it came to a glassed wall and a door, Moira called, "Wait! Let's go see what's inside, shall we?"

The fire demon bobbed in understanding, and Moira bustled over to it. She found the knob and turned, putting her weight against the door as it stubbornly refused to budge. No good.

"Hmph!" Moira reached into her handbag once more, felt about and pulled another thing from it. It was metal and spiky. She said to it, "See if you can make this door behave, please."

The fire demon flared brighter for a moment in greeting to the earth demon — technically a metal demon — before resuming its station. Moira pushed the little metal ball to the lock. In a moment, the metal demon had melted into a shape inside the lock and formed a convenient handle which wiggled to Moira invitingly.

"Well done," Moira said as she grasped the protruding end and twisted, like a key in a lock. "Really," she said to herself, "I don't know why people even *bother*." She slid the door open and gestured for the fire demon to explore while she retrieved the metal demon, which formed once more into a small spiky object and put it back into her purse, telling it, "You did well. I'll let you have a turn in the hearth tonight."

The fire demon hovered over a standing table, and Moira marched over to it. She glanced down, saw a large ledger and smiled to herself.

"There ought to be a lantern somewhere nearby," Moira said suggestively to the fire demon. "Be a dear and see if you can light it."

The demon streaked out of sight, dimmed, and a moment later a larger glow filled the room. Moira moved to take the lantern in her hand and bring in nearer the table. To the fire demon nestling smugly inside, she said, "There might be another brighter light overhead."

The demon needed no further prompting, flying from the lit lantern up into the heights above. Moments later a large spark flared and the whole room was bathed in light.

"If you want to stay up there for a while, I won't mind," Moira told the fire demon, and she peered down on the ledger. It was unlocked. She frowned. She looked about her and presently found a pile of scrap paper and a pencil. She felt in her purse, pulled out the metal demon and placed it on the table in a corner above the ledger, telling it, "I might need you to be a pen, if you don't mind."

The metal demon flowed with alacrity into her favorite pen shape. She smiled at it, reached into her purse and pulled out a small bottle of ink. "I can't guarantee it, mind."

Then she peered down at the ledger. She started with the last page. As she scanned it, she frowned. She sat on the tall stool and pulled it closer to the table.

"Oh, dear!" she said. "This won't do! This won't do at all!" A moment later, her frown deepened, and she muttered again, "Won't do at all."

"Well, how do we stand?" Colonel Lewis asked Captain Fawcett as he returned from his scan of the horizon at the bow of *Wasp*.

"Not good," Fawcett said glumly. "We probably have enough coal to make it to Korin's Pass."

"Probably?"

Fawcett shrugged. "It depends on the winds. If they continue to be this unhelpful, we'll find ourselves in a bit of a pickle."

"Out of coal?" Lewis guessed. "What do we do next?"

"Well, if we're near a house or a village, we might beg for some wood which we could burn in a pinch."

"Why didn't we get wood earlier, then?"

"It doesn't burn as well as coal, we'd need a great deal of it," Fawcett told him.

Lewis turned and pointed to the decking in front of them. "Why not just burn the ship?"

"Sir!" Fawcett protested hotly. "We could never do that!"

"Why not?"

"Well, how would we stand?" the airship captain asked reasonably. "And what if we had to fight?"

"The guns would work," Lewis replied with a shrug.

"Pull up the planking and the deck below is open to all the elements," Fawcett said with a sniff. "The men would freeze."

"Well, let's hope it doesn't come to it," Colonel Lewis said.

"If worse comes to worst, we can be a little late in getting back to the king," Fawcett said.

"If that worst comes to pass, I'll let *you* explain it to him," Lewis replied.

Captain Fawcett opened his mouth to reply, gaped at the colonel and shut it with a snap.

"Let's hope that we get fairer winds," Lewis said, taking pity on the young captain.

"Let me see if I understand what you're suggesting," Tracker said to Ibb and Rabel. "You're saying that the caravan was destroyed when it was forced to collapse on itself."

"Yes," Rabel said. "Somehow someone used the spells that allowed the caravan to hold many rooms at once to force the rooms to collapse on themselves." He waved at the corrupted caravan.

"And how would that spell work?" Angus asked, glancing between Ibb and Rabel.

"It seems like it'd be a very difficult spell to create," Pallas said. "And what sort of god would that magic follow?"

"Any number of gods," Rabel replied. "Ophidian —"

"Why would he allow such a thing?" Angus asked. "It doesn't seem to serve him."

"The dragon god is known to have a strange sense of humor," Tracker suggested.

"But if he knew how it was done, I don't think he set us this problem," Rabel said. He shook his head. "He's devious, but he's not *that* devious."

"Is it dragon magic?" Angus asked, glancing to Nestor Pallas.

"I doubt it is that," Ibb said. "It is simply a corruption of the magic that we used to create it."

"So how do we fix it?" Tracker asked.

"How do immortals do magic?" Angus wondered.

"Much the same way as humans," Rabel said flippantly.

"But humans believe in the gods," Angus said.

"Magic requires understanding the gods, not believing in them," Rabel said. He glanced toward Ibb thoughtfully. "That's right, isn't it?"

"What?" the metal man was staring off toward the warped caravan, apparently deep in thought. "Magic? Yes, we use it. It's not hard."

Rabel nodded, but his expression was reserved.

"How do we fix this, though?" Tracker asked. She glanced to Ibb. "*Can* we fix it?"

"The caravan, restore it to its original shape and purpose?" Ibb asked. Tracker nodded. Ibb shook his head. "No, I don't think we can. It is ruined. We can tear it apart and use the materials again, perhaps."

"Until we can understand how it was destroyed, we'll have little chance of figuring out how to prevent it again," Rabel warned.

"It must have been a god," Tracker said.

"It wasn't," Rabel said. The others looked to him. "Ophidian said so. There were other gods present, they would have felt it. Not only that, but the place where this occurred was close to a temple, all the gods would have felt it."

"I think it is perhaps better to consider *how* it was done than who did it, for the moment," Ibb said.

"My thinking, too," Rabel agreed. "If we know *how* we can guess who."

"So, once again, the question is: how was it destroyed?" Nestor said. The others glanced toward him and nodded. Then they glanced toward the caravan and frowned.

"Let us assume," Rabel said, "that your Lyric set the spell."

"She wasn't there when the caravan was destroyed," Angus said.

"A spell can be set to cast at a particular time," Rabel said.

"Or a particular set of circumstances," Pallas said. Nestor was always amazed at the way his voice changed when the female ice serpent spoke through it. He was also quite impressed with Pallas' extensive understanding of magic. In fact, they'd spent many profitable days working Pallas' magic with Nestor's body. Nestor felt that they were getting rather good.

*We are,* Pallas agreed. *You are a quick learner.*

Nestor felt a glow of pride flush through him.

Rabel raised a hand for attention. "I think," he began slowly, "that the spell used the spell of the caravan itself."

"Explain," Ibb said.

"Your caravans hold many places inside them," Rabel said. Ibb nodded creakily. With a grin, Rabel pulled a small oilcan from one of the many pockets in his overalls and tossed it to the metal man, miming the squeezing of some oil on the offending part.

Ibb's eyes flashed a brighter red, but the metal man did as suggested and tossed the oilcan back. "You were saying."

"So your spell overlays places on top of other places," Rabel said. "In the simplest form, your caravan contains its original structure and one other."

"Usually more than that," Ibb said, "but it is safe to proceed from that point."

"So for that to work, one of the spaces must be collapsed into the framework of the other."

"That is so," Ibb agreed.

"And all that Lyric's spell did was to cause *all* the spaces to collapse at once," Rabel said. "Quite simply, her spell used your spell to defeat itself."

"Yes," Ibb said, turning to Tracker for her opinion. The thin metal woman nodded her head down once.

"So the spell caused the already existing instability in the places to manifest itself, causing all the rooms to collapse at the same time, collapsing the caravan in on itself," Rabel said.

"So what we need is a spell that counters that collapse," Angus said, his eyes gleaming with excitement. "Something that keeps the caravan permanent."

"Yes, something that forces it to keep its state," Rabel agreed.

"That rather defeats the purpose, doesn't it?" Nestor asked. The others looked at him. "If you can only have one room, what's the point of bespelling many places into the same spot?"

"Actually," Rabel said thoughtfully, "I think we should be more concerned about where else this destabilizing spell could be used."

Ibb's red eyes flashed in alarm. "Fixer!"

# Chapter Three

Nothing! In three days riding, they had seen nothing out of hand. Villages were small, sparse, their inhabitants scared, hidden when they could be, cowed when they were forced to show themselves. Jaweer Elwes was pleased to take their tribute — it saved on their supplies — but disturbed by the poor lands around them.

At night the birdmen rose and allowed themselves to be catapulted into the sky where they turned into their eagle forms, screeched defiance, and disappeared into the darkness. When they returned and changed back into their human shape, it was always the same: nothing to report. At least not to the captain.

Gamdan Ikar was the leader and elder of the two. The other was Jaden Ostan, who nursed his jaw and shot dark looks at his leader when he thought the other wouldn't notice. Captain Elwes would not have turned his back on either of them.

They were looking for impossible things, things that no longer existed. Centaurs, and... what were *hexine*? But the Grand Duke had sent him on a mission and Captain Elwes knew the price of failure.

He spotted a hill rising in the distance and pointed it out to his lieutenant. "The sun will set soon enough, let's head there so that our feathered friends may have an easy launch."

"Alain Casman, well met," a voice spoke from behind him. Alain jumped and turned. There had been no one behind him the moment before. And now — now there were four. All girls. Alain took a second look and wondered if he should correct himself — perhaps there were three girls and one woman. Or...

*She's here!* Seena cried in triumph. *You must bow to her, she's a goddess!*

Alain's eyes widened, and he said, "You're a goddess?" He had only a moment to take in her amused expression before he fell to his knees. "How may I serve you?"

*Careful!* Seena warned. The hexine had become very comfortable talking to Alain even as the others — Mayse and Janzie — smouldered with resentment. His sister — thank goodness! — had calmed the two centaurs down, reminding them that his ancestry made him at least a duke.

"First, stand up," the goddess ordered. Alain rose quickly to his feet. He glanced at the other three — one was lying on the ground, asleep or drugged.

Alain's brows creased, and he demanded, "What have you done with her?" Before anyone could respond, Alain darted to the girl and put a hand to her head.

*You have the gift of your forebears*, Seena said in amazement.

Alain ignored her, concentrating on the unconscious girl. He took a deep breath, closed his eyes and probed. A moment later he stood up and turned to the goddess. "What happened?"

"Who *is* he?" the dark girl spoke up, giving Alain a fierce look.

"Tell me, youngling, what do you think happened?" the goddess asked.

"I am Alain Casman," he said with a bow to the goddess, "just recently arrived from the north with my sister."

"Your father was Pier Casman, Grand Duke of the Jasram Plain," the goddess said. "Your mother — " her brow creased as she looked thoughtfully at Alain "-- you do not know about your mother."

"My sister is a centaur," Alain said. He bowed low and, when he rose, said, "Might I know your name, fair goddess?"

"I am Kahlas."

*The goddess of the Moon, of dreams, mother of the centaurs, the hexine, and many others,* Leetar informed him.

Kahlas laughed, a loud pleasant chuckle from deep in her chest. She waved a hand toward the hexine. "And I see you are with child!"

*Indeed, oh wise one!* Seena replied.

Kahlas turned her gaze back to Alain and smiled. "For the others," she said, waving a hand toward the two girls standing and the unconscious one on the ground, "kindly relay what she said."

Alain glanced at the newcomers. The oldest was the dark-eyed girl. Next eldest was the girl on the ground. But both seemed dimmer than the third girl. His eyes narrowed as if blinded and his jaw gaped as he blurted, "There are *two* of you!"

The girl's eyes widened in surprise, and she glanced toward Kahlas in question.

"Alain!" Lisette called, running over. "Mayze says — " she broke off as she saw the others.

"Lisette, bow to the goddess!" Alain called urgently to her. Lisette stopped in her tracks, caught herself, and dipped in an elegant curtsy.

"Hello, mother," she said to the goddess. "I am Lisette Marie."

Kahlas eyed her and smiled. "I did not make you," she said, "but I greet you, daughter."

"Ellen Annabelle made me," Lisette said. "After I fell from the cliff high above."

"I know," Kahlas said. She waved a hand to the others behind her. "These are Bethany Margiss — a wyvern — Chandra her rider, and Barbara Garrett who is under my case." Her eyes cut to Alain in a strange look.

"What happened to her, may I ask?" Alain said.

"What do you think?" Kahlas asked.

"Her mind was hurt more than her body," Alain said instantly. He could not quite understand how he knew that.

*Because you are the same,* Leetar spoke up in his mind.

"Can she hear the hexine?" Alain asked Kahlas.

The goddess shook her head. "Her gift is with air; she is a mage."

"I see," Alain said, trying to hide the fact that he most certainly did *not* see.

"My magic is earth magic," Chandra spoke up, smiling at Lisette Marie and giving Alain a cautious look.

"May I tell him?" Margiss asked the goddess. Kahlas smiled and nodded. Margiss took a breath and said, "Our magic is healing, mostly of the mind, but we're new and don't know much."

"What can I do for you?" Alain asked the goddess. "You should know that I'm new here myself and —"

"Alain Casman! Just what do you — " Mayse's voice broke off as she came storming up to them. She stopped, looked at the newcomers, bristled at their presence and started to speak angrily when Alain cut her off with an upraised hand.

"Mayse, may I make you known to the goddess Kahlas?"

"You!" Mayse said, pointing to Kahlas. Suddenly she was crying, bawling, her face wet with tears. "Do you know how often we... we.."

Kahlas moved and grabbed the woman in her arms, hugging her tightly and pulling her head against her shoulder. "I know dear, I watched, and I heard, but I had to wait until the time was right."

Mayse pulled her head off the goddess' shoulder and wiped her tears. "And is it?"

"It is," Kahlas told her. "Now comes your time to decide. You and Janzie both."

"What's to decide?" Mayse said, drawing herself straight and then bowing deeply to the goddess.

"First the healing, then the war," Kahlas warned her.

"War?" Alain said.

"Yes," Kahlas said, turning to smile at him. "You *do* want your crown back, don't you?"

"It's not the crown," Alain told her firmly. "It's the people."

"Which is why, Your Highness, you will need your crown," Kahlas said.

"I don't know how to be a good ruler," Alain confessed, his misery apparent.

*Which is why you'll need to learn,* Leetar told him.

"I don't like it," Jacques Martel said sourly to Mage Tirpin as they stood beside their lamed, tired horses, eyeing a farmhouse in the distance. Snow was coming down steadily and it was hard to realize that it was still some hours before sunset. "There should be activity, some lights on — something!"

"Our horses are lame, our bellies are growling, we should approach the house and at least *see* what we can learn," Tirpin growled in reply.

"But if they're poor, they'll be able to do nothing for us," Martel protested.

"So?"

"So, my friend," Martel said in a biting tone, "if they are too poor to help us, they are perhaps desperate enough to sell information."

Tirpin frowned. "About us?"

Martel nodded.

"We can deal with that," Tirpin said. He started forward and turned around when Martel didn't follow. Walking backwards, Tirpin called, "Do you want to starve?"

With an irritated curse, the former airship captain grabbed the reins of the two lamed horses and tugged them into a walk.

Tirpin waited until the other caught up and then fell into step beside him. "Consider this," Tirpin offered diplomatically, pointing to the snow-filled sky above them, "if we still had the airship, we'd be *much* colder up there."

"If we still had an airship," Martel replied sourly, "we'd be *there* by now!"

"It will take us at least ten days, more likely two weeks to reach the border," Michael Armand, formerly general of the Sorian army, said to his companion as they rode westward through the falling snow.

"Yes," Ingam Oliver, mage and former chief of staff of the Sorian Army, agreed blandly. "And then we shall have to make some decisions."

"Oh?"

"Do we go north to Hjalvik or south to Nikjal?" Ingam asked. He pronounced the letter 'j' as a 'y' in the tradition of Vinik — actually the tradition of both Vinik and South Vinik, the two sundered kingdoms to the west. So Hjalvik was 'hee-yal-vik' and Nikjal was pronounced 'Neek-yal.'

"Hjalvik if we want to warn them, Nikjal if we want to join?" Michael Armand guessed.

"Say rather that Hjalvik will be more direct, but going to Nikjal might be more certain," Oliver said.

"Of course, the Emperor might decide that we need to lose weight," Armand said dryly, pointing a hand to his head for example.

Oliver chuckled. "Which is why it might be smarter to go to Hjalvik and see how things stand."

"We have time," Armand agreed. "I can't imagine King Markel planning an attack until the spring thaw at the earliest."

"But you didn't expect him to attack us in the winter," Oliver said. "It could be that his generals and mages have more surprises prepared."

"In which case our lives will be short," Michael Armand said. He waved a hand to the path ahead. "For now, we should keep going to the Pinch. We'll have plenty of time to think along the way."

"What do we do now?" Margaret asked Ellen Annabelle and Peter Hewlitt when she'd finished laying the track. The railcrew were busy hammering in the rail ties and would be busy for the rest of the day.

"We should go back to Kingsford," Thomas Walpish said. Skara Ningan nodded fervently beside him.

"But after?" Margaret asked. "The rail line here and the one from Korin's Pass — what about them?"

"I see your point," Hewlitt said, pursing his lips. He glanced to mage Margen and waved a hand at the laid tracks. "Could you do that?"

Margen shook his head and told Margaret Waters, "I have not such skill with air." Honestly, he added, "I doubt many others do."

"Barbara was good," Matt Evans chimed in loyally. Beside him, Freddie Fennimore nodded in agreement.

"And we have to consider you too," Hewlitt told the two youths.

"Moira, with the other team, she's pretty good," Margaret said. "They get the job done."

"Let us go back and see how things fare at the school," Margen said. He turned to Ellen Annabelle and waved a hand toward Matt and Freddie. "Could you make two trips so that we can bring these two with us?"

"No, she cannot," Margaret said firmly. The others turned to her. "She's done enough already this day and is more tired than she's willing to admit."

"She's right," Annabelle said with Ellen's voice. "Ellen would never admit it but…"

"Perhaps the mage and I could stay here the night," Peter suggested. "And if you couldn't return in the morning, perhaps Jarin Reedis would do us the favor?"

"Or you could take the train back to the capital," Margaret suggested. "And bring the railcrew with you." She nodded toward the workers in the distance. "In the morning, when they're done."

"I have no right to dictate — " Hewlitt began cautiously.

"Are you not a member of the King's court?" Thomas Walpish demanded. "And does that not give you power when none other is present?"

Hewlitt gave the ghost a thoughtful look.

"Our mission is to protect Ellen Annabelle," Skara added in agreement. She glanced fondly at the girl. "And she needs food, rest, and a chance to wind down."

"Very well," Hewlitt said. "Mage Margen, does this plan suit you?"

"I do believe, spymaster, that you had something you wished to discuss with me," Margan said in oblique agreement.

Hewlitt smiled and looked much, much younger than he had moments before. "Indeed, I do!"

# Chapter Four

"It might be a good idea not to mention us to Mrs. Kendral," Thomas Walpish said as he and Skara took guard positions around Margaret and Ellen Annabelle.

"She might surprise you," Annabelle said.

"But, all the same…" Skara said.

"I think they're right," Margaret said, nodding toward Ellen Annabelle. "It might frighten her out of her wits."

"Very well," Ellen said reluctantly. She raised her eyes to Margaret. "But I think you may be wrong about the innkeeper's wife."

They climbed the stairs leading into the school. Dusk had fallen, the last rays of the sun were glinting off the sea in the west. The interior of the school was well lit, and it was warm inside.

"I never knew this existed," Margaret said, eyeing the hall with interest.

"It's new," Thomas Walpish said. Skara eyed him warningly and he gave her an apologetic look.

"Hello!" Ellen yelled. "Jarin! Nelly! We're back!"

"We're in here!" a voice none of them recognized called back. "In the kitchen, come along, we've got leftovers!"

Ellen picked up her pace and was matched by Margaret at her side and Thomas and Skara — invisibly — at front and rear.

The room was just around the corner and not too large. A woman with her back to them was stirring a pot. Jarin Reedis and Nelly Kendral sat at a small table, smiling lovingly at each other. In front of them were two empty bowls. The smell from the pot on the stove revealed that they had previously held a marvelous spicy stew.

"Where's Margen?" Reedis asked as the party entered the room. He saw Thomas point at himself and wave his hand in warning. "And Hewlitt?"

"They stayed behind," Margaret said. "They're going to take the train back here in the morning."

"Oh? Sensible," Reedis allowed. "Are they bringing the two youngsters back with them?"

"Probably," Annabelle said with Ellen's voice.

"Good idea," the woman at the stove said. She turned and took in the two people she saw, her lips pursing as she took in Ellen Annabelle, then changing again when her eyes caught sight of Margaret. She grabbed a kitchen towel and wiped her hands, moving forward with her right hand extended to the smallest person in the room. "I'm Moira Kendral, Nelly's mother."

"We're pleased to meet you, ma'am," Annabelle said with Ellen's voice. Moira's eyes widened and then she glanced to her own daughter. "Nelly was right, you can tell the difference!"

"I'm Margaret Waters," the taller girl said, reaching to shake Mrs. Kendral's hand. She glanced past her to the pot on the stove. "Can I serve?"

"No, you'll do nothing of the sort," Mrs. Kendral said with a sniff. "Take those seats and I'll get you something immediately." She shot a sharp glance toward her daughter, and blushing, Nelly rose to help her.

In short order, the newcomers were seated with steaming bowls of stew in front of them.

"This looks marvelous!" Ellen exclaimed, diving in.

Mrs. Kendral tutted and said, "Did you not want to thank the gods first?"

"No," Ellen said, wolfing down her food, "they've done nothing for me."

"You've all the manners of an urchin!" Mrs. Kendral exclaimed.

"That's because she was," Annabelle said, taking control of Ellen's voice. "She would have died had it not been for Rabel."

"Rabel?" Mrs. Kendral said. "The smith?"

"Yes," Annabelle said. "He took her in."

"After his daughter turned into a wyvern?"

"After he was thrown in the jail," Ellen said, "and left to die."

"Oh!" Mrs. Kendral said in a much smaller voice. She turned back to the stove, grabbed some mugs from the shelf to the side and poured two cups of hot tea. "Here, there's honey on the table," she said as she served the two girls.

"Thank you," Ellen said, using both hands to grab the mug.

Babette Collet shivered in the cold. Night had fully fallen and there was nothing to keep her warm save the jacket that one prisoner had loaned her.

"You must wait until it is dark," Amuir had told her. "The power needed is in the dark."

Babette had nodded in understanding. The spell was simple, not too different from the one that had pulled her to Queen Airivik's burial mound — the place where she'd found the ghost of her murdered father.

"Look for one who is very drunk and very troubled," General Dartan had added. "Someone who feels guilt."

Babette had nodded once again.

Now, she stood huddled in the shadows outside a tavern which was packed with Kingsland soldiers. She'd spotted an officer going inside, pulled by his men, and had decided that he would be the one.

So she waited. And waited. The noise changed, there was an exclamation from inside and shouting and then the officer burst out of the doors, pulled up his collar and stormed off into the night.

Babette followed.

"Where's Krea?" Ellen asked as she sat back from the table, her half-empty mug in one hand and an empty bowl in front of her.

"Right here," Krea Wymarc said, coming into view from the hallway. She turned and waved a hand toward two girls behind her. "These ladies had some extra questions for me."

The two girls giggled, bobbed their heads nervously, and sped away.

"There's still some stew," Mrs. Kendral told her, gesturing her toward the table. "I can warm up some water for tea."

"Thank you," Krea said. She made a motioning hand behind her back. "And for Drake, too?"

"Drake?" Mrs. Kendral said.

A dark-haired lad ducked his head in the doorway behind Krea.

"My bodyguard when I'm human, rider when I'm a wyvern," Krea said.

Mrs. Kendral's eyebrows rose, and she turned to Jarin Reedis. "Is this the same for dragons, then?"

"It is," Reedis answered. He nodded toward Nelly. "The rider of a dragon or wyvern is security if anything happens to the mortal half of the twin soul."

"The mortal half?" Mrs. Kendral repeated. "That would be you."

"Yes," Reedis said. He gestured toward Nelly, who blushed. "I've asked Nelly if she'd accept the honor."

"And I've agreed," Nelly said, smiling back at him.

"Of course, we hope that nothing happens to either," Jarin said with Reedis' voice. "And I argued with both of them but… Reedis presented a powerful argument."

Nelly rose from the table and gestured for Krea Wymarc to take her place. Seeing this, Reedis also rose and waved Drake into his chair.

"I suppose if anything were to happen to you," Mrs. Kendral said, "it would be best to have the two who have the most hurt able to console each other."

"That was my thought, also," Reedis allowed. He bowed to her and grabbed Nelly's hand. "And now, if you will all forgive us, I have promised my intended some lessons on magic."

Nelly squeezed his hand and beamed with delight, turning and dragging him out of the room.

"Lessons!" Annabelle chortled.

Mrs. Kendral waved her ladle toward the twin soul. "You're too young to be talking that way!"

"Actually," Annabelle replied, "*I'm* not."

"Then she is," Mrs. Kendral responded immediately.

"Ugh!" Ellen said, catching on. "Although, Mrs. Kendral, I really do believe that Reedis means lessons, as in magic."

"He was the one who taught me balloon magic," Annabelle said in agreement.

"And the academy is named after him," Krea Wymarc added. "It's only fitting that the principal know the magic."

"We should clean up," Ellen Annabelle said, rising from her seat. Margaret joined her and the two put their dishes into the sink.

"Thank you, I appreciate that," Mrs. Kendral said.

"And how was your day?" Margaret asked. She sounded tired and worn out. Mrs. Kendral shot her a worried look.

"Not, no doubt, as tiring as yours, but intriguing," Mrs. Kendral replied. "I took a moment to examine your father's books."

"Books?" Margaret said. "Magic books?"

"In a way, yes," Mrs. Kendral said. "I went over his business records."

"And what did you find?" Drake asked, looking up from his stew.

"I think I'd best wait until I can talk with Mr. Hewlitt."

"Well, *that's* done," Crown Prince Sarsal muttered to himself as he closed the door to his royal chamber and threw off the ornately embroidered tunic that he'd been forced to wear throughout the damned proceedings. As it fell to the floor, he frowned, bent and picked it up, placing it on the back of one of the lounge chairs in his anteroom. "At least until tomorrow."

*Ah, yes, tomorrow!* The true coronation. He had survived the dress rehearsal, he'd probably survive the real thing.

"I'll survive," he muttered to himself, his lips curving upwards. "And then there'll be refreshments."

"Talking to oneself, even in one's own quarters, is never wise," a voice spoke from the shadows. "You never know who might be listening."

"Or, you might, if you're someone like myself who has trained from birth, have used a spell to sheath the room in a silence spell," Sarsal replied. He turned hooded eyes toward the speaker. "Did you get it?"

"I did," the woman replied, stepping out of the shadows. She was, if anything, prettier than her sister. Certainly she was smarter.

"And the plans?"

"As you desire, my prince," Melodie Gregory said, smiling at him. She reached up and moved to release the robe that was covering her nightgown. It slipped off. The nightgown underneath was thin and, with the light behind it, revealing.

"I desire much," Crown Prince Sarsal said. He gestured her toward the bed in the far room, pulling off his own shirt as he walked through the door.

She giggled as he grabbed her and threw her on the bed. She really was *much* prettier than Matilda.

"Quiet, wench," he said mockingly. "Have some respect for the dead."

The girl shook her head. "I know full well, Your Highness, that this is *not* the room in which my sister died. You changed quarters immediately afterwards."

"I didn't mean her," Sarsal said, unlacing his shoes and throwing them off. He rose to unhitch his trousers and threw them off, turning to her with a smile. "I mean those about to die."

"Oh, them!" Melodie snorted. "I'll stand beside you as they gasp their last, and I'll smile as they die."

"That's my girl," Sarsal said, turning back to the bed and throwing himself at her.

A long time later, as they languished beside each other, he said to her, "This time tomorrow, you'll be queen."

"What is the meaning of this?" Emperor Maximilian Kursk roared as the doors to his royal throne room burst open and two lifeless forms flew to land at his feet.

"It's an introduction," a man's voice came in reply. A figure lurched through the doors, a brilliant staff in one hand and the ear of a small child in the other. The child was still attached to the ear and squirming miserably. "A proof of power, as it were." The man threw the child by her ear as she skidded across the long floor of the throne room to come to rest near the two bodies. "Surely you recognize my calling card?"

"Guards!" Maximilian roared. His guards were already in motion — and then they weren't, standing frozen in mid-stride.

The man stopped and glowered at the Emperor. "I *said,* surely you recognize my calling card?" The girl was hunched over, her hands to her face, tears streaming endlessly. The man growled at her, "Stop snivelling." The girl flinched as if struck and fell in a heap.

"Who are you?" Emperor Maximilian of Vinik demanded.

"I'm your new mage," the man said with a crooked smile. He pointed his staff toward the larger of the two bodies on the floor. "I bested your last one and his apprentice." He frowned. "A son, I believe. Though not much of a son." He waved his staff toward the hunched girl. "That's his daughter, too. I shall take her in his stead."

The girl on the floor flinched at those words.

The man said confidentially, "I've had a great deal of success in raising children, you know."

"You are a mage," Maximilian decided. He glanced down at the two corpses in front of him. "And you think defeating my best mage gives you his position?"

"I could defeat the rest of them, but who would do the scut work then?" the man replied. "I like having apprentices."

"Who are you?"

"You may call me the Magemaster," the man replied. "I come bearing glorious news: soon you will be king."

"I am an Emperor!" Maximilian shouted. "Why would I want to be king?"

"You are emperor of one small slice of land," the Magemaster replied. "I am sent to offer you the whole land."

"South Vinik?" Maximilian guessed, licking his lips in anticipation.

"South Vinik, Soria, Kingsland, Palu — those are just names," the Magemaster replied. He caught the Emperor's eyes in his gaze. "I'm talking about Cuiyival. The entire continent." He shrugged. "Maybe more, if you please my master."

"Your master?"

"Often he is called the three-headed god," the Magemaster told him. "I'm sure you'll be happy to serve him."

"You must rest," mage Margen told Peter Hewlitt. "Magic is work and, like all work, unused muscles get the most tired and need the greatest rest."

"But I hardly did anything," Hewlitt said.

Margen grunted and pointed to the fireplace. "We need a fire."

Hewlitt's brow furrowed. "How?"

"Imagine the heat, the light," Margen told him. "And then make it be so."

"A huge roaring fire?"

"No," Margen said, laughing, "just a spark is all that's needed."

"Right," Hewlitt said, chagrined.

A moment later a small spark appeared, grew brighter, dimmed, and died.

"Try it again," Margen said.

"Very well," Hewlitt said. He took a deep breath and let it out slowly. As he did, the spark returned, grew brighter — and then a small flame appeared. Slowly it grew, growing to fill the fireplace.

"Good magic always begins small," Margen told him. "And a smart man uses just enough of it to do his will."

"I see," Hewlitt said, staring proudly into the fire. "It's much like spying."

"How so?"

"One only need learn enough to know something," Hewlitt said. "And usually all it takes is a simple question and a willing ear."

"Huh," Margen grunted. "I'd never thought of it that way."

"Most people think it requires threats, bribes, and treachery," Hewlitt said in agreement. "But often I learn the most by being quiet and listening honestly."

"Well, magic is *not* like that," Margen said. "It requires thought, study, and preparation." He stood and threw back the covers of the small bed nearest the fire. He gestured toward Hewlitt and the farther bed, the one nearest the window. "You can have that one."

Hewlitt nodded and went to the further bed, removed his boots and got under the inadequate blankets. "I think I shall like magic," Hewlitt said.

"Really?"

"Just like spying, it requires thought, study, and preparation," Hewlitt replied lightly.

"Hmph!"

# Chapter Five

"The wind is picking up, it's off our stern," Captain Fawcett said as Major Lewis came up on deck in the early morning. The airship *Wasp* was moving fast over the ground below.

"That's good?" Lewis guessed from the captain's cheerful tone.

"We might see Korin's Pass by this afternoon."

"Good, can't wait to get there," Lewis said.

"And if we don't it'll be a hard slog," Fawcett added more somberly. "We're almost out of coal."

"There's plenty of wood here to burn if we need it," Lewis said, eyeing the ship's timbers critically.

"It won't come to that," Captain Fawcett said.

"The king needs his treasure, captain," Lewis reminded him. "I'll do what it takes."

"She did *that*?" a young lad's voice exclaimed loudly in the morning air. "Why on Earth did you let her?"

"I was unconscious at the time, I didn't have any say in it," a girl's voice replied.

"Ahoy the gates!" a child's voice — a girl's — piped up.

"We come to offer help," a man's voice added. "Please send for Queen Diam and tell her that Ellen Annabelle and Jarin Reedis have come to redeem Chandra's word!"

From out of the ruins of the gate, a small form stepped forward. "Oh, it's you!" the figure said, his voice deeper than his height. "It's about time!"

"We had some distractions along the way," Jarin Reedis said with a delicate cough.

"Is that Granno?" Ellen asked.

"Ellen?" Granno replied, stepping into sight. "I might have known."

"Chandra's gone with Kahlas, so Freddie here is going to redeem her word," the small girl gestured to a taller lad, who nodded, eyes wide with amazement to the zwerg bodyguard.

"Why aren't you with Her Majesty?" Jarin Reedis asked.

"She's got more than one bodyguard," Granno grumbled. "And she asked me to see what could be done for this entrance."

"It is *rather* obvious at the moment," Freddie, the lad who had spoken first, agreed. He glanced toward a young woman and said, "Remind me never to get your sister angry."

"I remind everyone never to get Chandra angry," Margaret Waters assured him. She gestured toward the ruined gates and the crack splitting the entrance. "Can you fix it?"

Freddie gave her a dubious look in reply. "I've never seen such destruction."

"We could ask Mage Margen," Ellen Annabelle suggested evenly.

Freddie Fenimore's face clouded, and he shook his head. "Let me try, first." He nodded toward Granno. "How would you like me to fix it?"

"We need it buried, hidden, so no one can ever find it again," Granno told him.

"But how will you get out again?" Margaret asked worriedly.

Granno brought a finger to the side of his nose and said slyly, "Best you not know, miss."

"The zwerg like to keep their entrances hidden," Jarin explained. "There are too many humans hoping to steal their gold."

"You skytouchers are always tearing things up," Granno said.

Margaret stiffened in hurt. "Chandra was just trying to help me —"

Granno cut her off with a raised hand. "I wasn't talking about your sister, nor these others —" he waved his hand to include Ellen Annabelle and Jarin Reedis "-- neither of them have the gold sickness. But there've been others."

"So how far in do you wish us to bury this?" Jarin Reedis asked. "And are there any zwerg nearby that might need to be warned?"

"I'm the only one here," Granno said. "I was just trying to figure how best —"

The ground started shaking. Everyone turned to see that Freddie was kneeling down on one knee, his right hand resting on the ground, his brow taut with concentration. "I can do this," he said as the others looked at him. To Granno, he added, "Do you need to go inside or do you have another way?"

"Stop!" Granno barked. The ground stopped shaking. "First, lad, we're going to see what the queen desires."

"How will she know she's needed?" Margaret asked.

"I suspect the ground shaking will catch her attention," Jarin Reedis said with a small smile. "In the meantime, Granno, may I make you known to my fiance, the mage and teacher, Nelly Kendral?" He gestured to the woman clutching his arm tightly.

Granno bowed toward Nelly. "Congratulations, miss!" To Jarin he said, "How did you manage to get so lucky?"

"We'd met before I'd gone to the bitter north in the *Spite*," Reedis explained. "When I returned, I found that Nelly had set up a school of magic in my memory."

"Well, I'm thrilled for the both of you," Granno said enthusiastically. He bobbed his head toward Nelly. "Jarin Reedis are beloved in our kingdom, miss."

"They even allow me to nest in their gold," Jarin added.

"Well, now, Mister Jarin, I'm not sure that's the sort of thing we like others to know," Granno said in a soft, warning tone.

"Granno, she's going to be my wife!" Reedis said. "And she's agreed to be our rider."

"Rider?" Granno said, brows rising. "You mean, in case —"

"Exactly," Reedis said. He patted Nelly's hand. "If anything happens to me, I'll at least have the knowledge that she and Jarin will be safe."

"And nothing had better happen to you!" Nelly told him fiercely.

"I really don't understand why shaman Riess wasn't available," King Markel muttered as he and his new queen gathered before the doors to the royal temple.

"He wasn't feeling well, Your Majesty," Crown Prince Sarsal told him. "He sends his regrets, and he personally assured me that Meister Semple would be more than capable as his substitute."

"But this Meister Semple wasn't the one who crowned your father, was he?" Markel asked waspishly. He glanced toward Rassa. "Won't this cause talk?"

"If people talk, dear, we shall deal with it," Queen Rassa assured, patting his arm.

"In any case, Your Majesties, it's time," first minister Mannevy said as the guards swung open the huge double doors that led into the royal temple.

The royal trumpeters began their coronation processional. King Markel gave his new queen a wintry smile, raised a hand for hers and, together, the two started their royal progress down the aisle surrounded by nobles, statues of gods, and the whole of the new kingdom's royalty.

"No sign of General Armand?" General Gergen asked, popping up beside Mannevy's side.

"What?" Mannevy asked, distracted by the question from his attentive gaze on the king and queen as they made their stately way to the end of their walk and turned to face the approving roar of the crowd. Of course, the crowd was *paid* to roar approvingly, but Mannevy was the only one who knew that. He and Crown Prince Sarsal, of course. The young lad was quite obsequious and helpful. Mannevy appreciated that.

"What?" he asked again.

"General Armand," General Gergen said, his tone frosty. "I've been trying to find out who he's picked to lead the cavalry all day and I can't find him."

"He's in there, somewhere," Mannevy said, absently pointing to the thronging crowd in the temple. "Doubtless you'll find him later at the celebration."

"I suppose," Gergen said doubtfully. He turned away and then turned back. "And that's another thing —"

"Yes?" Mannevy interrupted, turning his gaze to the general.

"How are we going to house all the troops?" Gergen asked. "There can't be a hall large enough for the men of *both* armies."

"No," Mannevy agreed, "there isn't. You and your troops will be at one hall, Armand and his men in another."

Gergen gave him a look.

"It was the best we could do," Mannevy said. "If it hadn't been for Prince Sarsal, you'd all be eating in the stables."

"Sarsal found us a place?"

"Two places," Mannevy corrected absently. "Perhaps you should head there now."

"Not until I see them properly crowned," Gergen said.

"Of course," Mannevy agreed, turning his gaze back to the far end of the temple where Meister Semple was speaking inaudibly.

"I hope he doesn't make a mess of things," Gergen muttered, eyeing the coronation dubiously. "He's not their regular man, is he?"

"The other one is ill," Mannevy agreed absently. "But we only need this one for the next few minutes. When he's done, we'll be feasting for the rest of the day." He started forward, turning back to say to Gergen, "If you'll excuse me, this is a day I have awaited for a long time."

Gergen nodded and waved him away.

First minister Mannevy moved forward by way of the outside aisle, behind the nobles to the top of the temple. Shaman Semple, with white-frosted hair and eyebrows, looked none too steady as he shuffled forward to stand before and between Markel and Rassa.

Mannevy moved out of the shadows and took a place to the left of the queen, close enough to hear and beam encouragingly. But at the first words from the shaman, his face fell.

"Today, we ahr heah to unite these two souls in joyous harmony," the shaman said in a languid drawl, solemnly turning his head from Rassa to Markel and back again. "The sanctity of marriage brings us closer to the gods."

"The coronation," Mannevy hissed. "They're here for the coronation!"

"Not the wedding?" shaman Semple asked, eyes going wide. He licked his lips. "But I thought — I thought —"

"That, too," Mannevy said, moving closer to the raised dais. "The marriage, then the coronation."

"There ahr rings?" Semple asked seriously despite his drawl.

"Your Majesty, the rings," Mannevy said, nodding toward King Markel. Markel felt inside his rich cloak and pulled forth two rings, passing one to Rassa whose expression was beyond rage.

"With these rings, you exchange your pledges," Semple said, nodding to Markel who placed the ring on Rassa's finger. Rassa dimpled and curtsied before moving forward to place Markel's ring on his finger.

"Declare them man and wife," Mannevy urged, waving angrily at the shaman, "and then get on with the coronation?"

"Have you the crowns?" Semple asked Mannevy. With a strangled groan, Mannevy waved to the two crowns, fully visible, placed on the table behind the shaman. Semple turned at his urging and jerked in surprise when he spied them. "Good, then we should proceed."

"Man and wife!" Mannevy hissed to the shaman in reminder.

"Man and wife?" Semple repeated blankly, clearly thrown by the course of events.

"That'll do," Rassa growled, her eyes hooding her anger. "Get on with the coronation."

Semple nodded and turned back to pick up the King's crown.

"The Queen *first*," Mannevy growled at the man in frustration. He'd made it very clear to the shaman that the queen, as the former queen of Soria, must be crowned first.

Semple's eyes widened, and he nodded jerkily, moving forward and placing the King's crown on Queen Rassa's head. The crown, hastily re-sized the day before, slipped over Rassa's eyes.

"The *other* crown," Mannevy said with a groan.

Semple realized his mistake, pulled off the king's crown, moved and placed it on King Markel's head as though he were a hatstand and retrieved the queen's crown from the table.

"With this crown, receive the fealty of all Soria," Semple said, lowering the crown on Queen Rassa's head. He turned to the assembly and called out, "All rise for Queen Rassa!"

Mannevy stifled a groan: the shaman was supposed to call the assembly to their feet *after* King Markel had been crowned. Markel caught Mannevy's eyes with a baleful look; the first minister took a deep breath and let it out slowly, nodding to direct his king's attention back to the shaman.

"And now, *me*, if you would," Markel said in icy tones to the shaman.

"But you have already got your crown!" Semple said in purest confusion.

"Declare him king and oath-holder!" Mannevy ordered the shaman.

Semple looked at him as if seeing him for the first time, recovered and raised his arms above Markel.

"All rise for the new King of Sowia and give him fealty!" Shaman Semple called.

The assembly, already on their feet, looked at each other in confusion, trying to decide on their course of action.

"Long live the King!" Mannevy shouted. "Long live King Markel and Queen Rassa!"

"Long live the King!" the assembly dutifully bellowed back. Mannevy turned and gestured to the choir standing behind him. Several children in its midst were openly laughing. He glared at them and signalled the choirmaster to begin the recessional. The choir master nodded in understanding, raised his arms, and the choir sang the Sorian anthem.

The crowd turned and slowly filed out of the temple.

Rassa and Markel stood before them, beaming at each other with huge grins on their faces and holding hands.

"Well," Shaman Semple said as he tottered over to Mannevy, "I think that went rahtheh well."

"What's that noise?" Captain Welless called from his front office. "I say, Mr. Beck, what's that rumbling?"

"Outside!" Hamo Beck roared, putting action to his words, charging out of his inner office and dragging the Kingsland captain after him. "It is an earthquake!"

The booming sound dropped off just as the same time as the ground rippled up and down, causing buildings to shake and groan under the stresses.

Captain Welless looked around, turned southward and stared. "Something to do with your kin?" Welless asked, his brow creased. "Should we be worried?"

"No," Hamo Beck said after a moment. "I believe that was the gate being closed."

"I heard no explosion," Captain Welless said.

"No, that was magic," Hamo said in agreement. He gave the captain a wry look. "I suspect that perhaps our mage friends repaid the zwerg for their aid."

"Hmph," Welless said, looking thoughtful. He turned to Beck. "They might have warned us."

"They are rather impulsive and my kinsfolk were probably eager for the protection," Beck replied.

"Well, yes, I could understand that," Welless agreed. "Don't want every greedy gold hunter tracking them down." He pointed to the rising cloud of dust and added thoughtfully, "Though that might be hard to explain."

"Every mage in a hundred miles will have felt it," Beck said.

"Every *person* in a hundred miles will have felt *and* heard it," Welless corrected. He shrugged. "Well, there's nothing I can do about it."

"Call it an earthquake when asked," Hamo Beck suggested lightly.

"Oh, *that* was obvious!" Welless exclaimed. He turned back to their office and gestured for the mayor to precede him. "Let us hope we have no more excitement in the day."

"I haven't really had much chance to travel on the train," Mage Margen said to Peter Hewlitt as the train chugged steadily northwards.

Hewlitt sketched a quick smile. "I can well imagine."

"And how long until we reach the capital?"

Hewlitt looked up thoughtfully before answering, "About two hours."

"Hmm," Margen was clearly not impressed with the train's speed.

"We're pulling five cars," Hewlitt replied, "one with passengers and four with goods." He smiled at the mage. "That's about forty tons of goods."

"Hmm," and this time Margen's tone was entirely different, "*that's* something no mage would consider."

"Which is why I like the trains," Hewlitt agreed.

"I see," Margen said. He sat back for a moment, enjoying the scenery outside their window and the way it rushed by them. "Didn't you say you wanted to talk with me, earlier?"

Hewlitt smiled once more and nodded. "Indeed, I do."

"Something to do with your position and magic, I imagine."

"Not *quite*," Peter Hewlitt told him. "I was thinking more in terms of finance and profit."

"Please don't tell me you want to talk about turning lead into gold," Margen groaned.

"Nothing of the sort," Hewlitt said. "Gold is a nice metal and I respect it but I'm more… direct in my thinking: I want what it can buy and the power that comes with it."

"Hmm."

"I also want to help the magic community," Hewlitt said.

"Give yourself a good year of study and you'll be a mage yourself," Margen said, giving the spymaster a look of approval. "You're quite the study."

"Thank you," Hewlitt replied. "But I was thinking of city folk and the common man."

"City folk are not that common," Margen said with a sniff.

"But they are becoming more so," Hewlitt said. "We will always need food and those who harvest it but we have been moving for many centuries towards clusters of people. Those clusters have become the centers of trade, of commerce, and of learning."

"I quite agree," Margen said, somewhat surprised at the spymaster's philosophy. "In fact, it was one reason I came to work for the king."

"To teach magic," Hewlitt said. "That's a lofty goal, but it requires students."

"Miss Kendral seems to have not only recognized but capitalized on that," Margen said. "My class is just one of six at her academy." Margen cocked an eyebrow toward the spymaster. "And you've already talked with her about expansion and funding."

"Yes," Hewlitt agreed. "But my experience is that, even with this institute, there will always be more jobs for mages than there are mages."

"Yes," Margen agreed. "To become a mage takes time, dedication, and skill."

"As I'm learning," Hewlitt said.

"And so what has this to do with your proposition?"

"This train we're riding on results from the application of magic to a particular problem," Hewlitt said, waving a hand at the plush cushioned seats on which they were riding. "Mostly it was built by men who have no magic."

"Yes," Margen said encouragingly. "And?"

"The tracks could be laid without magic," Hewlitt said. He raised a hand to forestall Margen's reply, adding, "It would be slower but possible."

"Yes," Margen agreed reluctantly.

"The same cannot quite be said for the airships," Hewlitt continued, "because they need mages to provide the lift. But once aloft, the mechanical steam engines are their sole source of power."

"Are you suggesting that we could discover a non-magical way of raising airships?"

Hewlitt's eyes widened, and he shook his head. "I wasn't suggesting that although it is *quite* an interesting proposition, isn't it?"

"I suppose," Margen said, full of reluctance. "But then we'd need fewer mages, not more."

"We'd need fewer *airship* mages," Hewlitt countered, "which means we'd have more mages to employ elsewhere."

"And where might they be employed, then?"

"It's possible to store spells on certain metals and jewels, is it not?" Hewlitt asked.

"Of course," Margen agreed. "But a stored spell is never as good as a fresh one."

"But for people who don't have magic, it's much better than nothing," Hewlitt said. "And if we could come up with a number of sensible spells that people would want and create them in sufficient number, we would be performing a most useful service to the people of our land."

"Selling magic, is it?"

"Selling magic rings and amulets," Hewlitt said. "Consider this: a ring that could cast a light."

"People have torches and candles for that," Margen said.

"But there are many times when they don't," Hewlitt replied. "And times when it's windy or rainy, extinguishing those handy lanterns and candles."

"And if we could make enough of them, and cheap enough, the rings might prove more valuable than torches or candles," Margen muttered to himself. He raised his eyes to Hewlitt and gave the spymaster a firm nod. "Very well, what else?"

Peter Hewlitt suppressed a smile as he plunged into his list of possible ring spells, watching the mage grow more and more excited with each new revelation. Finally, he sat back in his chair and said, "So, do we have an agreement?"

"Oh, very much so!" Margen chortled, extending a hand to the spymaster who took it firmly. "I believe this marks the beginning of a glorious adventure!"

# Chapter Six

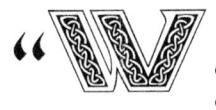"We heard nothing," the Kingsland officer told them, with misery in his eyes. He told them that he was Ensign Rivers. "We fired and fired and heard no sound."

"Why?" General Dartan asked, his voice hard. He had had one of his men take Babette Colette away to another tent so that she wouldn't be troubled by the interrogation. They'd had to wait until the afternoon to get the ensign sober enough to talk.

"The King said that your soldiers killed Queen Airivik, that you had forfeited all rights and that, because no one would take the blame, he would take a thousand lives for hers."

"And you didn't think to question this?" an officer shouted in outrage.

"Would you, sir, have questioned your King in front of your commanding officer?" the ensign asked. "And the king's mage was there, as were his apprentices." He shook his head. "It wasn't my place to question it."

"But you felt guilty," General Dartan said.

The hangdog man met his eyes for just an instant and dropped his head in shame, nodding slowly. "In war, that's one thing…"

"And you must have wondered, if he could do this to prisoners, what would he do to you if you disobeyed his order?"

"No," Ensign Rivers said, "I knew he'd kill me." He pursed his lips as if to say more, paused, then said in a rush, "I'd heard about the cavalry."

"Cavalry?"

"Colonel Walpish and his troopers," Traver said.

"What of them?"

"The king rewarded them for capturing the assassin," Rivers said.

"So they *caught* him!" one of the officers exclaimed.

"He wore the uniform of a Sorian colonel," Rivers said. "At least that's what I heard."

"You sound doubtful," Dartan said.

"Because the king gave the colonel and his best men new leather jackets, red leather," Rivers said.

"So?"

"And when the cavalry left to go north, every man wearing the new jackets was killed by an assassin," Rivers said.

"They were set up!"

"That's what I think now," Rivers agreed. "Before, my captain told me that it was probably a Sorian — " he gave the men surrounding him an apologetic look " — some holdout assassin."

"And now what do you think?" Murat, the soldier who'd been sent to guard little Babette Collet, asked.

"I think my captain was wrong," Rivers admitted miserably.

"If your king were to offer you a new jacket?" Dartan asked.

"I'd be happy to give it away," Rivers said.

"Listen," Dartan said, leaning in closer to the ensign, forcing him to meet his eyes, "your king betrayed his honor, he ordered you to kill innocent men. What are you going to do about it?"

"I don't know, what can I do?" Rivers asked, meeting the enemy general's eyes frankly.

"What would you do if it was our king, and he did that to your comrades?" Murat demanded heatedly.

"I'd kill him," Rivers said. "I would break my parole and get my men to revolt."

General Dartan waited a long moment before he asked, in a quiet voice, "Ensign, are you willing to regain your honor?"

"Ahoy the deck!" The lookout called from atop the central balloon of the airship *Wasp*. "Smoke cloud, dead ahead!"

"Get me my glass!" Captain Fawcett cried, moving to the bow of the airship. A sailor rushed the spyglass up to him and Fawcett snapped it out of his hands, bringing it to his eye and scanning the horizon. He was interrupted a moment later by someone jostling his shoulder and turned irritably to berate the idiot who'd disturbed him.

It was Lewis. "What do you see?"

"Smoke," Fawcett said, raising the glass to his eye once more. "A high plume."

A dull booming sound came to their ears.

"There's been an explosion," Lewis said. He gestured for Fawcett to pass him the looking glass. The airship captain passed it over without a word and waited, impatiently, while the cavalry officer completed his scan.

"Maybe an earthquake?" Lewis muttered to himself. He lowered the glass, passing it back to Fawcett and said, "Captain, the king will buy you a new ship. We *must* get to Korin's Pass now!"

"Stokers!" Fawcett shouted to the men working at the stern. "Full speed ahead!"

"We'll run out of fuel, sir!" the first mate called back.

"We'll feed the flames with whatever wood we can spare, have a crew armed with axes," Captain Fawcett shouted in reply. He turned back forward, raising his glass and muttering to Lewis, "We'll get there as soon as we can. I just hope you're right about the king."

"Well, the dust seems to be settling," Margaret said to Ellen Annabelle as she peered down from atop her wyvern friend. "I'd say that Freddie might not know his powers, really."

Beneath her, the twin-souled wyvern rumbled in agreement. The wyvern craned her neck around so that she could see Margaret, then dipped a wing down and started a marvelous curling descent.

"Wait!" Margaret cried, pulling on the wyvern's neck. "Over there!"

Wyvern and rider turned and then soared upwards high in the sky for a better view.

"What's that?" Margaret said, pointing to a dot in the distance, growing larger.

"How's the train line?" Moira Kendral asked spymaster Hewlitt when they met at the train station as the spymaster, mage Margen, and the railcrew returned.

"With Margaret's help, we managed to lay a full league," Peter Hewlitt told her. He raised an eyebrow. "Why do you ask?"

"We should talk about it later," Moira said. "Alone."

"In the meantime, the spymaster has come up with a brilliant idea," Margen said, rubbing his hands in glee. "An undertaking of the most profitable sort."

"Really?" Moira said, sounding doubtful.

Margen turned to Hewlitt. "Can I tell her?"

"Perhaps it's best if we wait to be certain of our production lines," Hewlitt said. He turned his attention to Mrs. Kendral. "May I ask, dear lady, why it is you greet us here at the train station and not, say, at the Reedis Memorial Academy?"

"I took a look at Brookes' accounts," Moira said, her expression harsh.

"Ah," Hewlitt said. He turned to Margen. "Mage Margen, perhaps it's best if you give me and this wonderful lady some time to confer alone." When Margen made to protest, Hewlitt cut him off with a raised hand, saying, "I suspect it will all be rather tedious for one such as you."

"And I'm *sure* your students will be eager for your return," Moira Kendral added enticingly. "There are cabs just outside, if you need."

"Of course," Margen said. He beamed at Hewlitt. "And perhaps I shall start the students on the new project when I get back."

"An excellent idea!" Hewlitt agreed. He waved Margen toward the exit and offered an arm for Mrs. Kendral, adding, "Where should we talk?"

"Mr. Brookes has an office," Moira Kendral said, ignoring Hewlitt's arm and, instead, leading the way. "I'm afraid it's desperately in need of a cleaning and it's rather dark."

"Some candles, perhaps?" Hewlitt suggested as Mrs. Kendral paused in front of a drab door.

Mrs. Kendral smiled and opened the door, while rummaging with her other hand in her purse. "I've got something better."

She pulled a small fire demon out and lofted it high into the room. Its brilliant light seemed overwhelmed by the size of the room.

"This is the front office, the books are back there," Mrs. Kendral said, pointing toward another door at the far end of the room.

"By all means, lead on," Hewlitt told her with a smile and a wave of his hand.

"On deck!" a voice called down from the crow's nest. "Strange sighting dead ahead!"

"Well, man, what is it?" Captain Fawcett called back irritably.

"It looks like—" the man faltered "—it looks like a small dragon, sir. Maybe a cloud."

"A cloud?"

"But it's moving toward us, sir," the nervous lookout called back.

"Let me see!" Fawcett grumbled, racing forward once more to the bow. A midshipman was sent trotting after him with the spyglass. Fawcett took it from him and trained it forward.

"I don't see — wait!" He lowered the glass and shouted the length of the deck. "Beat to quarters! Man all guns!"

"What is it?" Major Lewis asked, trotting toward Fawcett.

"I don't know, but I'd prefer to be prepared," Fawcett told him. He waved at the bow. "First, we see an immense cloud of smoke and now we see this."

"You're thinking maybe the dragon set fire to a village?" Lewis asked, his eyes going wide.

"Captain Ford in *Spite* hit one, I've no doubt we can, too," Fawcett said, his eyes going hard as he watched his men race to their stations. Captain Fawcett moved closer to the cavalry officer as he added in confidence, "I'd truly love to have *something* to fight right about now!"

Lewis gave him a worried look.

"What?" Captain Fawcett demanded.

"Well, wouldn't it be better to find out what's up before starting a battle?" The cavalry officer asked in reasonable tones.

"Do you suppose that dragon asked the village?" Fawcett snapped back, turning away from the cavalry officer and moving down the deck to encourage his sailors as they manned their guns.

"Fixer!" Ibb shouted as soon as he entered the cavernous halls of the metal immortal. "Fixer, show yourself!"

Silence.

"I shall make lights," Tracker said, raising her hands and moving them in intricate patterns. A moment later, two bulbs of light appeared where her hands had traced. She spoke to them and they ballooned into huge balls of brilliant light even as she sent them high up into the space above them.

Rabel and Angus both gasped at the sight that came to their eyes. The cavern was a ruin. Metal shards littered the floor, the high gantries and other edifices were all crashed upon each other, resting drunkenly atop other ruins. Hana glided up on a shaft of air and landed quietly behind them, her dark eyes taking in everything.

"We must find Fixer," Ibb said, plodding through the detritus in front of them.

"Wait!" Tracker called. The others stopped and turned toward the cylindrical immortal. "That is my job."

"Well, do not let us delay you," Ibb said tightly.

Tracker moved forward, scanned the area and pointed one thin arm decisively at a mound of broken metal. "That is Fixer." A moment later, she pointed in another direction. "And that." With an anguished cry, a second later she added, "And that, and that, and that, and that, and —"

"Shush now, Tracker, we get the picture," Angus said, moving up beside the distraught immortal and resting a hand lightly on her metal shoulder.

"Rabel, if you would help me collect her," Ibb said, moving forward to the last pile of scraps Tracker had indicated.

"We should be aware of traps," Rabel warned, waving his hands in a complex pattern in the air.

"Why would anyone do this?" Angus asked as he knelt down and started sorting through the largest pile of Fixer's remains.

"To cripple us," Ibb said. He picked up a small pile of gears and gently stepped back to deposit them with Angus' pile.

"Cripple or destroy?" Rabel asked, moving forward toward another pile of remains. "Who can rebuild Fixer?"

"Fixer," the two metal immortals said in unison.

"And, failing that," Rabel asked softly, "who else?"

The two metal men were silent. After a long moment Ibb spoke, turning to Tracker. "I believe we shall have to make a deal."

"Yes," Tracker said. "That is the obvious, predictable outcome."

Ibb's eyes flared brighter. "Are you saying this was planned to force our reaction?"

"I am not sure," Tracker said. "If this was meant to destroy us, a more thorough destruction would have been indicated. If meant only to cripple and force us into a bargain, then merely incapacitating Fixer beyond our own means of restoration would be sufficient."

"This seems more than that," Ibb said, gesturing at the destruction around them.

"Then, logically, the assailant wanted to do more," Tracker said.

"Not just cripple, but delay," Rabel guessed.

"Which," Tracker said in agreement, "means that delay is important."

"This is my hunt," Hana said. "Lyric — or whoever controls her — caused this to happen."

"And wants to delay you," Ibb said in agreement.

"I will go with you," Tracker declared.

"And I," Angus said, moving to stand beside the young woman, his hand within easy reach. Hana smiled and took it, clasping it tightly, even as she nodded toward Tracker, "I am grateful for your offer."

"Ibb and I will collect Fixer and get her to rights," Rabel declared.

"Sadly, I cannot," Ibb said.

"What?"

"I must warn the others," Ibb said. "What I have seen here may not be forgotten."

"Indeed," Tracker agreed. She looked at Rabel. "You are the best experienced among the humans in this sort of reconstruction."

"But it might take years!" Rabel protested.

"Thus making certain that it will be a job well done," Ibb agreed.

Rabel shot an exasperated look toward Angus, but the other was intent on Hana. With a groan, Rabel threw up his hands. "Fine! I'll get help from Ophidian."

"I cannot put Fixer in debt, I have not that right," Ibb said.

"You forget that we are already in debt, and that this was intended," Tracker reminded the other immortal softly. A moment later she added, "And who do you suppose arranged this debt, wise Memory?"

Ibb's chest rumbled in reflection of his irritation.

"You must get Jarin Reedis on this," Ibb said. "And the zwerg engineer, the one helping with the airship —"

"What airship?" Angus asked in surprise.

"She has the abilities, she worked with Fixer some decades back," Ibb continued, ignoring the young human.

"Yes, as did I," Rabel said, his humor returning. "Very well, before we separate, I ask that you all help me gather Fixer."

"Of course," Ibb said, moving forward toward the next pile of Fixer's ruined body.

"Ah, First Minister Mannevy," Prince Sarsal exclaimed when he caught sight of the man, "I was hoping to find you!"

"You were?" Mannevy asked in surprise. The Crown Prince was carrying a tray with two beautifully crafted glasses set upon it. In his other hand he had an old, dusty bottle — apparently some rare vintage of wine.

"I thought you should be the one," Sarsal said mysteriously.

"The one for what?"

"Why to give my mother and our new king the royal toast!" Sarsal said, cheerfully. He dipped his head to add conspiratorially, "You know, they've ducked out of sight and I imagine—" he broke off, reddening. "Well, let's just say that they will probably be less than excited if I were to interrupt them."

"And you want me to have that honor?"

"Well, it *is* the royal toast," Sarsal said in a huff. "Thousands of years of tradition that the king and queen drink from the royal goblets—" he dipped the tray suggestively "—and drink the special wine from the royal vaults."

"Oh, I see," Mannevy said, reaching for the tray, "very well, then."

"I've already opened the bottle, as you can see," Sarsal said helpfully. "Get them each to drink and wish them the health of their realm."

"Very well, my prince, I believe I can do that," Mannevy said, reaching for the bottle which the prince promptly passed to him.

"I'm sure you can," Crown Prince Sarsal said with a broad wink, turning away and rushing back to the festivities.

"Everything in order?" Melodie asked sweetly as she stepped out of the shadows and joined Sarsal as he entered the royal hall.

"Couldn't be better," Crown Prince Sarsal said, smiling at her. "And you?"

"All done," she replied primly. "Should be quite a show in about an hour."

"Really?"

"First, they all get roaring drunk, some will vomit —"

"Vomit?"

"— not enough to do any good," Melodie hastily assured him, "and then not long after that… they'll die."

"And thus ends the Kingsland Army," Crown Prince Sarsal said with a gleam in his eyes. He glanced toward Melodie. "And us?"

"Take this now and you'll be fine," she said, handing him two small pills.

"And you?"

"Already taken, my dear."

"Gunners, stand ready!" Captain Fawcett shouted as the flying beast zoomed toward them.

"Really, Captain—" Major Lewis began.

"I've already told you, sir, I'll not hazard my command on a hope!" Fawcett barked. "Now, if you continue to insist on making a nuisance of yourself, you may go below."

Major Lewis took a step back, furious. His hand went to the sword at his side. "May I remind you, sir, that this mission was assigned to me!"

"This has nothing to do with your mission!"

"Precisely!" Lewis replied, lowering his hand and moving closer to the airship captain. "We do not have the steam, nor the time, to engage in this frivolous —"

"On deck!" the lookout called from above. "There's someone *riding* the beast!"

Fawcett and Lewis both looked up and called back. "What?"

Fawcett gave Major Lewis a fulminating look and continued, "What sort of person?"

"It looks like—" the lookout returned slowly "—well, sir, it looks like a girl."

Fawcett glanced at Lewis. "Have you ever heard of someone riding a dragon?"

Lewis shook his head. "I'd never heard of dragons until that complete mess at Korin's Pass."

"And this dragon comes from Korin's Pass," Fawcett said.

"Lookout, is the beast a dragon or a wyvern?" Lewis called up, cupping his hands over his mouth for a loud-hailer. He added quickly, "Does it have two legs or four?"

"Two, sir," the lookout called down.

"So," Lewis said to Fawcett, "*not* a dragon."

"The beast is white with a tint of purple," the lookout added.

"The dragon was black with red," Lewis said to Fawcett. He gestured to the men tensely standing by their cannon. "Perhaps we should stand them down, to avoid any accidents."

Fawcett chewed his lip angrily and then, with an abrupt nod, called out, "Stand down but stand ready!"

"Sir, the beast is rising!" the lookout called. "I can't see it, the sun's blinding!"

Fawcett shot Lewis an angry look. "It could dive on us and we'd be defenseless."

"True," Lewis allowed with a shrug. "But having your men at the guns won't help in that case." He gestured for the air mage who came striding over to them. "If the wyvern attacks, can you defend us?"

Before the young mage could answer, there was a thump above them and the balloon sagged for a moment just as the lookout cried in alarm.

"Back to your guns!" Fawcett shouted to his men.

"Deck there!" the lookout called down. "Sir, you won't believe this. I've two girls here who want to talk with you."

"*Two* girls?" Fawcett repeated in surprise. He glanced at Lewis. "How will they get down? They can't climb the rigging!"

"They're coming down the rigging!" the lookout called from above. "They're requesting parley." A moment later, the lookout added in confusion, "The littlest one is the wyvern, sir."

Fawcett shot Lewis an accusing look, but the Major shrugged, unable to offer any advice.

The little girl scampered down the ratlines as though she'd been born on the sea — or in the air. The taller, older girl moved more carefully, but when she stumbled and seemed doomed to fall to her death, she merely squeaked and bounced back to the lines, holding on more tightly.

"Really, Margaret, why don't you just *float* down?" the little girl's piping voice carried down to the deck where the crew were milling nearby, looking both worried and amazed.

"Are you an air mage?" Lewis called up.

"I know you, you're the one Vistos called 'useless'!" Fawcett's young air mage, Marsters, exclaimed. The other air mage climbed out of the hatchway and Marsters called to him, "Here, Warren, isn't that the one Vistos called useless?"

Mage Warren gave Margaret a cursory inspection and nodded.

"Vistos is dead," the little girl called back, jumping on the deck. She turned and scanned the crew. A moment later she smiled and moved straight toward Major Lewis. "You're Major Lewis, aren't you?"

Lewis didn't reply, an expression of terror on his face. "Sir, sir! What are you doing here?"

"Lewis," Fawcett said in a worried tone, "what is it?"

"Don't you see?" Lewis said, turning back to Fawcett and waving toward the little girl. "Don't you see him?"

"What I'd like to know, Major Lewis, is how *you* can see him," the little girl said. "I was told I'd have to make introductions."

"I'd know Colonel Walpish anywhere, miss," Lewis told her firmly. "But, sir, they said you were dead!"

"I'm afraid he is," the little girl said. "Tell me," she asked out of curiosity, "can you see her, too?"

"See who, miss?" Lewis asked. He seemed to recover, "And, may I ask, who are you?"

"Thomas Walpish is my protector," the girl said. "Ophidian tasked him with guarding me, along with Skara Ningan." She gestured to a spot of thin air just to the right of her, and Lewis gasped. The girl smiled grimly. "Mage Vistos killed them."

"Lewis?" Captain Fawcett began in a small voice. "Are you saying that you're seeing ghosts?"

"I'm Margaret Waters," the taller girl said, moving forward in front of the child. "I'm the wyvern rider." She smiled down at the girl. "And this is Ellen Annabelle, the wyvern."

"What about the ghosts?" Fawcett said, taking the older girl to be the most sensible at the moment. "Can you see them, too?"

"Of course," Margaret said with a smile. She nodded to her left. "Colonel Walpish, may I make you known to—" she broke off and her brows creased as she said, "Sir, whom am I addressing?"

"That's Captain Walter Fawcett," Major Lewis said with a wave of his hand. "And this is His Majesty's Airship, *Wasp*."

"Captain Fawcett," Margaret said with a nod and a quirk of her lips, clearly she was enjoying herself, "This is Thomas Walpish, late of the Kingsland Cavalry —"

Fawcett gasped as the air in front of him seemed to ripple and a figure appeared out of it.

Margaret continued, her dimple growing, as she waved to her right, "And this is Skara Ningan, formerly assassin in the King's employ."

Fawcett gaped at the woman who'd appeared out of nothing.

"They are dead, sir," Ellen Annabelle said. "They died destroying mage Vistos." She stretched out her hands to Skara and Thomas, who smiled and took them in return. "Ophidian has asked them to guard me."

"Against what?" Mage Warren asked in amazement.

"The three-headed god wants her dead," Margaret Waters said, moving to stand before Ellen Annabelle. She gave the two other mages a grim smile. "That will not happen while I live."

# Chapter Seven

"You understand what you're to do?" General Dartan said to the Ensign Rivers.

The young Kingsland officer nodded grimly. He looked down at Babette Colette. "I can't say that I like involving the child in this —"

"It's not your choice, sir," Babette told him defiantly. "It was not your father who was murdered."

Rivers started to reply, but the fierce look in the girl's eyes made him think better of it and he settled for a mere nod of his head.

"You with the girl could gain entrance where you with any other could not," General Dartan reminded him softly.

"And as soon as we're in, the soldiers will come for the weapons," Babette said with wicked satisfaction.

General Dartan gave her a sharp look. "Be careful, child, that you do not become that which you despise."

"I will do anything to see these Kingsland scum get what they deserve!"

General Dartan chewed his lip, wondering whether to reply.

"General, we haven't much time," Colonel Molet reminded him. "We need to move before the sun sets."

General Dartan sighed and nodded in agreement. "Very well, go and may the gods bless you!"

"And how much will you sell these rings for?" Moira Kendral asked as mage Margen proudly jiggled a handful of new-spelled copper rings in his cupped hands.

"How much?" Margen made a face and turned to Hewlitt.

"Mrs. Kendral, I was hoping I could enlist your aid in that project," Hewlitt responded with a suave bow of his head. "You have much talent in that arena."

"Hmph!" Moira snorted, not taken in by the flattery. She narrowed her eyes at the rings thoughtfully, then said, "Ten percent."

"Five," Hewlitt replied immediately.

"Eight."

"Seven and a half."

"Deal," Moira said, extending her hand. Hewlitt shook it gladly. The innkeeper's wife and Nelly's mother smiled as she confessed, "I was willing to go as low as six."

"And I was willing to go as high as nine," Hewlitt told her with a grin.

Moira shook her head and turned her attention back to mage Margen. "So how many of these can you make a day?"

"Actually, I'm more interested in *what* we can make each day," Hewlitt said.

"You say seven and a half," Margen said, ignoring the two. They blinked. "Then the students must get twenty."

"Ten!" Moira and Hewlitt roared in unison.

The mage blinked in surprise. "I suppose ten per cent isn't too bad —"

"Mage Margen, I'm afraid you have not the right to negotiate on behalf of students of my college," Nelly Kendral said as she entered the kitchen. She shot a glance toward her mother and waved a hand towards Margen's handful of rings. "Am I right in guessing this has to do with those?"

"Oh, now you've done it!" Moira told the two men with a cackle. Margen looked confused, but Hewlitt looked thoughtful. "I'm not a *patch* on her!"

"Uh, yes, we *were* talking about the spell rings," Margen said.

"Made in *my* school, with *my* materials, and on *my* time," Nelly said, moving closer and closer to Margen with each word. At the end, she scooped the rings out of his cupped hands and spilled them into a wide pocket at her side. "So those rings are *mine*."

"But they wouldn't have made them if I hadn't taught them," Margen complained.

Nelly turned on Hewlitt. "And why did he have the students make them?"

"Well," Hewlitt replied slowly, "because we wanted to make a lot in a hurry."

"A *lot?*" Nelly shouted, glancing toward her mother for support. "Do you know *nothing* about supply and demand?"

"Pardon?" Margen said, with an owlish blink.

"And you?" Nelly demanded of Hewlitt.

"This is just the first batch," the spymaster replied with just a touch of panic in his voice.

"And the *last* batch!' Nelly said.

"But, my dear—" Margen began.

"And how many students will I lose tomorrow?" Nelly demanded of him. "Now that they know how to do it, what's to keep them from doing it themselves?"

"Um… nothing," Margen admitted.

Nelly turned flashing eyes on Hewlitt. "Supply and demand!"

"Actually, I think it's a good thing," a new voice spoke up. Nelly spun toward the owner and took a step back in shock. "Jarin? Reedis?"

"Both of us," Reedis admitted as the twin-souled mage entered the room.

"Where have you been?" Nelly demanded.

"Listening," Reedis said, pointing to the corridor.

"And you think it's a good thing?"

"Yes," Reedis said. "Consider, how many people have you taught balloon magic?"

"That's… that's *beside* the point!" Nelly protested.

"No, my love," Reedis said, moving to engulf her in a hug, "that's exactly the point."

"Explain," Nelly said, allowing her tone to soften.

"We really want more people to know this," Reedis told her, "just as we want more people to know balloon magic. So that we can make more spell rings, so that we can lift more airships." He turned his head to Hewlitt. "And so we can build more rail lines and steam engines."

"To make Kingsland richer," Hewlitt said, nodding in understanding.

Reedis smiled at the spymaster. He looked down to his fiance. "And if you lose all your students tomorrow, just how many *new* students will be at your door in the morning?"

Nelly's eyes grew wide and then thoughtful.

"But what about the gods," Reedis continued thoughtfully. "I wonder how they will feel?"

"Well, some of them will be delighted," Ophidian spoke up, appearing instantly just beside the kitchen stove.

"Which means that others will be appalled," Margen added in a thoughtful voice. He turned to Ophidian. "Has this ever happened before?"

Ophidian's eyes grew dark. "In the God's War."

# Epilog

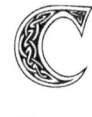

Crown Prince Sarsal slammed open the double doors to the royal chambers uninvited. He smiled as he saw the shocked looks on the faces of the King and his mother, the Queen.

"Oh, sorry! I hope I'm not interrupting anything," he said as he moved toward them.

King Markel, eyes bulging, hand to his throat, face flushed and red, waved his free hand excitedly. Beside him, Queen Rassa's eyes widened even as she gestured imploringly to her one and only son.

"Oh," Sarsal said, with a huge grin, "perhaps I *am*." He was close enough now to bat his mother's hand down. "I wonder whatever could it be?" He turned to King Markel. "Certainly not what you were hoping for, I see."

The King turned to Queen Rassa.

"What's that?" Sarsal asked, leaning forward with a hand cupped to his ear. "Speak up, I can't hear you!"

The Queen fell backwards onto the bed, her arms limp. Markel gave his stepson one horrified look and tried to raise a hand toward him, but failed.

"Oh, that's it!" Sarsal said. "You're dying!" He nodded toward the King. "I was told that this is a most painful poison, and it gives you a lingering death." He pursed his lips. "Won't be much longer, though."

He turned toward the door and raised his voice. "Guards! Guards!"

A figure raced into the room and stopped, eyes wide.

"Yes," Sarsal said, "first minister Mannevy. Perfect."

"What is it?" Mannevy cried in alarm, moving toward the stricken royals.

Sarsal raised an arm to restrain him. "Don't tell me you don't know!" He waved at the King who had finally succumbed and joined his wife in death. "After all, you were the one who served them the wine!"

Mannevy's eyes went wide, and he licked his lips. "The wine? But you —"

"Poisoned them?" Sarsal asked. He nodded happily. "But, you see, dear first minister, no one will ever know. Because we all know that you brought them the drink."

"You're mad!"

"No," Sarsal said, pulling his dagger from its sheath and grabbing the first minister, "I'm King."

And he slashed Mannevy's throat with one quick motion. As the first minister crumpled to the floor, Sarsal buried the point of his blade in the dying man's heart. He took a moment to relish the tableau, then turned to the door and raised his voice.

"Guards! Guards! Come quickly! The King! The Queen!"

"It is night, you asked to be told," a guard called from outside the darkened caravan.

"How fares the weather?" Gamden Ikar called back, turning his sore body over and pushing himself out from under his sleeping furs.

"There is a mist on the ground and the moon is full," the guard replied.

"And our height?" Gamden demanded with a growl. It was easier to get into the air from a height. He lashed out with his foot and struck the backside of the other eagleman, Jaden Ostan. "Get up!"

"Captain Elwes says you'll be able," the guard replied. Gamden allowed himself a bitter smile: the guard was more scared of his captain than of the eaglemen — that needed fixing.

"My compliments to the captain and tell him that he's an ignorant dog not fit to lick my boots," Gamden replied.

The guard had no answer to that.

Ten minutes later, Gamden and Jaden were on top of the caravan, looking down into a valley — the captain had selected a good campsite and launching point.

The moon was full, and the ground covered in a low fog.

"A perfect night for flying," Gamden declared. He cocked his head at Jaden. "Isn't it?"

"Do we have enough height?" Jaden asked, glancing to the valley below.

"If you can't fly from this height, you deserve to die," Gamden told him contemptuously. "Come on, we have to look around." He saw Captain Elwes below and the rest of the guards lounging. To Jaden he added, "We'll show these ground-hoggers what it's like to soar."

He stepped back to the rear of the caravan, turned, and raced toward the far edge and the valley below. He hurled himself off the edge, roared with delight —

— and soared up into the cold air above.

A moment later, another shape joined him, flapping hard and steadily to gain height.

With his eagle eyes, Gamden Ikar glanced out over the valley, straining for any hint of light or encampment. He cawed to Jaden Ostan, indicating that they should spread out to cover more ground.

Ostan shrieked back and twisted down and away in a bank, widening the gap between them.

Gamden soared upwards, his eyes straining over the ground below, when something caught his attention. He turned it. There! Light!

From a dim spark it became a brilliant flash, then a flare, a beacon of light. The light was purple-white, burning his eyes. He screeched in pain but arced toward it, determined to attack.

Shapes were rising from the ground!

He caught sight of wings, something flying. A challenge! He roared with delight and dove toward the ascending creature.

It was not a bird. It was not an eagle. With a flash of fear, Gamden Ikar spread his wings wide, straining desperately to avoid the intruder.

Another shape rose from the ground. And another. He recognized them. *Hexine!* The Duke was right!

With an angry cry, he dove again, determined to attack the hexine.

A warning shriek rose toward him, and a flash of purple-white grew brighter and larger.

*Wait!* A voice called. It seemed to shake the air and the very center of his being. Suddenly Gamden was blinded by a brilliant light. *This one will do no harm.*

"It is an eagleman!" A worried voice shouted in reply.

*Yes,* the voice agreed, *and much injured in its own way.* There was a pause, as if the voice were thinking. *Come with us, there is much to learn.*

Gamden screeched in protest.

"He's here to hurt the hexine!"

*He does not have my permission,* the voice replied.

A moment later, Gamden found a hand grabbing his wingtip, tugging at him. In amazement, he looked to see a young girl mounted on a flying shape — a wyvern. "Climb on," the girl called, tugging him closer. "You don't have the strength to fly all the way yourself."

Gamden cawed in protest, but it died in his throat. Fly where?

*To my home, of course.*

"That's the goddess Kahlas," the girl's voice explained. "I don't know why she wants you, but I think you don't really have a choice." The girl tugged again. "Let me pull you close and then you can change back. Bethany Margiss can carry us both."

Bethany Margiss?

"She's the wyvern," the girl explained. "I'm Chandra. People call me Earthshaker." She tugged again. "Really, you don't have a choice."

Goddess. Gamden could feel the truth in that. Kahlas was the goddess of the moon. Were they going to the Moon?

*Yes.*

## END

# Acknowledgements

No book gets done without a lot of outside help.

We are so grateful to Jeff Winner for his marvelous cover art work.

We'd like to thank all our first readers for their support, encouragement, and valuable feedback.

Any mistakes or omissions are, of course, all our own.

# About the Authors

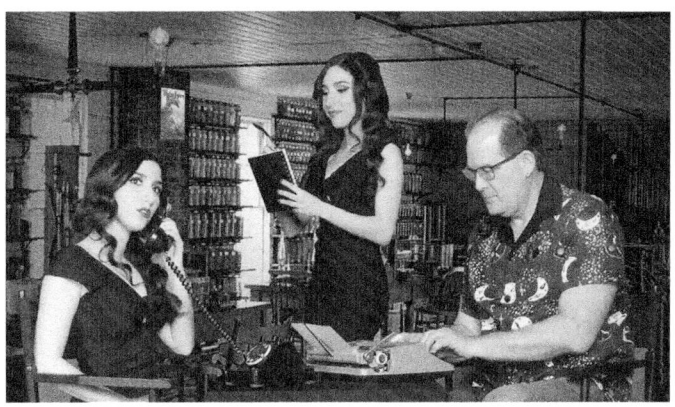

AWARD-WINNING AUTHORS THE WINNER TWINS, BRIT AND BRIANNA, HAVE been writing for over ten years, with their first novel (*The Strand*) published when they were twelve years old.

*NEW YORK TIMES* BESTSELLING AUTHOR TODD MCCAFFREY HAS WRITTEN OVER A dozen books, including eight in the Dragonriders of Pern® universe.

http://www.twinsoulseries.com

Printed in Great Britain
by Amazon

75818472R10132